OXFORD SPECIALTY TRAINING

**Structured Oral Examinat
Practice for the Final FRCA**

OXFORD SPECIALTY TRAINING

Structured Oral Examination Practice for the Final FRCA

EDITED BY

Rakesh Tandon
Consultant Anaesthetist, Addenbrooke's Hospital, Cambridge University Hospitals, Cambridge, UK

OXFORD
UNIVERSITY PRESS

OXFORD
UNIVERSITY PRESS

Great Clarendon Street, Oxford OX2 6DP
Oxford University Press is a department of the University of Oxford.
It furthers the University's objective of excellence in research, scholarship,
and education by publishing worldwide in

Oxford   New York
Auckland Cape Town Dar es Salaam Hong Kong Karachi
Kuala Lumpur Madrid Melbourne Mexico City Nairobi
New Delhi Shanghai Taipei Toronto

With offices in
Argentina Austria Brazil Chile Czech Republic France Greece
Guatemala Hungary Italy Japan Poland Portugal Singapore
South Korea Switzerland Thailand Turkey Ukraine Vietnam

Oxford is a registered trade mark of Oxford University Press
in the UK and in certain other countries

Published in the United States
by Oxford University Press Inc., New York

© Oxford University Press, 2012
The moral rights of the author have been asserted
Database right Oxford University Press (maker)

First published 2012

All rights reserved. No part of this publication may be reproduced,
stored in a retrieval system, or transmitted, in any form or by any means,
without the prior permission in writing of Oxford University Press,
or as expressly permitted by law, or under terms agreed with the appropriate
reprographics rights organization. Enquiries concerning reproduction
outside the scope of the above should be sent to the Rights Department,
Oxford University Press, at the address above
You must not circulate this book in any other binding or cover
and you must impose the same condition on any acquirer

British Library Cataloguing in Publication Data
Data available

Library of Congress Cataloging in Publication Data
Data available

Typeset in GillSans by Cenveo, Bangalore, India
Printed in Great Britain
on acid-free paper by
CPI Group (UK) Ltd, Croydon, CR0 4YY

ISBN 978–0–19–958401–7

10 9 8 7 6 5 4 3 2 1

Oxford University Press makes no representation, express or implied, that the
drug dosages in this book are correct. Readers must therefore always check the
product information and clinical procedures with the most up-to-date published
product information and data sheets provided by the manufacturers and the most
recent codes of conduct and safety regulations. The authors and publishers do not
accept responsibility or legal liability for any errors in the text or for the misuse or
misapplication of material in this work. Except where otherwise stated, drug dosages
and recommendations are for the non-pregnant adult who is not breastfeeding.

This book is dedicated to my amazing parents for making me what I am today

and

To my wife Kavita and lovely kids Aman, Devika, and Ansh for being so supportive and understanding

Acknowledgements

Recently the format of the Structured Oral Examination (SOE) of The Royal College of Anaesthetists, intended to test the safe practice of anaesthesia, has changed considerably. This book is based on the SOE as set out by the most recent requirements and guidance from Royal College of Anaesthetists.

We are grateful to Chris Reid, Commissioning Editor for Medicine at Oxford University Press, who had the foresight to see instantly that a new book was needed to help the trainees prepare for this novel method of assessment. Once the proposal was accepted a team of writers willing to take on the challenge was assembled, and the task was steered to completion. We are all grateful to him for this initiative.

I wish to express my personal gratitude to the individual contributors with their massive wealth of experience and expertise. To all of them I record my thanks, not only for their thoughtful contributions, but also for their promptness when manuscripts have been returned for amendments. I would particularly like to thank Dr Penelope Moyle, Consultant Radiologist, for her assistance in providing the required X-rays.

Our grateful thanks also go to Dr Nic Williams for her efficient copy-editing.

Finally, to Sian Jenkins, Production Editor, who has put in the extra effort to go through the manuscript in great detail and to produce the book in record time. We are grateful for her overseeing the project through to publication.

We extend our thanks to all the trainees who have attended the Cambridge Final FRCA viva course and provided us with the suggestions and feedback which are incorporated into this book.

Rakesh Tandon

Contents

List of abbreviations xi

List of contributors xv

Introduction xvii

Chapter 1 1

Clinical anaesthesia 3
   Long case: A case for craniotomy 3
   Short cases 8
      Questions 8
      Answers 9
Clinical science 19
   Questions 19
   Answers 20

Chapter 2 29

Clinical anaesthesia 31
   Long case: A case for total thyroidectomy 31
   Short cases 35
      Questions 35
      Answers 37
Clinical science 41
   Questions 41
   Answers 42

Chapter 3 47

Clinical anaesthesia 49
   Long case: A case for elective colectomy 49
   Short cases 54
      Questions 54
      Answers 56
Clinical science 60
   Questions 60
   Answers 61

Chapter 4 67

Clinical anaesthesia 69
   Long case: A patient with carcinoma of the sigmoid colon 69
   Short cases 73

Contents

    Questions   73
    Answers   75
Clinical science   80
  Questions   80
  Answers   81

Chapter 5   87

Clinical anaesthesia   89
  Long case: A patient for total hip replacement   89
  Short cases   95
    Questions   95
    Answers   97
Clinical science   103
  Questions   103
  Answers   104

Chapter 6   111

Clinical anaesthesia   113
  Long case: A patient with spinal stenosis   113
  Short cases   119
    Questions   119
    Answers   121
Clinical science   126
  Questions   126
  Answers   127

Chapter 7   135

Clinical anaesthesia   137
  Long case: A case of hiatus hernia   137
  Short cases   142
    Questions   142
    Answers   144
Clinical science   150
  Questions   150
  Answers   151

Chapter 8   161

Clinical anaesthesia   163
  Long case: A young boy with Guillain–Barré syndrome   163
  Short cases   168
    Questions   168
    Answers   169

Clinical science   176
    Questions   176
    Answers   177

Chapter 9   185

Clinical anaesthesia   187
    Long case: A patient for elective open AAA repair   187
    Short cases   192
        Questions   192
        Answers   193
Clinical science   200
    Questions   200
    Answers   201

Chapter 10   211

Clinical anaesthesia   213
    Long case: A patient in Accident and Emergency   213
    Short cases   219
        Questions   219
        Answers   220
Clinical science   225
    Questions   225
    Answers   226

Chapter 11   233

Clinical anaesthesia   235
    Long case: A patient with multiple medical issues   235
    Short cases   240
        Questions   240
        Answers   241
Clinical science   245
    Questions   245
    Answers   246

Chapter 12   253

Clinical anaesthesia   255
    Long case: A patient for dental clearance as day-case procedure   255
    Short cases   261
        Questions   261
        Answers   263

Clinical science   269
   Questions   269
   Answers   270

Chapter 13   279

Clinical anaesthesia   281
   Long case: A patient for major cancer surgery   281
   Short cases   287
      Questions   287
      Answers   288
Clinical science   295
   Questions   295
   Answers   296

Chapter 14   305

Clinical anaesthesia   307
   Long case: A patient with epilepsy on emergency operating list   307
   Short cases   313
      Questions   313
      Answers   314
Clinical science   319
   Questions   319
   Answers   320

Chapter 15   327

A child with upper respiratory tract infection   329
Anaesthetic management of a patient with severe sepsis   331
Smoking and drinking alcohol and anaesthesia   334
Fast tracking in anaesthesia   336
What is ziconotide?   337
What is dabigatran?   338
What is sugammadex?   339
Applications of transdermal drug delivery   340
Role of cell salvage in anaesthesia   342
Sedation in children and young people: current recommendations   344
Failed spinal anaesthesia: mechanisms, management, and prevention   347
Ultrasound-guided or peripheral nerve stimulation for peripheral nerve blocks   349
Rapid sequence induction and intubation: current controversy   351
The current findings of The Centre for Maternal and Child Enquiries (CMACE)   354

List of abbreviations

A&E	accident and emergency
AAA	abdominal aortic aneurysm
AAGBI	Association of Anaesthetists of Great Britain & Ireland
ABC	airway, breathing, circulation
ABCDE	airway, breathing, circulation, disability, exposure
ABG	arterial blood gas
ACE	angiotensin-converting enzyme
ACh	acetylcholine
ACTH	adrenocorticotropic hormone
AF	atrial fibrillation
AL	axial length
ALI	acute lung injury
ALP	alkaline phosphatase
APH	antepartum haemorrhage
aPTT	activated partial thromboplastin time
ARDS	acute respiratory distress syndrome
ARF	acute renal failure
ASA	American Society of Anesthesiologists
ATP	adenosine triphosphate
AVB	atrioventricular conduction block
AVPU	alert, voice, pain, unresponsive (scale)
AVPU	atrioventricular
BAL	bronchoalveolar lavage
BP	blood pressure
BTS	British Thoracic Society
cAMP	cyclic adenosine monophosphate
CBF	cerebral blood flow
CHB	complete heart block
CMACE	Centre for Maternal and Child Enquiries
$CMRO_2$	cerebral metabolic requirement of O_2
CN	cranial nerve
CNS	central nervous system
CO	carbon monoxide
CO_2	carbon dioxide
COHb	carboxyhaemoglobin
COPD	chronic obstructive pulmonary disease
CPAP	continuous positive airway pressure
CPP	cerebral perfusion pressure
CPR	cardiopulmonary resuscitation
CRP	C-reactive protein
CSA	central sleep apnoea
CSF	cerebrospinal fluid
CT	computed tomography
CVP	central venous pressure
CVS	cardiovascular system

DDAVP	desmopressin acetate
dL	decilitre/s
DVT	deep vein thrombosis
EBM	evidence-based medicine
ECG	electrocardiogram
ECMO	extracorporeal membrane oxygenation
ECT	electroconvulsive therapy
EEG	electroencephalogram
ELMS	Eaton–Lambert myasthenic syndrome
ERC	European Resuscitation Council
ERV	expiratory reserve volume
$ETCO_2$	end-tidal carbon dioxide
ETT	endotrachael tube
FDA	Food and Drug Administration
FEV_1	forced expiratory volume in 1 second
FFP	fresh frozen plasma
FGF	fresh gas flow
FRC	functional residual capacity
FVC	forced vital capacity
GABA	gamma-aminobutyric acid
GCS	Glasgow Coma Scale
GFR	glomerular filtration rate
GI	gastrointestinal
GIT	gastrointestinal tract
GP	general practitioner
GTN	glyceryl trinitrate
Hb	haemoglobin
HbA	adult haemoglobin
HbF	fetal haemoglobin
HDU	high dependency unit
HPA	hypothalamo–pitutary–adrenal
HR	heart rate
IC	inspiratory capacity
ICP	intracranial pressure
ICU	intensive care unit
IHD	ischaemic heart disease
IM	intramuscular
IO	intraosseous
IRV	inspiratory reserve volume
IU	international units
IV	intravenous
IVRA	intravenous regional anaesthesia
J	joule/s
K	potassium

LMA	laryngeal mask airway
LMWH	low-molecular-weight heparin
LOC	loss of consciousness
LVH	left ventricular hypertrophy
MAC	minimum alveolar concentration
MAP	mean arterial pressure
mcg	microgram/s
MCV	mean cell volume
ml	millilitre/s
MLT	microlaryngeal tube
mmHg	millimetres of mercury
MRI	magnetic resonance imaging
ms	millisecond/s
MTCT	mother-to-child transmission
Na	sodium
Nd:YAG	neodymium-doped yttrium aluminium garnet
NICE	National Institute for Health and Clinical Excellence
NMBD	neuromuscular blocking drug
NSAID	non-steroidal anti-inflammatory drug
O_2	oxygen
OER	oxygen extraction ratio
ORIF	open reduction and internal fixation
OSA	obstructive sleep apnoea
PCA	patient-controlled analgesia
PCO_2	carbon dioxide partial pressure
PDA	posterior descending artery
PE	pulmonary embolism
PEEP	positive end-expiratory pressure
PEFR	peak expiratory flow rate
PFT	pulmonary function test
PO_2	oxygen partial pressure
PONV	postoperative nausea and vomiting
PR	per rectum
PT	prothrombin time
PTH	parathyroid hormone
RAD	right axis deviation
RAE	Ring, Adair, and Elwyn
RBC	red blood cell
RCA	right coronary artery
RCT	randomized controlled trial
RCT	randomized control trial
RSII	rapid sequence induction and intubation
RV	residual volume
SAE	subarachnoid haemorrhage
SAE	sinoatrial

sec	second/s
SIADH	syndrome of inappropriate antidiuretic hormone secretion
SIRS	systemic inflammatory response syndrome
SVR	systemic vascular resistance
SVT	subventricular tachycardia
T_3	triiodothyronine
T_4	thyroxine
TAP	transversus abdominis plane
TBSA	total body surface area
TIA	transient ischaemic attack
TIVA	total intravenous anaesthesia
TKR	total knee replacement
TLC	total lung capacity
TOE	trans-oesophageal echocardiography
TRH	thyrotropin-releasing hormone
TSH	thyroid-stimulating hormone
TURP	transurethral resection of prostate
U&E	urea and electrolytes
URTI	upper respiratory tract infection
V	volt/s
VAP	ventilator-associated pneumonia
VC	vital capacity
VF	ventricular fibrillation
VT	ventricular tachycardia
VTE	venous thromboembolism
WBC	white blood cell
WPW	Wolff–Parkinson–White
Ω	ohm/s

List of contributors

Amr Abdelaal
Consultant Anaesthetist,
Cambridge University Hospitals NHS Foundation Trust

Sam Bass
Consultant Anaesthetist,
Cambridge University Hospitals NHS Foundation Trust

Ajit Bhat
Anaesthesia Registrar,
Cambridge University Hospitals NHS Foundation Trust

Nathaniel Broughton
Anaesthetic Registrar,
Cambridge University Hospitals NHS Foundation Trust

Ari Ercole
Clinical Lecturer in Anaesthesia,
Cambridge University Hospitals NHS Foundation Trust

Ravi Kare
Anaesthetic Registrar,
Cambridge University Hospitals NHS Foundation Trust

Lucy Pearmain
Anaesthesia Registrar,
Cambridge University Hospitals NHS Foundation Trust

Karim Shoukrey
Anaesthesia Registrar,
Cambridge University Hospitals NHS Foundation Trust

Claire Williams
Consultant Anaesthetist,
Cambridge University Hospitals NHS Foundation Trust

Imaging:

Penelope Moyle
Consultant Radiologist, Hinchingbrook and Cambridge University Hospitals

Introduction

The format of the Structured Oral Examination (SOE) of The Royal College of Anaesthetists has changed considerably since its inception in 1996. This book is based on the SOE as set out by the most recent requirements and guidance from the Royal College of Anaesthetists, and as such it offers updated and highly relevant content for anyone preparing for this examination.

We have produced this book after almost 8 years of experience in examination practice. The book combines aspects of clinical anaesthesia as well as clinical sciences. The pattern of questions in this book is designed to be like the real examination. In addition we have included some questions which specifically focus on current issues and recent development in anaesthesia, to better equip the examination candidate.

The book is structured to specifically follow the pattern of examination as set out by the Royal College of Anaesthetists. The book is arranged in 15 chapters, with the first 14 chapters each representing one complete examination. The clinical anaesthesia SOE consists of one long case with the relevant laboratory results, X-ray, and ECG. This information is followed by a set of questions based on the clinical scenario. The questions are answered individually with evidence-based answers. The short cases are scenario-based with questions which are also followed by model answers. The SOE for clinical sciences also follows a similar pattern as the examination covering applied aspects of anatomy, physiology, pharmacology, physics, and clinical measurements. The questions are separated by subject and answers are provided individually by topic.

A special feature of this book is the inclusion of X-rays which are individually reported by the radiologist, and anatomy diagrams which are simplified and can be reproduced easily. The graphs are simple to understand as well as simple to reproduce.

The last chapter in the book is called 'Hot topics in anaesthesia'. This is specially written in view of the changing and evolving role of anaesthetists, who are expected to deliver evidence-based practice with full patient safety in mind. Moreover, recently there are new recommendations from the National Audit Project of the Royal College of Anaesthetists, the National Patient Safety Agency, the Association of Anaesthetists, and the Centre for Maternal and Child Enquiries. Such information as well as new knowledge from scientific publications are quite topical for the examination, and are included in this last chapter of the book.

Marking

Structured Oral Examination I

Clinical anaesthesia is of 50 minutes' duration, comprising 10 minutes to view clinical material, 20 minutes of questions on clinical material, and 20 minutes of questions on clinical anaesthesia unrelated to the clinical material.

Structured Oral Examination II

Clinical science lasts for 30 minutes on the application of basic science to anaesthesia, intensive care medicine, and pain management.

The marking system
The College uses a five-point closed-marking system in its examinations, the marks being:

2+	Outstanding performance
2	Pass
1+	Fail
1	Poor fail
0	Veto (if a candidate fails to answer a compulsory question in the SAQ paper of the Final Fellowship of Royal College of Anaesthetists examination)

To pass the oral examination the examinee requires a minimum score of 2 or 2+. The 2+ plus examinee is a potential medal winner.

Structured Oral Examination I: Clinical anaesthesia

The SOE for clinical anaesthesia (SOE-I) lasts for 50 minutes, and comprises 10 minutes to view clinical material, 20 minutes of questions on the clinical material, and 20 minutes of questions on clinical anaesthesia unrelated to the clinical material as three short cases.

The aim of the clinical anaesthesia section of the examination is to test the ability to manage a real scenario appropriately. This means assessing a patient in an orderly manner, carefully analysing and interpreting the given investigations, presenting coherent justification for any further information that may be required, planning the perioperative management, and perhaps most importantly, communicating effectively.

Structured Oral Examination I: Long case

- Preparation time 10 minutes:
  - Read the scenario carefully and prioritize important issues.
  - Go through the investigations.
  - Based on the clinical scenario, analyse and interpret the findings.
- Organize your thoughts. Divide your answer into three parts that are based around the perioperative stages:
  - Preoperative stage: assessment and investigation.
  - Intraoperative stage:
    - Induction of anaesthesia and airway management plan.
    - Monitoring during surgery.
  - Postoperative stage:
    - Pain relief.
    - Recovery.
- How to 'Summarize the long case':
  - The opening sentence is quite important as this sets the tone of the viva. This should be well prepared, short, and well structured.
  - It is important that you follow a simple rule of one to two sentences.
  - Important information you convey should include age and sex of the patient, your diagnosis, planned procedure and the urgency of the case.
  - Outline the important issues particularly highlighting important preoperative morbidities.

- **Long case investigations:** analyse/interpret all the investigations available, formulate your differential diagnosis or specific diagnosis, and provide the rationale for your conclusion. You should make this response short and specific.
  - Chest X-ray: detailed discussion and differential diagnosis as appropriate.
  - Electrocardiograph (ECG) diagnosis based on findings.
  - Arterial blood gas analysis: systematic report with your inference.
  - Alveolar gas equation likely to be asked to explain the $P(A-a)O_2$ difference.
  - Pulmonary function tests (PFTs): FVC (forced vital capacity) graph, flow–volume loops (differentiating between obstructive and restrictive disease).
  - Echo: explain the information you seek and its effect on patient management.
  - Justify any further investigations you require.
- **Anaesthetic management:** for all the long case questions you will be asked about your plan of anaesthetic management. There is no right or wrong answer per se—the important thing is that you need to think and formulate a structure and technique with appropriate justification. Patient safety is paramount and the answers should cover all aspects of patient safety.
- **What anaesthetic monitoring?** Monitoring is based on the Association of Anaesthetists of Great Britain and Ireland recommendations:
  - ECG
  - NIBP and IBP, CVP catheter
  - Pulse oximetry
  - Capnography including inhalational agent
  - Urine output
  - Temperature, and
  - Neuromuscular junction monitoring

Structured Oral Examination I: Short cases

At the end of the first 20 minutes the examiners will change, and the second examiner will discuss three short cases. These cases could include anything from a list of clinical issues with anaesthetic problems or ECG or radiological image to begin a discussion. The discussion could be based on the management of the situation based upon the findings.

On a regular basis in your day-to-day practice of anaesthesia you should incorporate certain routine habits like interpreting the ECG and chest X-ray. This would certainly improve your practice of communication skills as well as that of interpretation of results presented to you. There are certain common situations in anaesthesia which can be practised on regular basis. An example is shown below.

Phraseology to be used/opening gambits:

- Patient with type 2 diabetes and a gangrenous leg requiring amputation.
  'My main concerns in this case would be the effect of diabetes on the various organ systems, the perioperative control of blood glucose, and the urgency of the operation.'
- How do you manage a difficult airway?
  'Difficult airway is a serious problem in anaesthetic practice. I would like to discuss its definition, prediction, and management of unexpected and anticipated situations.'

Structured Oral Examination II: Clinical science

The SOE in clinical science is intended to assess the examinee's understanding of the applied basic science to the practice of clinical anaesthesia, critical care, and chronic pain management. This part of the examination takes 30 minutes and is divided into a 15-minute session with each of the two examiners.

This is further divided into 7 minutes per topic with each examiner. All the candidates in the room are asked the same question and these questions would not be repeated in SAQ.

Applied anatomy

The applied anatomy relevant to clinical anaesthesia practice is a fair subject to be examined. The common clinical practice of anaesthesia of intravenous cannulation, regional anaesthesia, and intubation all require the applied knowledge of clinical anatomy. The anatomy is best described with a good line diagram and knowledge of relationships to adjacent structures. A typical question could be, for instance, about the blood supply of the heart followed by the clinical application of the applied knowledge. Types of anatomy question can be divided into a theoretical anatomy question or a practical anatomy question. This means that a question about coronary circulation is an example of a theoretical question but this knowledge is essential as we can alter the circulation. Similarly, cerebral circulation and spinal circulation is purely a theoretical concept but it is in the management of the head injury patient that one requires specific understanding of applied anatomy. The question on practical anatomy will be simple to address if you have experience of femoral or brachial plexus nerve block, or radial artery cannulation. The theoretical anatomy question has to be memorized for the examination and the best method is to pick-up the questions which are relevant to anaesthesia and practice with the help of line diagrams. The practical anatomy questions are the ones which can be practised every day while you are performing the procedures. For instance, if you are performing the brachial plexus block you can practise taking a colleague completely through each and every step of the block including the nerves you are blocking with their roots. Once you get in the habit of doing this a few times you will have sufficient knowledge and will not have to spend time reading it from a book. This means you can revise applied anatomy for the final FRCA in your day-to-day practice of anaesthesia.

It is good practice to draw some line diagrams of common anatomical structures which we come across in day-to-day practice. The anatomy diagram should be practised and memorized. This not only improves the performance but also has the advantage of increasing one's confidence too.

Applied physiology

The understanding of anaesthesia is very much dependent on the knowledge of physiology. A safe practice of perioperative medicine, anaesthesia, critical care, and pain is only possible when there is sound knowledge of physiology. The different aspects of applied physiology could be explored leading into the clinical manifestation of the disease and its management. A thorough understanding of cardiorespiratory physiology is essential.

Applied pharmacology

The practice of anaesthesia is not possible without the knowledge of applied pharmacology. The examinees are expected to be familiar with the applied pharmacology of all the commonly used drugs. This includes the application of pharmacodynamics and pharmacokinetics. Individual patients could be on multiple drugs and it is important to consider potential drug interactions. There has to be an understanding of geriatric changes along with effects of disease processes on anaesthetic drug administration, especially in critical care and pain management.

The number of drugs used in anaesthesia as such is limited. The drugs include anaesthesia induction agents, neuromuscular blockers, volatile analgesics, and local anaesthetic drugs. Hence, as an anaesthetist, there should be complete knowledge of these topics. Apart from this, the receptor functions and hormones as drugs are also quite important. The understanding of pharmacodynamics and pharmacokinetics is also a fair examination topic.

The pharmacological exam question also covers the principles of applied statistics and clinical trials which are common in the anaesthetic literature. Fundamental understanding of basic statistics and clinical research is expected. The current practice recommendations for the National Health Service come generally come from National Institute for Health and Clinical Excellence (NICE) guidelines which help you to deliver the best practice. The understanding of evidence-based medicine based on an understanding of the hierarchy of evidence, including evidence from meta-analysis, would be quite topical.

Applied physics

The anaesthetic speciality has evolved over the years based on various physical principles, hence the knowledge of these represent a basic expectation from the examinee. It is important to understand the basic principles of the gas laws, and at the same time it is important to demonstrate that there is essential clinical awareness and safety implication.

General guide to the Structured Oral Examination

The SOE viva for the final FRCA is intended to test the understanding of the safe practice of anaesthesia. Once the written part is completed, there is a time gap prior to the oral examination. It is very difficult, and potentially stressful for some, to get motivated into the full swing of revision needed for the oral examination when the result is not posted for the preceding written examination. In many instances, 2 weeks down the line when one discovers the results of the written examination, panic sets in and one wonders how best to utilize the limited time appropriately. This book will equip you and help you to prepare and organize your answers. The knack of passing examinations of this kind is to possess techniques which enable one to appear knowledgeable, confident, and safe.

The preparation for the clinical oral examination normally begins when an examinee is aware of the results of the written examination. This preparation is very simple as the examination is based on the day-to-day practice of any trainee. Once the written examination is passed it is clear that the knowledge has been tested but the application of this knowledge for the broad understanding of clinical anaesthesia is also required. The other skills which are required are assessment of the patient, interpretation of investigations, prioritization, planning of the management plan, good judgement, and communication. These skills can be gained with clinical experience and specific preparation.

Such skills can largely be achieved with the planning of day-to-day clinical work, particularly if you get into a habit of considering your normal theatre list as problem-based learning. So when you go to see your patient preoperatively take some more time and carefully assess the patient, and look at the investigations with a view to interpreting the results, including the radiograph. Summarize the case with important issues and possible options of management. Then request a senior colleague to go through the case and provide you with feedback. In doing so, you develop the all important presentation skills which represent another facet of the examination.

Similarly, during the module in critical care you could take the opportunity to work-up a patient fully and make sure you present such cases during the ward rounds. Regular examination of laboratory results, assessment of ECGs, chest X-ray and magnetic resonance imaging (MRI) should be part of your routine practice. You should specifically learn how to interpret and present the ECG and chest radiograph. The cornerstone of clinical practice is effective communication and if this is repeated regularly and routinely, it will improve the performance during a formal examination.

The time you have spent as a trainee gaining real experience, when combined with the knowledge you have attained will equip you to answer most of the questions. However, it is very important to communicate the confidence of your knowledge that will be needed to impress the examiners.

Structured Oral Examinations require a different approach to revision

Some of the techniques that are very useful in preparation are summarized below.
- A general idea of the syllabus and important core topics.
- Problem-based learning.
- Case-based discussion.

- Regular practice and discussion.
- Reflective learning.
- Organizing your answer.

The syllabus for the final fellowship examination is vast and can be both very daunting and a considerable task, but this book will help you with specific skills to get through this with a level of confidence.

The book can be used as an examination guide for a single candidate or a group of candidates using a question and answer pattern. This will enable candidates to assess their knowledge and skills within the time limit, and will provide thorough revision for the examination which will enable the trainee to identify their strengths and weakness in areas of clinical knowledge, clinical skills, problem solving, and organization.

We sincerely hope that the information provided in this book will be beneficial to candidates preparing for the final fellowship examination.

Chapter 1

Clinical anaesthesia

Long case: A case for craniotomy   3

Short cases   8
  Questions   8
  Answers   9
    Short case 1: Morbid obesity   9
    Short case 2: Patient retrieved from house fire   11
    Short case 3: Septic shock   14

Clinical science

Questions   19
Answers   20
  Anatomy: Trigeminal nerve   20
  Physiology: Lung volumes   22
  Pharmacology: Thiopentone   24
  Physics and clinical measurements: Electricity   26

Clinical anaesthesia

Long case: A case for craniotomy

A 38-year-old male patient presented to his GP with visual disturbance. A head CT scan demonstrated a tumour in the occipital region. He had one episode of seizure after the CT scan and needs an urgent craniotomy for biopsy of the occipital lesion. His past medical history includes neurofibromatosis. He smokes about 20 cigarettes per day and consumes alcohol in moderate to large amounts.

Clinical examination	Temperature: 38.2°C; weight: 85 kg; height: 160 cm			
	Pulse: 78/min, regular; BP: 138/70 mmHg; respiratory rate: 12/min			
	Chest: bilateral decreased air entry at bases, vesicular breath sound, wheeze and crackles are heard on auscultation			
	Cardiovascular system: normal heart sound with no murmurs			
	Central nervous system: no neurological deficit apart from visual field defects			
Laboratory investigations	Hb	16.0 g/dL	Na	142 mEq/L
	MCV	109 fL	K	3.7 mEq/L
	WBC	14.0×10^9/L	Urea	6.6 mmol/L
	Platelets	351×10^9/L	Creatinine	107 μmol/L
	CRP	110	Glucose	5.2 mmol/L
			Alkaline phos.	400 IU/L
Pulmonary function tests			Predicted	
	FEV_1	1.5 L	2.6 L	
	FVC	2.3 L	3.5 L	
	FEV_1/FVC	65%	74%	

QUESTIONS

1. Summarize the key features of this case.
2. What do you think—is this case elective or emergency?
3. How can you say someone is alcoholic? What is the recommended maximum weekly alcohol intake?
4. Comment on the mean corpuscular volume (MCV).
5. What are the causes of high MCV?
6. Comment on alkaline phosphatase and C-reactive protein (CRP).
7. Discuss the chest X-ray.
8. Read the ECG.
9. What are the causes for the raised ST?
10. What do you see from the flow–volume loop of this patient?
11. What is the differential diagnosis for the cause of seizure in this patient?
12. What is the cause of right inferior homonymous hemianopia?

Structured Oral Examination Practice for the Final FRCA

13. What other investigations would you need?
14. Will you proceed with the case?

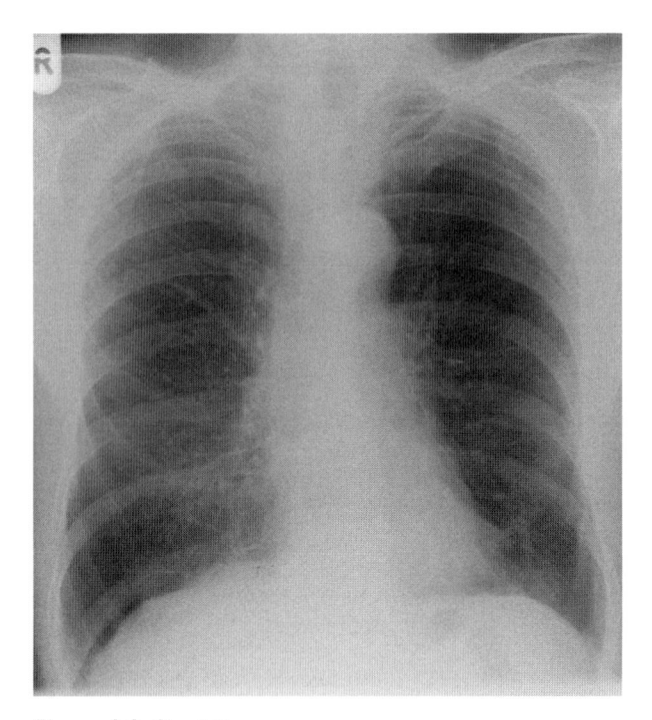

Figure 1.1 Chest X-ray.

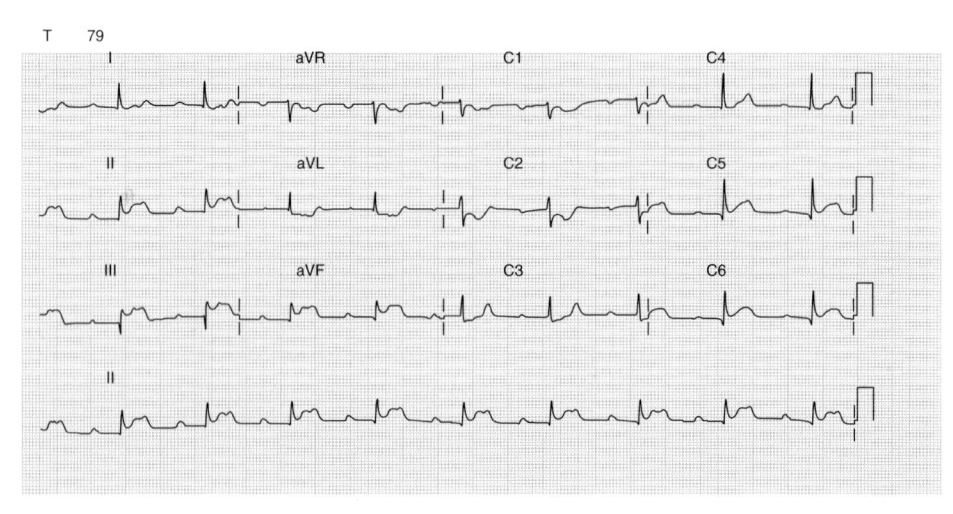

Figure 1.2 ECG.

Chapter 1

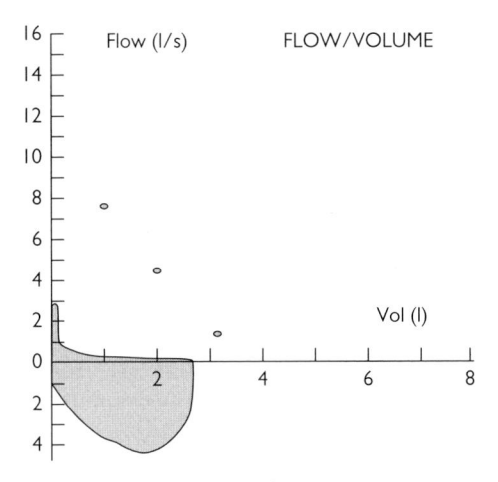

Figure 1.3 Flow–volume loop.

ANSWERS

1. Summarize the key features of this case.
We have a 38-year-old male patient who is obese (BMI 33) with an intracranial lesion in occipital region. He has presenting symptoms of visual disturbance and seizure with associated history of neurofibromatosis. He has a significant alcohol intake and is a smoker. There is pyrexia with signs of chest infection.

2. What do you think—is this case elective or emergency?
The case describes his need for urgent craniotomy rather than emergency. However, I do not consider it elective due to the nature of the gentleman's symptoms and need for biopsy.

3. How can you say someone is alcoholic? What is the recommended maximum weekly alcohol intake?
Well 1 unit of alcohol is 10 ml by volume or 8 g by weight of pure alcohol. The recommendation for males is not more than 21 units of alcohol in one week (and four units per day). For females not more than 14 units per week (and three units per day) are recommended.

4. Comment on the mean corpuscular volume (MCV).
The MCV relates to the size of the red blood cells (RBCs) and the normal range is 76–96 fL. The MCV is elevated when RBCs are larger than normal (macrocytic), for example in anaemia caused by vitamin B_{12} deficiency. When the MCV is decreased, RBCs are smaller than normal (microcytic) as is seen in iron deficiency anaemia or thalassaemias.

This patient has raised MCV. The cause could be explained on the basis of chronic alcohol intake.

5. What are the causes of high MCV?
The causes of high MCV are:

- Liver disease
- Hypothyroidism
- Alcohol abuse
- Hereditary anaemia(s).

- Drugs (anticonvulsants)
- Zidovidune treatment (AIDS)
- Megaloblastic anaemias (pernicious, folic acid deficiency, B$_{12}$ deficiency)
- Reticulocytosis (acute blood loss response; reticulocytes are immature cells with a relatively large size compared to a mature RBC)
- Artefact (aplasia, myelofibrosis, hyperglycaemia, cold agglutinins)

6. Comment on alkaline phosphatase and C-reactive protein (CRP).

Looking at the investigation the alkaline phosphatase is 400 IU/L which is raised. The normal level is 30 to 300 IU/L in adults. In this case the raised level indicates the liver disease.

C-reactive protein is raised in this patient which is an indication of infection. CRP is a pentraxin protein synthesised in liver and found in the blood. The levels rise in response to inflammations. The physiological role of CRP is to bind to phosphocholine which is expressed on the surface of dead or dying cells which activates the complement system.

7. Discuss the chest X-ray.

It is a posterior-anterior chest X-ray with the lungs hyperexpanded and flattening of the hemidiaphragms. There are disorganized vascular markings and paucity of lung markings especially in the right upper lobe. No focal collapse or consolidation is seen. The appearances are in keeping with COPD. Cardiomediastinal contour is normal with normal heart size.

8. Read the ECG.

Sinus rhythm (HR: 1500/25 = 60), normal PR interval, characteristic large Q waves in lead III, ST elevation in II, III, and aVF and reciprocal ST segment depression in lead aVL (may also see in anterior leads). Inferior wall MI with normal axis. My impression is inferior wall myocardial infarction—acute.

9. What are the causes for the raised ST?

Causes of raised ST are:
- Normal ST-segment elevation and normal variants
- Acute myocardial infarction
- Left bundle-branch block
- Acute pericarditis and myocarditis
- Hyperkalaemia
- Arrhythmogenic right ventricular cardiomyopathy
- Pulmonary embolism
- Transthoracic cardioversion
- Prinzmetal's angina
- Brugada syndrome

10. What do you see from the flow–volume loop of this patient?

Flow–volume loops provide a graphical illustration of a patient's spirometric efforts. Flow is plotted against volume to display a continuous loop from inspiration to expiration. The overall shape of the flow–volume loop for this patient indicates chronic obstructive disease.

11. What is the differential diagnosis for the cause of seizure in this patient?

The causes of seizure can be divided into:

- Central nervous system:
  - Brain tumour (primary or secondary)
  - Head trauma (high alcohol intake)
  - Cerebral infection—encephalitis, meningitis, HIV
- Vascular causes:
  - Intracerebral bleed/subarachnoid haemorrhage
  - Arteriovenous malformation
- Metabolic:
  - Fever
  - Electrolyte disturbance
  - Hypo/hyperglycaemia
  - Thyroid disease
  - Hepatic failure
  - Drugs and toxins
  - Alcohol withdrawal
- Congenital/inherited disorders: neurofibromatosis
- Idiopathic epilepsy

12. What is the cause of right inferior homonymous hemianopia?

The mass in the patient's left occipital lobe could account for this. In addition, vascular and neoplastic lesions of the optic tract, visual cortex, or uncal herniation can cause a contralateral homonymous hemianopia.

13. What other investigations would you need?

I would like to investigate the following:

- Troponin level
- Echocardiography
- Lung function tests and arterial blood gas
- Sepsis screen
- Liver function test
- Ultrasound of liver
- Coagulation studies
- Group and save

14. Will you proceed with the case?

I will not proceed with the case but would pre-optimize the patient prior to surgery. He has evidence of possible chest infection on a background of chronic obstructive respiratory disease. He requires a sepsis screen, antimicrobial therapy, bronchodilators, and chest physiotherapy. In addition, antiepileptics should be considered prior to a general anaesthesia in order to reduce the likelihood of further seizures.

Further reading

Allman, K.G. and Wilson, I.H. *Oxford Handbook of Anaesthesia*, 2nd edn. Chapter 7: Hepatic disease: Anaesthetic management of the patient with liver failure, pp. 133–49. Oxford: Oxford University Press, 2006.

Wang, K., Asinger, R.W., and Marriott, H.J.L. ST-segment elevation in conditions other than acute myocardial infarction. *New England Journal of Medicine* 2003; **349**:2128–35.

Short cases

QUESTIONS

Short case 1: Morbid obesity

A 156-cm tall man weighing 120 kg is on the list for knee arthroscopy.

1. When do you consider a patient to be morbidly obese? Classify obesity.
2. What are the pathophysiological changes in the obese patient?
3. What are the pharmacokinetic effects of morbid obesity on the body?
4. What are the possible problems during anaesthetic management of this patient?
5. How would you proceed in this patient (anaesthetic management)?

Short case 2: Patient retrieved from house fire

A young man is retrieved from retrieved from a house fire and is coming to Accident and Emergency. You are on-call and have been bleeped to assess the patient. On arrival his oxygen saturation is 99%, he appears a little disoriented and soot can be seen on his face and nostrils.

1. What are the things going through your mind?
2. What do you need to know from the patient?
3. What are the signs of inhalational injury?
4. How would you manage the patient for inhalational injury?
5. What are the signs and symptoms of carbon monoxide poisoning?
6. What are the effects of carbon monoxide on haemoglobin and why?
7. What would be your management plan?

Short case 3: Septic shock

You are called by the intensive care nurse to see a patient who had a laprotomy last night. The patient is tachycardic, their oxygen requirement is increasing and their airway pressure is up.

1. What do you think is going on? Define sepsis.
2. What are the principles of the management of sepsis?
3. What fluids you would use to resuscitate and how much?
4. If the blood pressure is not responding to fluids how you would choose the Inotropes? Which inotrope and why and doses for each?
5. How would you assessment of tissue oxygenation?
6. What would be your mode of ventilation in a severe sepsis?

Chapter 1

ANSWERS

Short case 1: Morbid obesity

1. When do you consider a patient to be morbidly obese? Classify obesity.

An individual is considered obese when the body mass index (BMI) is >30. BMI is defined as weight in kilograms divided by height (m²).

A BMI <25 kg/m² is normal; 25–30 kg/m² is considered overweight; and it is obesity when BMI is ≥30 kg/m². This is further classified as:

- Class I: BMI 30.0–34.9
- Class II (severe obesity): BMI 35.0–39.9
- Class III (morbid obesity): BMI ≥40.0
- Super-morbid obesity: BMI ≥50.0

2. What are the pathophysiological changes in the obese patient?

- **Cardiovascular system:** There is an increase in blood volume, cardiac output, ventricular workload, O_2 consumption, and CO_2 production. These may lead to systemic and pulmonary hypertension and later cor pulmonale leading to right ventricular failure. There is an association of hypertension, left ventricular hypertrophy, and coronary artery disease with risk of thromboembolism.
- **Respiratory:** There is decreased compliance (35%) and functional residual capacity (FRC) with increased work of breathing, hypoxaemia, and hypercapnia. There can be obstructive sleep apnoea and pulmonary hypertension. The combination of reduced chest wall and diaphragmatic tone during general anaesthesia, the increased incidence of atelectasis, and retention of secretion resulting from reduced expiratory reserve volume and FRC renders the morbidly obese patient at risk of rapid desaturation during hypoventilation or apnoea. These problems can persist into the postoperative period.
- **Airway:** There is mask ventilation with difficult intubation and extubation.
- **Gastrointestinal system:** There is increased acidity and volume of gastric contents, hiatus hernia, with higher risk of regurgitation and aspiration.
- **Fatty liver**.
- **Endocrine:** There is increased incidence of diabetes mellitus likely

3. What are the pharmacokinetic effects of morbid obesity on the body?

Factors affecting drug pharmacokinetics in obesity include:

Volume of distribution

- Decreased fraction of total body water
- Increased adipose tissue
- Increased lean body mass
- Altered tissue protein binding
- Increased blood volume and cardiac output
- Increased concentration free fatty acids, cholesterol, alpha-1-acid glycoprotein
- Organomegaly

Plasma protein binding

- Adsorption of lipophilic drugs to lipoproteins so increased free drug available
- Plasma albumin unchanged
- Increased alpha-1-2-acid glycoprotein-acid glycoprotein

Drug clearance
- Increased renal blood flow
- Increased glomerular filtration rate (GFR)
- Increased tubular secretion
- Decreased hepatic blood flow in congestive cardiac failure

4. How would you proceed in this case (anaesthetic plan)?

Team plan
- Senior anaesthetic staff
- Trained and experienced staff in theatre

Appropriate equipment
- Appropriate operating table and large sphygmomanometer cuff. Invasive BP monitoring may be required.
- Support for arm, leg, and body. Patient may require strapping to prevent falling or slipping.
- Calf compression devices should be used to prevent venous thromboembolism.
- Particular care should be taken to prevent pressure sores and nerve injury.
- Difficult airway trolley checked and ready to use.

Conduct of anaesthesia
- Pre-oxygenation with intubation in all cases even if it is a short procedure.
- Induce anaesthesia on the operating table with an appropriate maximum weight allowance.
- Standard monitoring with correct-sized BP cuff.
- A patient with difficult venous access should have a central venous line cannulation.
- Obesity with comorbid conditions should have direct intra-arterial monitoring.
- Patient positioning is paramount in view of difficult airway and nerve injury.
- For bariatric surgery awake fibreoptic intubation should be routine.
- Ventilation should be pressured controlled with positive end-expiratory pressure (PEEP). Increased I:E (inspiratory-to-expiratory time) ratio may reduce the airway pressures.
- The short-acting muscle relaxant with the use of total intravenous anaesthesia (TIVA) would ensure rapid recovery.
- Aortocaval compression can be avoided with a tilt.
- Effective temperature maintenance using forced warm air over-blankets are extremely effective along with fluid warmers.
- Precaution should be taken for fluid balance; blood loss should be replaced.

Postoperative care
- Patients fit enough for extubation should be extubated wide-awake in the sitting position and transferred to appropriate postoperative care.
- Postoperative shivering, which increases oxygen consumption, prolongs the effects of some anaesthetic agents and increases cardiovascular stress.
- Pain relief.
    - Morphine patient-controlled analgesia (PCA) with postoperative oxygen.
    - NSAIDs are extremely effective as part of a multimodal postoperative analgesic regimen, but they should be used judiciously as they may increase the incidence of postoperative renal dysfunction.
- Thromboprophylaxis should be prescribed.
- HDU care should be available for higher-risk patients with pre-existing respiratory disease, especially those undergoing thoracic or abdominal surgery.

Chapter 1

Further reading
Allman, K.G. and Wilson, I.H. *Oxford Handbook of Anaesthesia*, 2nd edn. Chapter 8: Obesity, pp.182–4. Oxford: Oxford University Press, 2006.
Association of Anaesthetists of Great Britain and Ireland. *Peri-operative management of the morbidly obese patient*. London: AAGBI, 2007.
Lotia, S. and Bellamy, M.C. Anaesthesia and morbid obesity. *Continuing Education in Anaesthesia, Critical Care & Pain* 2008; **8**:151–6.

Short case 2: Patient retrieved from house fire

1. What are the things going through your mind?
This is a serious life-threatening situation where I have to assess the patient and start immediate management. My management plan would be along the lines of trauma and burn, adopting the Airway, Breathing, and Circulation (ABC) approach.

If the patients are able to speak then I would take a full history of the mechanism and time of the burn. I would also speak to paramedics and the family. I'd look for coexisting injuries—perhaps indicating an explosion, fall from a height, etc.

2. What do you need to know from the patient?
I would require a full history of the mechanism and timing of the burn. Also, I would like to know:
- If the patient was trapped in an enclosed space.
- Any inhalation of fumes/smoke, length of time of exposure.
- If they have experienced coughing, dyspnoea, soot in sputum, a change in their voice or stridor.
- History of symptoms suggestive of elevated carboxyhaemoglobin (COHb)—headache, shortness of breath, irritability, dizziness, visual changes, palpations, chest pain.
- Patient background: pre-existing illnesses, drug therapy, allergies and drug sensitivities are also important; previous exposure to general anaesthetics and family history. (Possibility of being pregnant if female!).
- Establish the patient's tetanus immunization status.

3. What are the signs of inhalational injury?
- Face and/or neck burns.
- Singeing of the eyebrows and around the nose.
- Carbon deposits and acute inflammatory changes in the oropharynx.
- Carbon-particles seen in sputum.
- Hoarseness.
- History of impaired awareness, e.g. alcohol or head injury, and/or confinement in a burning environment.
- Explosion, with burns to head and torso.
- COHb level greater than 10% if the patient is involved in a fire.

4. How would you manage the patient for inhalational injury?
- Early management may require endotracheal intubation and mechanical ventilation.
- Transfer to a burn centre.

- Stridor is an indication for immediate endotracheal intubation.
- Circumferential burns of the neck may lead to swelling of the tissues around the airway and so require early intubation.

5. What are the signs and symptoms of carbon monoxide poisoning?

The clinical course of CO poisoning is directly related to the degree and duration of exposure. In the majority of cases those with a COHb level in the blood of less than 10% will have no symptoms whereas in those with a level of 50% of greater are likely to suffer from coma, cardiac depression, or cardiac arrest. Myocardial injury is common and a predictor of mortality. Some patient may also develop rhabdomyolysis and renal failure.

The classical cherry pink discoloration of the skin caused by large amounts of COHb is in practice rarely seen. Skin pallor and cyanosis are more usual. Skin blisters may occur as a result of tissue hypoxia.

COHb level (%)	Clinical signs and symptoms
0–10	In general no symptoms
10–20	Mild headache, slight shortness of breath
20–30	Moderate headache, weakness, difficulty with concentration
30–40	Irritability, nausea/vomiting, dizziness, visual changes
40–50	Tachycardia, tachypnoea, arrhythmias, ataxia, confusion
50–60	Stupor, convulsions, often fatal
60–70	Coma, cardiac depression

6. What are the effects of the carbon monoxide on haemoglobin and why?

Carbon monoxide inhibits oxygen binding to haemoglobin during gas exchange in the lung. Carbon monoxide has a 240 times greater affinity for haemoglobin than oxygen. Carbon monoxide competitively inhibits oxygen binding to haemoglobin. Carbon monoxide shifts the oxygen dissociation curve to the left (decreasing oxygen delivery to tissues). This is because carboxyhaemoglobin changes the configuration of the protein, preventing the release of bound oxygen. In addition, it also appears that carbon monoxide (under hypoxic conditions) inhibits cellular respiration, possibly through binding to other haem-containing proteins, e.g. cytochrome A3. These tissue effects may be the main cause of clinical toxicity due to net cellular hypoxia.

7. What would be your management plan?

Immediate management

- I will treat immediate life-threatening injury with the ABC approach.
- Fire is almost always associated with other injuries.
- Burns are associated with alcohol intoxication and epilepsy.
- Mortality is related to age, total body surface area (TBSA), and depth of burn.

Airway and control of cervical spine

Evidence of airway compromise is decreased consciousness; look for injury to airway. If intubation is required at this early stage, it is rarely technically difficult. Beware the use of fibreoptic scope for induction if there is evidence of airway swelling as this makes it difficult to anaesthetize and airway instrumentation is likely to cause bleeding and further trauma—consider inhalational induction with senior present. Suxamethonium can be used in the first few hours following major burn.

Breathing

High-flow O_2, 15 L/min (inspiratory reservoir on the mask). Intubation may be required if patients have reduced conscious, trauma, chest injury, smoke inhalation. Check tracheal position, tension pneumothorax is a common life-threatening injury in blast trauma injuries.

Circulation and control of bleeding

Burns >25% TBSA produce a marked systemic inflammatory response resulting in oedema. Resuscitation should start immediately based on BP, pulse, capillary refill (check in both burned and unburned limbs), conscious level. Seek cause of hypovolaemic shock as initially never due to burn itself.

- Large-bore intravenous access.
- Monitor glucose particularly in children.

Fluids and Foley catheter

Fluid resuscitation will be required if the TBSA of the burn is >10% in a child and >15% in an adult. Various formulae exist. The Parkland formulae continue to be widely used: 3–4 ml/kg/%burn of crystalloid to be given over 24 hours from the time of burn (half in the first 8 hours and the remaining half in the next 16 hours).

Urine output should be closely monitored— the aim is for >0.5 ml/kg/hour for adults and 1.0 ml/kg/hour for children.

Nutrition should also be considered as these patients are catabolic.

Measure carboxyhaemoglobin

Standard pulse oximetry infrared cannot distinguish between COHb and oxyhaemoglobin and will over-read. Co-oximetry represents the definitive test. A blood sample is exposed to six different wavelengths of light to quantify each fraction of reduced haemoglobin (oxy-haemoglobin, methaemoglobin, carboxyhaemoglobin).

Circumferential burns of chest will require escharotomies.

Disability

Glasgow Coma Score or AVPU. Provide analgesia as required.

Exposure and estimation of burn

Keep the patient warm. Use specific burns chart or rule of nines to estimate burn.

Treatment of carbon monoxide poisoning

Continue high-flow oxygen therapy. Intubate and ventilate if required. In severe cases the risk of cerebral oedema should be recognized and treated.

The value of hyperbaric oxygen therapy is controversial. Several randomized controlled trials have failed to conclude the effectiveness of this therapy. The theoretical basis of this therapy is that it increases the amount of dissolved oxygen in blood as well as decreasing the elimination half-life of COHb. According to Henry's law, 100 ml of blood contains 0.3 ml of dissolved oxygen at a PO_2 of 13.3 kPa whereas, for 100% O_2 at 3 atm the dissolved O_2 is 5.7 ml. The elimination half-life of CO is reduced from 250 min when breathing air to 59 min when breathing 100% O_2 and 22 min when breathing 100% at 2.2 atmosphere.

The current recommendations for considering hyperbaric oxygen therapy include:

- Recovery of consciousness after an initial high COHb concentration.
- Neurological or psychiatric features other than headache.
- Evidence of myocardial ischaemia.
- Pregnancy (greater susceptibility of fetus to CO, risk of fetal mortality if COHb levels >20%).

Contraindications to this therapy are mainly logistic. The transfer of patients to centres with hyperbaric facilities can be long and difficult. In addition, many chambers are only single-person chambers thus contraindicating patients who are mechanically ventilated, unable to maintain their own airway, requiring inotropic support, or suffering from conditions which may require urgent intervention, e.g. asthma, arrhythmias.

Predictors of poor outcome
- Increased length of exposure and minute ventilation. Trapped in an enclosed space—resence of industrial and household chemicals.
- Age >50 years increases mortality form burns. Increased extent of burn body surface area increases likelihood of inhalation injury and mortality.
- COHb levels correlate poorly with clinical outcome and treatment should be based on clinical signs. Myocardial injury is a predictor of long-term mortality.

Further reading
Allman, K.G and Wilson, I.H. *Oxford Handbook of Anaesthesia*, 2nd edn. Chapter 34, pp. 838–43. Oxford: Oxford University Press, 2006.
Enoch, S., Roshan, A., and Shah, M. Emergency and early management of burns and scalds. *British Medical Journal* 2009; **338**:b1037.
Hinds, C. and Watson, D. *Intensive Care A Concise Textbook*, 3rd edition. Philadelphia, PA: Saunders, 2008.
Hilton, P.J. and Hepp, M. The immediate care of the burns patient. *British Journal of Anaesthesia CEPD Reviews* 2001; **1**(4):113–16.

Short case 3: Septic shock

1. What do you think is going on? Define sepsis.
In my view this situation directs towards sepsis. Sepsis is a condition where there is infection with systemic manifestation, and when there is sepsis-induced hypotension persisting despite fluid resuscitation it is considered septic shock. I would consider this sepsis when:
- Temperature >38.3°C or <36°C.
- Heart rate >90 bpm
- Respiratory rate of >20 per minute or $PaCO_2$ <4.4 kPa
- White cell count >12 × 10^9/ L or < 4 × 10^9/L
- Loss of consciousness
- Hyperglycaemia in non-diabetic

2. What are the principles of the management of sepsis?
Sepsis six:
1. High-flow oxygen
2. Take blood cultures
3. Give IV antibiotics
4. Start IV fluid resuscitation
5. Check haemoglobin and lactate
6. Monitor hourly urine output

Chapter 1

These goals could be achieved by following:
- An ABCDE approach started immediately and transferred to intensive care unit.
- Delivery of oxygen to the tissues should be restored rapidly and completely to prevent organ damage.
- Ensure adequate oxygenation and ventilation.
- Restore cardiac output and BP.
- Investigations, with treatment of the underlying cause.
- Identify source of infection.
- Treat complications.
- Administer analgesia.
- Consider adjunctive therapy (activated protein C, steroids).

Investigations
- FBC, glucose, coagulation, U&E, liver biochemistry, blood gases, acid–base state, 12-lead ECG. Consider the following: blood cultures, culture of sputum, urine, pus, CSF. Blood lactate, D-dimmers.
- Identify source of infection: clinical examination, chest and abdominal X-ray, ultrasound, CT, labelled white cell scan.
- Treat underlying cause: treat infection—consider appropriate antibiotics, antifungals, removal of indwelling catheters, surgical exploration and drainage.
- Treat the complications: coagulopathy, renal failure, acidosis, hyperglycaemia.

3. What fluids would you consider and how much?

Immediate fluid resuscitation is needed in hypotensive patients and those with a lactate greater than 4 mmol/L.

The surviving sepsis guideline recommends the use of either crystalloid or colloid. Give 1000 ml (crystalloid) or 300–500 ml (colloid) fluid challenges over 30 min associated with haemodynamic improvement whilst aiming for:

- CVP 8–12 mmHg (12–15 mmHg if mechanical ventilation or pre-existing low ventricular compliance)
- Mean arterial BP ≥65 mmHg
- Urine output ≥0.5 mls/kg/hour
- Central venous oxygen saturations ≥70% or mixed venous ≥65%
- The rate of fluid replacement should be slowed if cardiac filling pressures increase without concurrent haemodynamic improvement.
- If venous oxygen saturation target not achieved:
  - Consider further fluid: transfuse to a haematocrit ≥30% and/or
  - Commence dobutamine (max. 20 micrograms/kg/min)

4. If the blood pressure is not responding to fluids how you would choose the Inotropes? Which inotrope and why and doses for each?

Persistent hypotension remains despite adequate fluid resuscitation; the patient either has inadequate myocardial 'pump' function or has a degree of vasodilatation which cannot be overcome by fluid therapy alone.

- If the patient appears vasodilated with a hyperdynamic circulation, an agent with vasopressor (adrenoreceptor agonist) properties, such as noradrenaline (norepinephrine), is appropriate to elevate the BP.

- If the patient is cool peripherally (has a large core to peripheral temperature difference), has signs of poor organ perfusion, and/or a low BP then an agent with more positive inotropic properties is the best choice. Examples are dopamine, adrenaline (epinephrine), dobutamine.

Inotropes should be given through a central venous catheter and direct intra-arterial BP measurement should be started as soon as possible.

The surviving sepsis campaign guidelines recommend that a MAP of ≥65mmHg should be maintained and that cardiac output should not be increased to supramaximal levels. Noradrenaline and dopamine are the centrally administrated vasopressors of choice. Low-dose dopamine should not be used for renal protection. Adrenaline can be used as a first-line alternative in shock when noradrenaline and dopamine have failed.

Infusions of inotropic and vasopressor drugs

Adrenaline and noradrenaline	Mix 5 mg in 50 ml 5% glucose. This gives a mixture of 1 in 10,000 adrenaline. Start at low dose (1–5 ml/hour) and titrate to the desired BP
	Noradrenaline may be available in 4-mg vials: mix 4 mg in 40 ml 5% glucose and use as above
Dobutamine and dopamine	Multiply the patient's weight in kg by 3. Make this number of milligrams of dobutamine or dopamine up to 50 ml in dextrose or saline. Infusion of this solution at a particular rate in ml/hour gives the same number in mcg/kg/min (e.g. 2 ml/hour = 2mcg/kg/min.)

5. Oxygenation is important, how are you going to assessment of tissue oxygenation?

Clinical evaluation: signs of poor tissue perfusion are cold, pale, dusky blue skin with delayed capillary refill and absence of veins in hands and feet. In seriously unwell patients the extremities may be clammy due to profuse sweating. The pulse volume and BP may be normal or low. Oliguria may be present. In septic patients, however, clinical examination can often be misleading, with warm, pink peripheries and rapid capillary refill.

Core-peripheral temperature gradient: the difference between the core temperature (usually nasopharyngeal or thermistor of PA catheter) and the peripheral temperature (often extensor surface of great toe). The fall in peripheral temperature can represent the first sign of deterioration in cardiovascular function; however, this does not correlate well in the septic patient.

Central and mixed venous oxygen saturation; arteriovenous oxygen content difference and oxygen extraction ratio: central venous oxygenation can only be measured from the pulmonary artery but the mixed central venous oxygen saturation can be taken from the superior vena cava. In critically ill patients these two measurements are not interchangeable.

The mixed central venous oxygenation is a reflection of tissue oxygenation; its normal range is 70–85%. A fall in its value suggests that the supply of oxygen to tissues is inadequate and if below 50% that anaerobic metabolism is occurring. Evidence suggests that changes in the mixed venous oxygen level occur earlier than other measured variables and can be a useful guide to decompensation. Rearranging the Fick principle allows the causes of these changes to be considered:

$$CvO_2 = CaO_2 - VO_2/Qt \qquad DO_2 = CO \times Hb \times \text{oxygen saturation}$$

Tissue oxygenation can depend on arterial hypoxia, anaemia, fall in cardiac output, or an increase in oxygen consumption.

The main flaw in using mixed central venous oxygenation as a method of assessing tissue perfusion in septic patients is that cellular hypoxia occurs notably due to impaired extraction or utilization of oxygen despite adequate delivery. Pathological supply dependency explains when at and below a critical level of oxygen delivery, despite further reductions in the supply of oxygen, cells are unable to extract further oxygen, therefore the mixed venous oxygen level does not fall and VO_2 decreases. It should also be noted that it is an average; hypoxia in one region may be compensated for by luxury perfusion in another. The presence of an intracardiac shunt left-to-right will give very high mixed venous oxygen readings.

The oxygen extraction ratio (OER) is the proportion of blood extracted by the tissues ($CaO_2 - CvO_2$)/CaO_2. The normal value is 0.22–0.3. This value is influenced only by changes in cardiac output and oxygen consumption. An increased OER indicates inadequate oxygen supply; a decreased OER suggest reduced metabolic rate or impaired oxygen extraction or utilization.

Gastric tonometry: intra-mucosal pH and the development acidosis may herald the first sign of compensated shock and therefore allow rapid detection of a decrease in tissue perfusion. A persistent acidosis has been suggested to indicate the development of gut ischaemia and subsequent multiorgan failure in septic patients.

Lactic acidosis is a relatively late and non-specific marker of impaired tissue perfusion as a consequence of cellular hypoxia leading to anaerobic glycolysis and the production of lactate. It should also be noted that in the critically unwell, lactate levels can rise due to reduced clearance due to hepatic and renal dysfunction.

Criteria for organ dysfunction
- Respiratory: a new or increased O_2 requirement to maintain SpO_2>90%.
- Renal: creatinine >177 μmol/L or UO <0.5 ml/kg/hour for 2 hours.
- Hepatic: bilirubin >34 μmol/L.
- Coagulation: platelets <100, INR >1.5, or activated partial thromboplastin time (aPTT) >60s.

Criteria for tissue hypoperfusion as organ dysfunction
- BP systolic <90 or mean <65 mmHg.
- A reduction of >40 mmHg from the patient's normal systolic BP.
- Lactate >2 mmol/L.
- A single organ dysfunction criterion or a single hypoperfusion criterion is sufficient to define severe sepsis. It is common for more than one organ dysfunction to coexist—identification of one dysfunction should prompt evaluation of other systems.

6. What would be your mode of ventilation in a severe sepsis?

Mechanical ventilation abolishes or minimizes the work of breathing, reduces oxygen consumption, and improves oxygenation. Mechanical ventilation of sepsis-induced acute respiratory distress syndrome (ARDS) has been investigated by the ARDSNet group and the following recommendations suggested in the 2008 surviving sepsis campaign:

Protective mechanical ventilation and recruitment manoeuvres
- Target a tidal volume of 6 ml/kg (predicted) body weight in patients with acute lung injury (ALI)/ARDS
- Target an initial upper limit plateau pressure ≤30 cmH$_2$O. Consider chest wall compliance when assessing plateau pressure.
- Allow PaCO$_2$ to increase above normal, if needed, to minimize plateau pressures and tidal volumes.
- Set PEEP to avoid extensive lung collapse at end-expiration.

Prone position ventilation
- Consider using the prone position for ARDS patients requiring potentially injurious levels of FiO$_2$ or plateau pressure, provided they are not put at risk from positional changes.

- Maintain mechanically ventilated patients in a semi-recumbent position (head of the bed raised to 45°) unless contraindicated.
- Non-invasive ventilation may be considered in the minority of ALI/ARDS patients with mild to moderate hypoxaemic respiratory failure. The patients need to be haemodynamically stable, comfortable, easily arousable, able to protect/clear their airway, and expected to recover rapidly.

High frequency oscillatory ventilation
HFOV delivers small tidal volume, with use of higher constant mean airway pressure to promote alveolar recruitment with minimizing trauma.

Inhaled pulmonary vasodilators
Inhaled pulmonary vasodilators are considered to improve ventilation–perfusion mismatch. nhaled nitric oxide and prostacyclin are commonly used.

Extracorporeal membrane oxygenation (ECMO)
ECMO is expensive but works to provide gas exchange across synthetic membrane outside body providing time to improve lung recovery.

Weaning
Use a weaning protocol and an SBT (spontaneous breathing trial) regularly to evaluate the potential for discontinuing mechanical ventilation. SBT options include a low level of pressure support with continuous positive airway pressure 5 cm H_2O or a T-piece.

Before the SBT, patients should:

- Be arousable.
- Be haemodynamically stable without vasopressors.
- Have no new potentially serious conditions.
- Have low ventilatory and end-expiratory pressure requirement.
- Require FiO_2 levels that can be safely delivered with a face mask or nasal cannula.

Further reading
Allman, K.G., and Wilson, I.H. *Oxford Handbook of Anaesthesia*, 2nd edn. Chapter 34; pp. 848–55. Oxford: Oxford University Press, 2006.

Dellinger, R.P., Levy, M.M., Carlet, J.M., et al. Surviving Sepsis Campaign: International guidelines for management of severe sepsis and septic shock: 2008. Special Article. *Critical Care Medicine* 2008; **36**(1):296–327.

Vincent, J.-L., Sakr, Y., Sprung, C., et al. Sepsis in European Intensive Care Units: Results of the SOAP Study. *Critical Care Medicine* 2006; **34**(2):344–53.

Clinical science

QUESTIONS

Anatomy: Trigeminal nerve

1. Describe the anatomy of the trigeminal ganglion. What is its aetiology?
2. What is trigeminal neuralgia?
3. What is the pathophysiology of trigeminal neuralgia?
4. What treatment options do you have?

Physiology: Lung volumes

1. What tests of respiratory function are commonly used?
2. Draw a diagram representing lung volumes.
3. How do you measure FRC? What factors affect FRC?
4. What is dead space? How is it measured?
5. What is closing capacity?
6. What is commonly measured in force expiration?
7. What affects the FEV_1/FVC ratio?
8. Draw flow loops: normal, obstructive lung disease, restrictive lung disease, laryngeal obstruction.

Pharmacology: Thiopentone

1. Draw the structure of thiopentone. What is its chemical group? What is the recommended dosage for thiopentone?
2. What is its mechanism of action?
3. What is the effect of thiopentone on cerebral blood flow?
4. What are the implications of using thiopentone in patients with hypovolaemia?
5. What are the effects of thiopentone on the respiratory system?
6. How does thiopentone lead to porphyria?

Physics and clinical measurements: Electricity

1. Define the terms: resistance, inductance, and capacitance. What are their units?
2. What are the effects of an electric current transmitted through the body?
3. What do you understand by the term microshock?
4. Explain the principle of diathermy.
5. What is the difference between unipolar and bipolar diathermy?
6. What are the safety mechanisms to prevent electrocution from a cautery?

ANSWERS

Anatomy: Trigeminal nerve

1. Describe the anatomy of the trigeminal ganglion. What is its aetiology?

Anatomy

The ganglion is at the floor of the middle cranial fossa and the branches are:

- Ophthalmic via superior orbital fissure: (sensory only) lacrimal, nasociliary, frontal, supraorbital, supratrochlear nerve.
- Maxillary via foramen rotundum: (sensory only) buccal, nasal and palatine; infraorbital, superior alveolar nerve.
- Mandibular via foramen ovate: (mainly sensory) buccal, auriculotemporal, lingual, inf. alveolar, mental never motor to muscles of mastication.

Aetiology

Tumour	Vascular	Inflammatory
Acoustic neuroma	Pontine infarct	Multiple sclerosis
Chordoma at the level of the clivus	Arteriovenous malformation in the vicinity	Sarcoidosis
Pontine glioma	Persistence of a primitive trigeminal artery	Paraneoplastic
Epidermoid		
Metastases	Pulsatile compression by the adjacent superior cerebellar artery	

2. What is trigeminal neuralgia?

Trigeminal neuralgia is a severe, lancinating pain in the trigeminal nerve territory that can be triggered by various stimuli (e.g. touch). The type of pain could be allodynia, hyperalgesia, triggers.

The International Headache Society has diagnostic criteria for idiopathic trigeminal neuralgia as paroxysmal attacks of facial or frontal pain, lasting a few seconds to less than 2 min.

The pain has at least four of the following characteristics:

- Distribution along one or more divisions of the trigeminal nerve.
- Sudden, intense, sharp, superficial, stabbing or burning in quality.
- Severe pain intensity.
- Precipitation from trigger areas or by certain daily activities (e.g. eating, talking, washing the face, cleaning the teeth).
- No symptoms between paroxysms.
- No neurological deficit is present.

Other causes of facial pain are excluded by history, physical examination, and special investigations (when necessary). In symptomatic cases, a persistence of aching can occur between paroxysms, as well as signs of sensory impairment in the trigeminal division. A cause is then demonstrated by appropriate investigation.

3. What is the pathophysiology of trigeminal neuralgia?

Trigeminal neuralgia is a typical example of neuropathic pain as the pain mechanisms are altered. There is evidence of both small and large fibre damage is present, as suggested by the potential for vibration to trigger an attack. The primary or secondary demyelination of the nerve, leads to uncontrolled firing of small unmyelinated trigeminal nerve fibres. This occurs, in part, because of the lack of inhibitory inputs from large myelinated nerve fibres. However, features also suggest a partly central mechanism (e.g. delay between stimulation and pain, refractory period).

4. What treatment options do you have?

Medical treatment

- Carbamazepine: has proven its efficacy in numerous studies and treatment of choice.
- Phenytoin has a lower rate of success, but a patient occasionally responds to it.
- Baclofen has proven efficacy in this condition.
- Clonazepam has moderate efficacy not very commonly used due to side effects and dependence.
- Amitriptyline has been used, but the success rate is low.
- Gabapentin seems to be effective.
- Lamotrigine has been proven more effective than placebo. The dosage should be increased slowly for better tolerance (e.g. 25 mg daily dose each week; up to 250 mg twice a day).

Surgical treatment

- **Microvascular decompression (MVD)**: this procedure consists of opening a keyhole in the mastoid area and freeing the trigeminal nerve from the compression/pulsating artery; then, a piece of Teflon is placed between them. Large series have been published, and the initial efficacy is >80%. Recurrence rates are among the lowest compared with other invasive treatments. Usually, it requires the demonstration of true contact and compression by the artery on the nerve, but series are published that show an almost equally effective result without any demonstrated abnormality on imaging or even frank compression shown preoperatively.
- **Alcohol injection** of the trigeminus can be performed at various locations along the nerve and is aimed at destroying selective pain fibres. Although it is an easy procedure, the success rate is low, in part because of a low selectivity of effect on the fibre type with this substance.
- **Glycerol injection** of the gasserian ganglion to selectively destroy the pain-transmitting fibres has been used for a long time. This injection has a higher efficacy rate and a lower recurrence rate than the alcohol injection.

Recently introduced, **gamma-knife treatment** consists of multiple rays (over 200) of high-energy photons concentrated with high accuracy on the target.

Further reading

Bennetto, L., Patel, N.K., and Fuller, G. Trigeminal neuralgia and its management *British Medical Journal* 2007; **334**:201–5.

Cruccu, G., Gronseth, G., Alksne, J., et al. AAN-EFNS guidelines on trigeminal neuralgia management. (European Federation of Neurological Societies Guidelines). *European Journal of Neurology* 2008; **15**:1013–28.

NICE. *Stereotactic radiosurgery for trigeminal neuralgia using the gamma knife*. London: NICE, 2004.

Trigeminal neuralgia. Clinical Knowledge Summaries (November 2008). Available at: http://www.cks.nhs.uk/trigeminal_neuralgia

Physiology: Lung volumes

1. What tests of respiratory function are commonly used?

The common respiratory function tests are:

Tests of static volumes	Tests of dynamic volumes	Gas exchange	Pulmonary circulation
Spirometry	Forced expiratory spirometry	Blood gas—ABG	Radioisotope scanning
Dead space	Peak expiratory flow rates	Pulse oximetry	Angiogram
Closing capacity	Flow loops	Diffusing capacity	
Compliance			
Maximal voluntary ventilation			

2. Draw a diagram representing lung volumes.

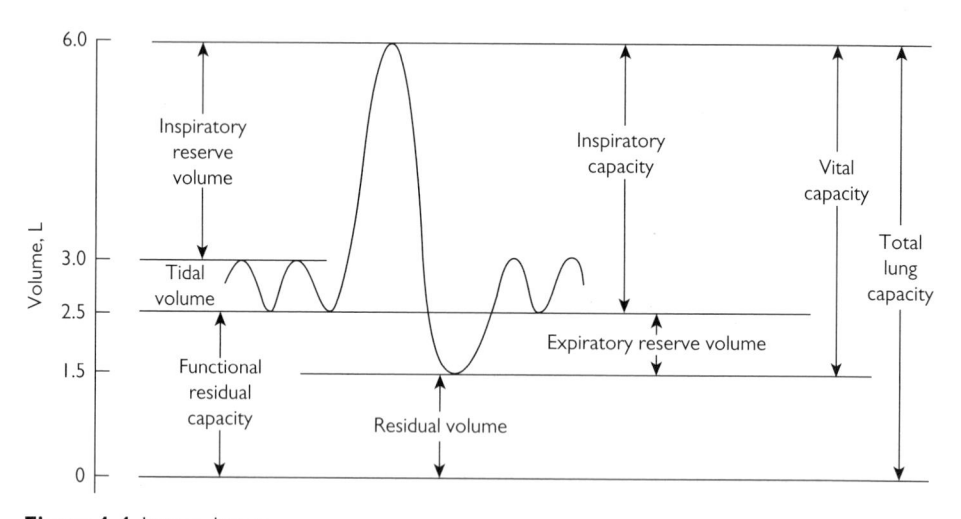

Figure 1.4 Lung volumes.

Volumes: Vt 500 ml; IRV 2500ml; ERV 1500 ml; RV 1500 ml.

Capacities: IC 3000 ml; FRC 3000 ml; VC 4500 ml; TLC 6000 ml.

3. How do you measure FRC? What factors affect FRC?

The FRC is measured by helium dilution, nitrogen washout, and body plethysmography.

The factors affecting the FRC are:
- Height and sex (male > female by 10%)
- FRC reduced by: obesity, pregnancy, supine position, restrictive lung disorders, anaesthesia.
- FRC increased by: asthma, PEEP/CPAP.

4. What is dead space? How is it measured?

This is a volume of air inhaled but does not taking part in gas exchange.

- **Anatomical**: mouth, nose, pharynx to large airways not lined with respiratory epithelium.
- **Alveolar**: ventilated lung which is not perfused. An extreme of V/Q mismatch.
- **Physiological**: anatomical + alveolar dead space.

The dead spaces are measured by:

- Anatomical: Fowler's method—nitrogen washout.
- Physiological: Bohr method:

$$\frac{Vd}{Vt} = \frac{PaCO_2 - PeCO_2}{PaCO_2}$$

5. What is closing capacity?

The closing capacity (CC) is the lung volume at which small airways in the dependent parts of the lung begins to close. CC= closing volume (CV)+ residual volume (RV). It is measured with single breath nitrogen washout out—sharp rise in expired nitrogen.

CC usually considerably less than FRC in fit young adults:

- CC = FRC in neonates and infants.
- CC = FRC in supine position at 44 years.
- CC = FRC in upright position at 66 years.

6. What is commonly measured in force expiration?

Using the forced expiration we can measure FEV_1, FVC, FEV_1/FVC ratio, peak expiratory flow rate.

7. What affects FEV_1/FVC ratio?

The FEV_1/FVC ratio are affected by:

Ratio is reduced in obstructive lesions, e.g. asthma, COPD.

Ratio is increased in restrictive lesions, e.g. pulmonary fibrosis, kyphoscoliosis.

8. Draw flow loops : normal, obstructive lung disease, restrictive lung disease, laryngeal obstruction

- Normal: from TLC (6–7 L) to RV (3 L); PEFR ~8–10 L/sec.
- Obstructive: greater TLC due to hyperinflation, greater RV; low flow rates and scooped out appearance.
- Restrictive: reduced maximum flow rate total volume exhaled reduced; reduced TLC normal RV.
- Upper airway obstruction: RV normal, TLC reduced flow rates low and constant.

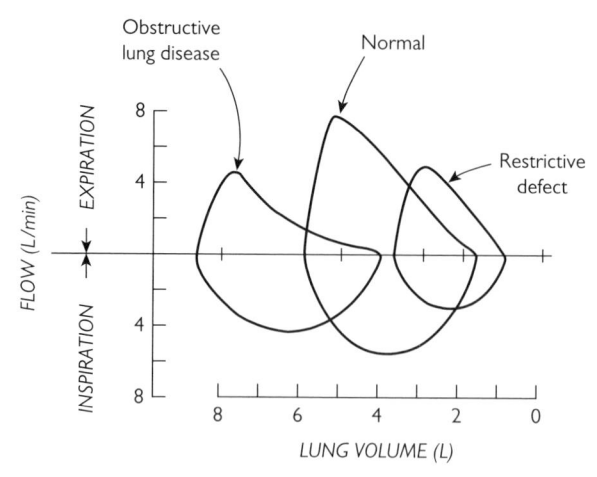

Figure 1.5 Flow loops.
Reproduced from *Physiology for Anaesthesiologists* by J.P. Howard Fee and James G. Bovill with kind permission of Taylor and Francis.

Pharmacology: Thiopentone

1. Draw the structure of thiopentone. What is its chemical group?

Figure 1.6 Structure of thiopentone.

Sodium thiopentone (also known as thiopental or pentothal) is prepared by dissolving a yellowish powder in sterile water to provide a 2.5% solution (i.e. 25 mg/ml). The solution should be used within 24 hours of preparation and kept cool.

The solution is alkaline with a pH of greater than 10, and can be irritating and painful if accidentally injected into tissues. Because of the alkalinity, thiopentone should not be mixed in the same syringe as other drugs, as it may cause formation of a cloudy precipitate and inactivate the drug. Thiopental has a pKA ~7.6 (~40% ionized at physiological pH).

Thiopentone is metabolized in the liver; less than 1% of the drug appears in the urine unchanged. The recommended dosage for a healthy adult is 3–5 mg/kg. The paediatric dosage is 5–7 mg/kg. The dosage for geriatric age group is reduced to 2–2.5 mg/kg.

2. What is its mechanism of action?

This is a barbiturate with the capability of depressing the reticular activating system. The response may reflect the ability of barbiturates to decrease the rate of dissociation of the inhibitory neurotransmitter gamma-aminobutyric acid (GABA) from its receptors. GABA causes an increase in chloride conductance through ion channels, resulting in hyperpolarization and, consequently, inhibition of postsynaptic neurons.

Barbiturates selectively depress transmission in the sympathetic ganglia, which may contribute to the drug-associated decrease in BP.

Mechanisms of action

Barbiturates both enhance and mimic the action of GABA; by binding to the receptor they:

- Decrease the rate of GABA dissociation.
- Increase the duration of GABA-activated Cl^- channel opening.
- At higher concentrations directly activate Cl^- channel.

3. What is the effect of thiopentone on cerebral blood flow?

Decrease of cerebral blood flow (CBF ~50%) and cerebral metabolism ($CMRO_2$ ~ 50%) with anaesthetic doses of thiopentone in patients with decreased intracranial compliance, or increased intracranial pressure (ICP), the barbiturates increase the cerebral perfusion pressure:

$$CPP = MAP - ICP$$

- This is due to their greater effect on decreasing ICP than arterial BP.
- This profound cerebral vasoconstriction may be offset by increases in $PaCO_2$.
- Therefore, in the absence of controlled ventilation and normocapnia, thiopentone may increase CBF secondary to decreased respiration.

4. What are the implications of using thiopentone in patients with hypovolaemia?

Thiopentone causes:

- Further fall in BP.
- The decreased central compartment leads to increased concentration of the drug reaching the brain and heart, with resulting severe respiratory and cardiovascular system depression.
- There is also a decreased rate of redistribution.

5. What are the effects of thiopentone on the respiratory system?

- Two or three hyperapnoeic breaths followed by apnoea.
- Respiratory depression is dose related, with reduction in ventilatory responsiveness to CO_2 and hypoxia.
- The respiratory pattern rapidly returns to normal; however, the CO_2/O_2 response curves remain depressed for some time.
- Hypoxic pulmonary vasoconstriction is unaffected.
- There is a low incidence of laryngospasm and bronchospasm, unless the upper airways are stimulated.
- Laryngeal reflexes are not depressed until deep levels of anaesthesia.

6. How does thiopentone leads to porphyria?

Porphyrias are inborn errors of metabolism with abnormal porphyrin metabolism. Porphyrin consists of 4 pyrrole rings linked by –CH– bridges found in haemoglobin, plus some of the cytochrome and peroxidase enzymes. The rate limiting reaction for its synthesis is catalysed by d-aminolevulinic acid synthetase, this is responsible for the production of delta-ALA from succinate and glycine within the mitochondria; this enzyme is induced by the barbiturates and is increased in certain types of porphyria.

Further reading

Hayashi, M., Kobayashi, H., Kawano, H., et al. Treatment of systemic hypertension and intracranial hypertension in cases of brain hemorrhage. *Stroke* 1988; **19**: 314–21.

Homer, T.D. and Stanski, D.R. The effect of increasing age on thiopental disposition and anesthetic requirement. *Anesthesiology* 1985; **62**:714–24.

James, M.F.M. and Hift, R.J. Porphyrias. *British Journal of Anaesthesia* 2000; **85**:143–53.

Mustajoki, P. and Heinonen, J. General anesthesia in 'inducible' porphyrias. *Anesthesiology* 1980; **53:**15–20.

Wood, M. and Wood, A.J. (eds). *Drugs and anesthesia: pharmacology for anesthesiologists*, pp. 200–19. Baltimore, MD: Williams & Wilkins, 1983.

Physics and clinical measurements: Electricity

1. Define the terms: resistance, inductance, and capacitance. What are their units?

Resistance: The resistance along a conductor to the flow of current. It is measured in Ohms. It is defined as the resistance which allows a current of one ampere to flow under the influence of a potential of one volt.

Capacitance: The measure of the capability of a conductor or a system to store charge. The farad is the capacitance of an object when its electric potential increases by one volt when one coulomb of charge is added to it.

Inductance: inductance is a measure of the amount of magnetic flux produced for a given electric current. The SI unit is Henry (H).

2. What are the effects of an electric current transmitted through the body?

- 1 mA: tingling pain
- 5 mA: pain
- 15 mA: tonic muscle contraction
- 50 mA: tonic contraction of respiratory muscles and respiratory arrest
- 100 mA: ventricular fibrillation

3. What do you understand by the term microshock?

Currents of small strength (0.05–0.1 mA) can cause ventricular fibrillation (VF) when applied directly to the myocardium (like leakage from an intracardiac catheter). This small current is called microshock.

4. Explain the principle of diathermy.

Diathermy uses high frequency electric current to produce heat. It is used in surgery for coagulation and cutting. The principle is based on Ohm's law which states that:

$$\text{Voltage} = \text{current} \times \text{resistance} \ (V = IR).$$

$$\text{The heat energy produced} = (\text{current})^2 \times \text{resistance} \ (E = I^2R).$$

5. What is the difference between unipolar and bipolar diathermy?

Unipolar diathermy has an active electrode where there is a high current density due to the small area of the electrode. This leads to generation of heat energy and cautery. The passive electrode (diathermy plate) used with unipolar diathermy has a large area and so the current density (and hence the heat produced) is small. The diathermy plate and hence the patient is kept at earth potential. However, if the contact is poor then either there is a reduced area of contact (with a higher current density) or increased resistance. Both these faults lead to an increased risk of burning.

Bipolar diathermy does not have a passive electrode, and the current passes from an active electrode to a return electrode; these are the two blades of the diathermy forceps. Here there is no diathermy plate and the circuit is not earthed. Bipolar diathermy uses lower power than monopolar, and this limits its efficacy in coagulation of all but the smallest vessels.

6. What are the safety mechanisms to prevent electrocution from a cautery?

In diathermy a high-frequency current is used (500,000–1000,000 Hz). This high-frequency current passes directly through the body without causing VF, unlike low-frequency (50 Hz) current from standard electric connections.

- An isolating capacitor is located between the patient plate and the earth. This capacitor has high impedance to low-frequency 50 Hz current, thus protecting the heart against electric shock.
- Risks from flow of current to earth are reduced if the circuit is completely isolated from earth, i.e. floating. This is achieved by use of transformers.
- Audio alarm activation if diathermy plate incorrectly applied.
- Using a quiver for the active electrode when not in use.

Further reading

Magee, P. and Tooley, M. *The Physics, Clinical Measurement and Equipment of Anaesthetic Practice for the FRCA*, 2nd edn. Oxford: Oxford University Press, 2011.

Chapter 2

Clinical anaesthesia

Long case: A case for total thyroidectomy 31
Short cases 35
   Questions 35
   Answers 37
      Short case 1: Fracture mandible for ORIF 37
      Short case 2: Awareness under anaesthesia 38
      Short case 3: Hypothermic elderly lady 39

Clinical science

Questions 41
Answers 42
   Anatomy: Cardiac conduction 42
   Physiology: One-lung anaesthesia 43
   Pharmacology: Renal failure and pharmacodynamics 44
   Physics and clinical measurements: Anaesthesia circuits 45

Clinical anaesthesia

Long case: A case for total thyroidectomy

On your list there is a 55-year-old West African gentleman for a total thyroidectomy. He has a large goitre. He has a history of hypertension, controlled with atenolol, and is known to be sickle cell trait positive.

Clinical examination	Temperature: 38.2°C; weight: 110 kg; height 170 cm				
	Pulse: 65/min, regular; BP: 138/85 mmHg; respiratory rate: 12/min				
	Chest: bilateral air entry, vesicular sounds, no crepitations/rhonchi				
	Cardiovascular system: normal heart sound with no murmurs				
	Large goitre with tracheal deviation to the right				
Laboratory investigations	Hb	14.4 g/dL	Na	142 mmol/L	
	MCV	90 fL	K	4.7 mmol/L	
	WBC	4.1 × 10⁹/L	Urea	3.9 mmol/L	
	Platelets	261 × 10⁹/L	Creatinine	96 μmol/L	
	TSH	1.5 mu/L	T_4	75 mmol/L	

QUESTIONS

1. Summarize the case.
2. What are the main issues concerning you?
3. What more information do you need from the history and examination?
4. Comment on the blood results. What other investigations would you like?
5. What are the implications of sickle cell trait?
6. Comment on the ECG. What is the pathophysiology of Wolff–Parkinson–White syndrome (WPW) syndrome? What are the implications for anaesthesia?
7. How should an intraoperative SVT be managed?
8. What are the abnormalities on the chest X-ray and CT scan of the neck?
9. How would you proceed with the induction of anaesthesia in this patient?
10. What are the likely causes of airway obstruction in the immediate postoperative period?
11. How would you manage hypocalcaemia?

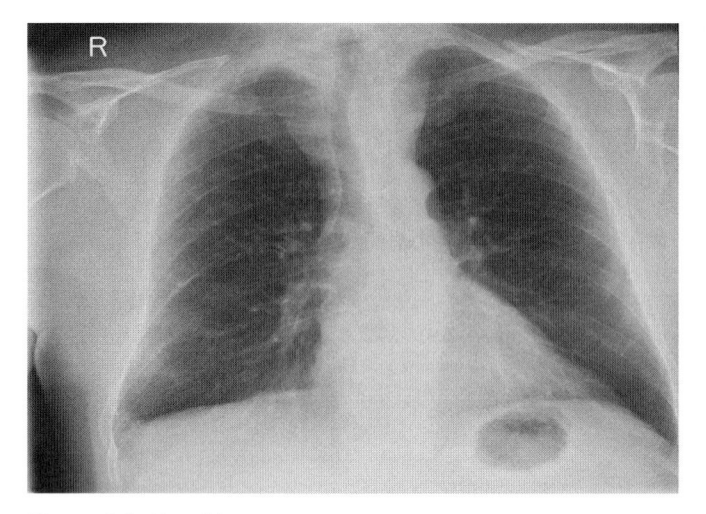

Structured Oral Examination Practice for the Final FRCA

Figure 2.1 Chest X-ray.

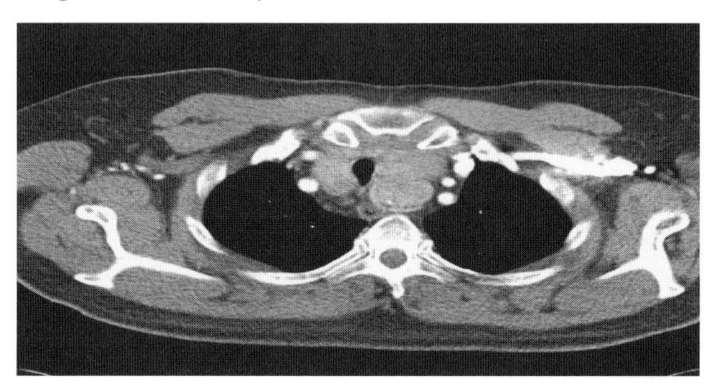

Figure 2.2 CT.

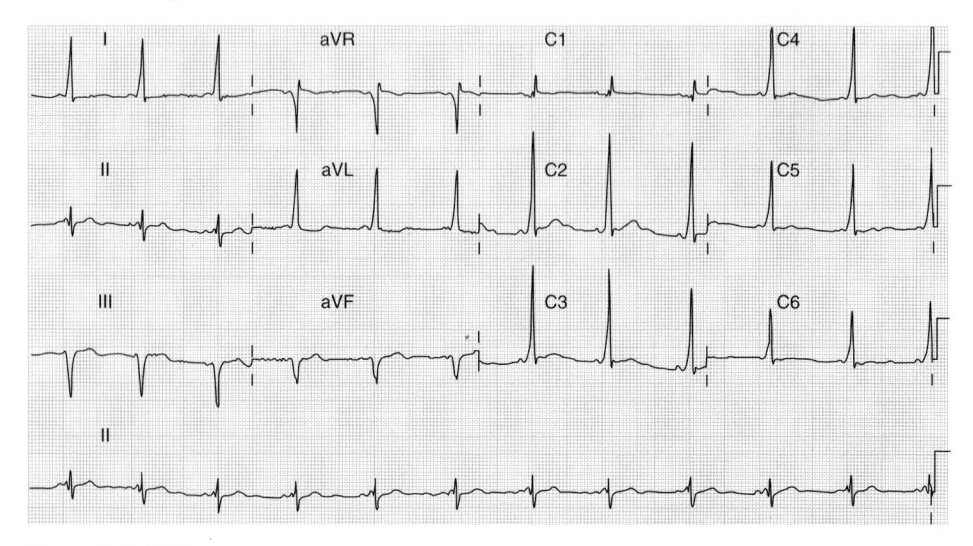

Figure 2.3 ECG.

ANSWERS

1. Summarize the case.

We have a middle-aged man for elective thyroid surgery. The patient is biochemically euthyroid but has the comorbidities of obesity, hypertension, WPW syndrome, and sickle cell trait. This case involves a potentially difficult airway with imaging showing a deviated trachea.

2. What are the main issues concerning you?

- Thyroid status
- Airway management
- Cardiovascular instability
- Preventing a sickle crisis

3. What more information do you need from the history and examination?

- Goitre:
    - Thyroid status
    - Cause of the goitre
    - Any other associated autoimmune disorders
    - Duration of the goitre—if chronic may have tracheomalacia
    - Any symptoms or signs of positional airway compromise
    - Presence of malignancy
    - Full airway assessment including any retrosternal spread of the goitre
    - Any signs of SVC obstruction
- Sickle trait: HbS level
- WPW: any history of SVT

4. Comment on the blood results. What other investigations would you like?

- FBC: all values within normal ranges
- U&Es: all values within normal ranges
- Thyroid function test: biochemically euthyroid

Other investigations I would like are:

- Nasendoscopy: to assess vocal cord movement and laryngeal displacement
- Serum calcium
- Electrophoresis: HbS level

5. What are the implications of sickle cell trait?

- Patients with trait have HbS levels <50%, sickling is uncommon
- Patients usually have a Hb level within the normal range

Measures to prevent sickling

- Avoid hypothermia
- Keep hydrated
- Provide analgesia
- Normocarbia to prevent acidosis
- Give prophylactic antibiotics

6. Comment on the ECG. What is the pathophysiology of WPW syndrome? What are the implications for anaesthesia?

HR 65 bpm in sinus rhythm and the presence of δ waves suggest WPW. Given the patient is on atenolol a HR of 65 is expected. The pathophysiology of WPW syndrome is due to the congenital accessory pathway which permits more rapid conduction than the usual pathway via the atrioventricular node which allows circular conduction and is prone to SVT and AF. The implications under anaesthesia could be SVT which can be prevented by avoiding hypoxia and electrolyte imbalance and the anaesthetist must be alert to the possibility of SVT and be ready to treat it if it occurs.

7. How should an intraoperative SVT be managed?

- If hypotension—DC cardioversion
- Adenosine
- Beta-blocker such as esmolol
- Do not give digoxin—may increase accessory conduction and lead to VF

8. What are the abnormalities on the chest X-ray and CT scan of the neck?

- **Chest X-ray**: there is well-defined widening of the superior mediastinum and deviation of the trachea to the right which suggests a thyroid goitre. Blunting of the right costophrenic angle.
- **CT**: there is a large multinodular goitre with retrosternal extension. This is causing tracheal deviation to the right and tracheal compression.

9. How would you proceed with the induction of anaesthesia in this patient?

- Induction is usually straightforward but if there are any concerns involve a senior anaesthetist
- Check equipment.
- Ensure a surgeon is immediately available.
- Antisialogue medication if considering awake intubation.
- Induction:
  - Can use IV, inhalational, or awake fibreoptic.
  - Be able to discuss and justify your chosen technique.
- Tracheostomy under local anaesthetic in cases of profound airway compromise.
- May need a smaller tube—can estimate trachea size from CT scan.

10. What are the likely causes of airway obstruction in the immediate postoperative period?

- Haematoma
- Tracheomalacia
- Recurrent laryngeal nerve palsy
- Laryngeal oedema
- Pneumothorax
- Inadequate reversal of muscle relaxation
- (Tetany is rare)

11. How would you manage hypocalcaemia?

- If >2 mmol/L give oral calcium supplementation.
- If <2 mmol/L give IV calcium—10 ml 10% calcium gluconate over 3 min.

Further reading

Allman, K.G. and Wilson, I.H. *Oxford Handbook of Anaesthesia*, 2nd edn. Chapter 22: Endocrine surgery; Thyroidectomy, pp. 554–7. Oxford: Oxford University Press, 2006.

Malhotra, S. and Sodhi, V. Anaesthesia for thyroid and parathyroid surgery. *Continuing Education in Anaesthesia, Critical Care & Pain* 2007; **7**(2):55–8.

Short cases

QUESTIONS

Short case 1: Fracture mandible for ORIF

A 19-year-old male who had a fight in a pub and has fractured his mandible is on your emergency list for an ORIF.

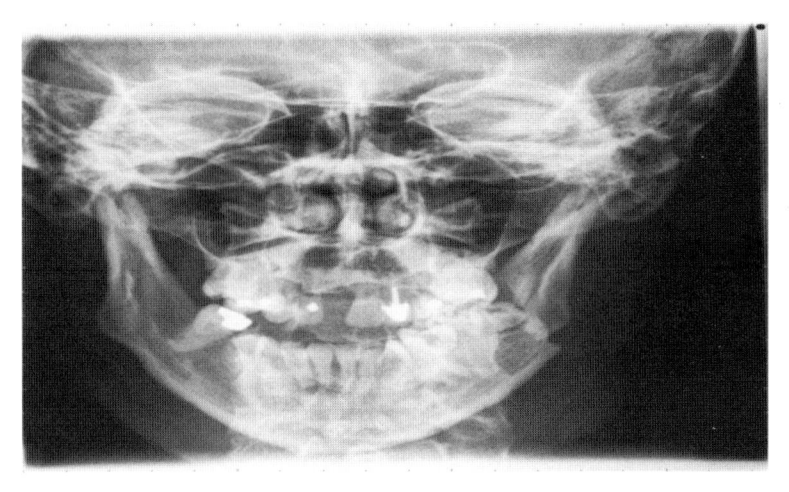

Figure 2.4a X-ray of fractured mandible.

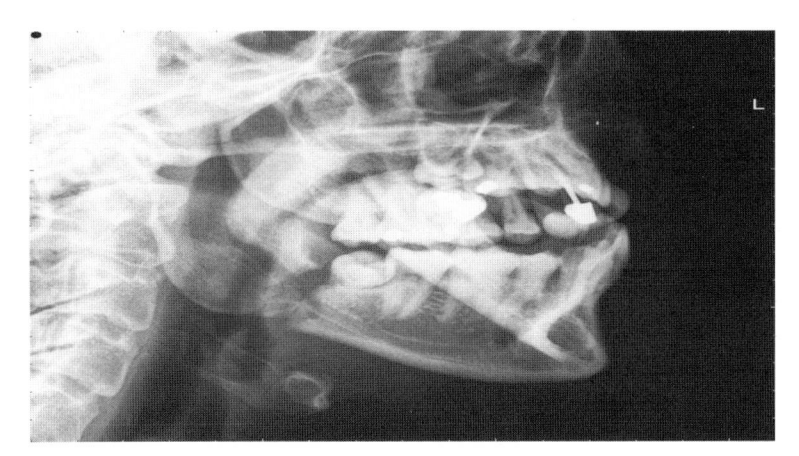

Figure 2.4b X-ray of fractured mandible.

1. What do you see on the X-ray?
2. What are the main issues regarding this patient?
3. How will you assess his airway? (The patient's mouth opening is limited to 1 cm.)
4. What investigations may be helpful in this case?
5. How would you clear his C-spine?
6. How would you proceed?

Short case 2: Awareness under anaesthesia

A recovery nurse calls you to assess a patient who has just woken up from anaesthesia. The patient has had a diagnostic laparoscopy. She is complaining that she heard everything during the procedure.

1. How would you proceed?
2. Define implicit and explicit awareness.
3. What is the incidence of awareness?
4. What patient groups are at high risk for awareness?
5. How do you prevent awareness?
6. What is likely to mask it?
7. Should we routinely use BIS monitoring?

Short case 3: Hypothermic elderly lady

In the middle of a Sunday night you are called to the emergency department to see an elderly female patient who has been brought to hospital after being found unconscious in bed. She has a temperature of 29°C.

1. How would you classify this degree of hypothermia?
2. What mortality is associated with severe hypothermia?
3. What are the cardiovascular effects of hypothermia?
4. How would you go about warming this lady?
5. Where would be the most appropriate place to measure her temperature?
6. When might hypothermia be advantageous?

Chapter 2

ANSWERS

Short case 1: Fracture mandible for ORIF

1. What do you see on the X-ray?
There is a fracture of the body of the left mandible with minor displacement of the fracture fragments. There are no other fractures.

2. What are the main issues regarding this patient?
- Potential difficult airway.
- Intoxication: timing of surgery, effect of alcohol on stomach emptying.
- Associated injuries: potential for head or neck injury.

Be prepared for questions on base of skull fracture and clearing the c-spine.

3. How will you assess his airway? (The patient's mouth opening is limited to 1 cm.)
- Mouth opening may be limited by pain, trismus, or mechanical disruption of the temporomandibular joint.
- Assess and document damage to any teeth.
- Mallampati score.
- Thyromental distance (Patil's test).
- Body habitus and facial hair.
- Mandible protrusion.
- It is always good to check the size and patency of the nostrils as this will be helpful in nasal intubation. However, nasal intubation is contraindicated in base of skull fracture.

4. What investigations may be helpful in this case?
- If any suggestion of a head injury or loss of consciousness then CT head is helpful.
- Lateral C-spine X-ray or CT neck if any concern about a neck injury.

5. How would you clear his C-spine?

History
- Mechanism of injury
- Neck pain

Examination
- Pain on palpation
- 'Step' in the alignment of the vertebrae
- Controlled active movement

Imaging
- Lateral C-spine X-ray or CT neck
- Reported by an experienced radiologist or neurosurgeon

6. How would you proceed?
- This operation is rarely an emergency so there is time for an adequate period of fasting (may need increased time as alcohol delays gastric emptying).
- Consider an antacid premed if concerned about aspiration.
- Antisialogue medication if considering awake intubation.

- In reality it is often easy to intubate these patients.
- Decide what is your method of choice—be able to discuss it and justify it.

Further reading
Allman, K.G. and Wilson, I.H. *Oxford Handbook of Anaesthesia*, 2nd edn. Chapter 36; Airway assessment and management, pp. 917–52. Oxford: Oxford University Press, 2006.

Short case 2: Awareness under anaesthesia

1. How would you proceed?
Patient awareness during general anaesthesia has considerable potential for severe emotional distress in the patient as well as professional, personal, and financial consequences for the anaesthetist. It is a serious consequence of relaxant anaesthesia with an incidence of around 1 in 1000. The incidents are due to errors in anaesthetic administration.

I will take a detailed account of events and record them in the patient's notes. Assure the patient and visit the patient daily after the event. It is important to involve a senior colleague. Consider referral to a psychologist or psychiatrist.

2. Define implicit and explicit awareness.
- **Explicit:** a memory may be recalled spontaneously.
- **Implicit:** memory is not recalled spontaneously but might affect mood and behaviour.

3. What is the incidence of awareness?
- Explicit recall of pain the incidence is 1 in 3000 for general anaesthesia.
- Awareness without recall of pain the incidence is 1 in 142–1000 for general anaesthesia.

4. What patient groups are at high risk for awareness?
Awareness is due to too light a plane of anaesthesia. It is more likely where muscle relaxants are used. This may be due to:
- Inadequate dose:
    - Omission of anaesthesia
    - Reduced dose during hypotensive episodes
    - Emergency surgery
    - Cardiac surgery
    - Obstetric surgery
    - Normal variability in minimum alveolar concentration (MAC)
    - Inability to monitor dose in TIVA
- Resistance:
    - Hypermetabolic states
    - Obesity
    - Smokers
    - Regular, heavy drinkers
- Equipment malfunction: breathing circuits, vaporizers, and TIVA line disconnection may occur

5. How do you prevent awareness?
- Recognise the at-risk patients
- Know exactly how the anaesthetic machine works and check before use
- Benzodiazepines at induction
- Periodically check the vaporizer level and provide adequate MAC levels
- Only use muscle relaxants where necessary

6. What is likely to mask the signs of awareness?
The signs of awareness are due to sympathetic nervous system activity. Many drugs or medical conditions may mask these signs. For example, beta-blockers may mask a tachycardia.

7. Should we routinely use BIS monitoring?
Its use has been recommended in high-risk groups but as yet there is no evidence it reduces the incidence or awareness.

Further reading
Hardman, J.G. and Aitkenhead, A.R. Awareness during anaesthesia. *Continuing Education in Anaesthesia, Critical Care & Pain* 2005; **5**(6):183–6.

Ranta, S.O.V., Laurila, R., Saario, J., *et al.* Awareness with recall during general anesthesia: incidence and risk factors. *Anesthesia & Analgesia* 1998; **86**:1084–9.

Short case 3: Hypothermic elderly lady

1. How would you classify this degree of hypothermia?
Hypothermia is a core temperature below 35°C and classified as:
- Mild hypothermia: 32–35°C
- Moderate hypothermia: 30–32°C
- Severe hypothermia: below 30°C

2. What mortality is associated with severe hypothermia?
One-third of patients with a core temperature below 28°C do not survive.

3. What are the cardiovascular effects of hypothermia?
- Bradycardia: combined with decreased metabolic rate this leads to decreased oxygen demand and therefore decreased cardiac output.
- Systemic vascular resistance is increased so this maintains MAP.
- The ECG shows an increased PR interval, widened QRS complex, and J waves.
- J waves, or Osborne waves, are a notch on the downstroke of the QRS complex.
- Arrhythmias occur below 30°C. Initially this is AF but it develops in to refractory VF below 28°C.
- There is increased blood viscosity and haematocrit below 30°C.

4. How would you go about warming this lady?

Where the onset of the hypothermia was gradual, the aim is to increase core temperature by 1°C every hour. The methods are:
- Forced air warmer
- Warmed IV fluids
- Irrigate body cavities with warmed fluids
- Humidify and warm inspiratory gases

5. Where would be the most appropriate place to measure her temperature?

Core temperature can be measured in the:
- Ear: tympanic membrane
- Oral/nasopharynx, bladder, or rectum
- Pulmonary artery via PA catheter

6. When might hypothermia be advantageous?

- Postventricular fibrillation cardiac arrest
- Following head injury
- During cardiac surgery
- In newborn hypoxic-ischaemic encephalopathy

Further reading

Kirkbride, D.A. and Buggy, D.J. Thermo-regulation and mild peri-operative hypothermia. *Continuing Education in Anaesthesia Critical Care & Pain* 2003; **3**:24–8.

Luscombe, M. Clinical applications of induced hypothermia. *Continuing Education in Anaesthesia, Critical Care & Pain* 2006; **6**(1):23–7.

Clinical science

QUESTIONS

Anatomy: Cardiac conduction

1. Describe the heart's conduction system.
2. How do you calculate the QT interval?
3. What is long QT syndrome?
4. What might cause QT syndrome?
5. How do you treat QT syndrome?
6. What are the important points to remember when anaesthetizing a patient for insertion of an implantable cardiodefibrillator?

Physiology: One-lung anaesthesia

1. When might you want to use one-lung ventilation?
2. What do you know about double lumen tubes?
3. What physiological changes occur in a spontaneously breathing patient in the lateral position?
4. What physiological changes occur during one-lung ventilation?
5. What will you do if a patient de-saturates when on one-lung ventilation?

Pharmacology: Renal failure and pharmacodynamics

1. What are the physiological implications of renal failure?
2. What are the pharmacological effects of renal failure?
3. What muscle relaxant would you use in a patient with renal failure?
4. What would determine your choice of opiate in a patient with renal failure?
5. Why might a patient with renal failure be at increased risk of postoperative bleeding?

Physics and clinical measurements: Anaesthesia circuits

1. How can you classify breathing circuits?
2. Please draw the Mapleson circuits.
3. You have a 1-year-old patient for repair of hernia who weighs 12 kg. What breathing circuit would you use?
4. Tell me more about the Mapleson E (Ayres T-piece).
5. In order to maintain the respiration what fresh gas flow is required?
6. What is the Jackson–Rees modification?

ANSWERS

Anatomy: Cardiac conduction

1. Describe the heart's conduction system.
- Sinoatrial node is at the junction of SVC and right atrium.
- Atrioventricular node conducts through to the ventricles.
- Bundle of His has right and left bundle branches on each side of the septum.
- Bundle branches become Purkinje fibres which spread into the myocardial tissue.
- Both nodes receive vagal and sympathetic input.
- Ventricular depolarization spreads from the apex.

2. How do you calculate the QT interval?

$$\text{Bazette's formula: } QTc = QT/\sqrt{RR}$$

Normal range is 0.30–0.44 sec.

3. What is long QT syndrome?
- Long QT syndrome is a familial condition associated with recurrent syncope and sudden cardiac death resulting from ventricular arrhythmias.
- A variety of conditions cause prolongation of the QT interval.
- There is impaired ventricular repolarization.
- Predisposes to torsades de pointes, a polymorphic ventricular tachycardia.

4. What might cause QT syndrome?
- **Congenital:**
  - Autosomal dominant inheritance
  - Genetic mutation in cardiac ion channels
- **Acquired:**
  - Drugs
  - Metabolic abnormalities: starvation, electrolyte imbalance, neurological injury

5. How do you treat it?
Treat any underlying condition; keep serum potassium greater than 4.5mmol/L.

Long QT can be managed by:
- Pharmacology: beta-blockers.
- Surgery: left cardiac sympathetic denervation.
- Electrophysiology: cardiac pacing, implantable cardiac defibrillator.
- Torsades de pointes is often self-terminating but can be treated with cardioversion or prevented with magnesium sulphate.

6. What are the important points to remember when anaesthetizing a patient for insertion of an implantable cardiodefibrillator?
- Sedation required for periods of induced VF.
- Existing pacemakers—caution with diathermy.
- Have external defibrillator/pacer available.

Chapter 2

Further reading

Abrams, D.J., Perkin, M.A., and Skinner, J.R. Long QT syndrome. *British Medical Journal* 2010; **340**:b4815.

Allman, K.G. and Wilson, I.H. *Oxford Handbook of Anaesthesia*, 2nd edn. Chapter 4: Perioperative arrhythmias, pp. 77–90. Oxford: Oxford University Press, 2006.

Hunter, J.D., Sharma, P., and Rathi, S. Long QT syndrome. *Continuing Education in Anaesthesia, Critical care & Pain* 2007; **8**(2):67–70.

Physiology: One-lung anaesthesia

1. When might you want to use one-lung ventilation?

Indications:

- **Absolute:**
  - To avoid lung contamination, e.g. in bronchopleural fistula.
  - Surgical opening of a major airway. Giant unilateral cyst or bulla.
- **Relative:** to improve surgical access, e.g. in oesophageal or pulmonary surgery.

2. What do you know about double lumen tubes?

The double lumen tubes are used in thoracic surgery to isolate the lungs. They are right- or left-sided according to the main bronchus they are designed to intubate. Usual practice is to use a left tube where possible. Size given in Charriere gauge, this is external diameter. Double lumen tubes have a small internal diameter.

Contraindication to use is distorted tracheobronchial anatomy.

Names of tubes are Carlens, Whites, Robertshaw, and bronchocath.

3. What physiological changes occur in a spontaneously breathing patient in the lateral position?

The dependent lung is compressed by the mediastinum and abdominal contents. The FRC is lower in the dependent lung which leads to increased compliance. The dependent lung receives the largest portion of ventilation and has increased perfusion due to a gravitational effect.

4. What physiological changes occur during one-lung ventilation?

The essential change is the presence of a shunt whereby the upper lung is perfused but not ventilated. Hypoxic pulmonary vasoconstriction occurs in an effort to decrease perfusion and thereby reduce the effect of this shunt.

5. What will you do if a patient de-saturates when on one-lung ventilation?

- Increase the FiO_2 but this might be ineffective in the presence of a large shunt.
- Ensure there is an adequate cardiac output.
- Check the position of the double lumen tube and suction both ports.
- Apply PEEP to the lower lung.
- After warning the surgeon, apply CPAP to the upper lung or insufflate with a few litres of oxygen.
- Try intermittent lung inflation.
- If all these measures fail, return to two-lung ventilation.

Further reading
Allman, K.G. and Wilson, I.H. *Oxford Handbook of Anaesthesia*, 2nd edn. Chapter 15: Thoracic surgery, pp. 351–80. Oxford: Oxford University Press, 2006.

Pharmacology: Renal failure and pharmacodynamics

1. What are the physiological implications of renal failure?
Renal failure produces multisystem effects:
- Hypertension
- Ischaemic heart disease
- Autonomic neuropathy
- Hyperparathyroidism
- Hyperphosphataemia
- Anaemia
- Delayed gastric emptying
- Uraemia cause immunosuppression and prolonged bleeding times

2. What are the pharmacological effects of renal failure?
- The majority of drugs are excreted via the kidney therefore they accumulate in renal failure.
- The loading dose of a drug often remains the same but there is an increased dose interval.
- Patients may have an increased volume of distribution—due to fluid retention—so may require an increased loading dose to achieve the same effect site concentration.
- Decreased protein binding may contribute to an increased volume of distribution.
- An increased volume of distribution reduces drug clearance.

3. What muscle relaxant would you use in a patient with renal failure?
- Atracurium is an ester and undergoes Hoffman degradation. This is a pH- and temperature-dependent process that occurs in plasma and is independent of renal function.
- Rocuronium and vecuronium are aminosteroids; there is concern that their metabolism and excretion is affected in renal failure.

4. What would determine your choice of opiate in a patient with renal failure?
- Morphine undergoes glucuronidation to morphine-6-glucuronide. This accumulates in renal failure leading to a prolonged duration of action.
- This effect does not seem to occur with fentanyl.
- Remifentanil is metabolized and excreted independent of renal function.

5. Why might a patient with renal failure be at increased risk of postoperative bleeding?
Uraemia impairs platelet function and leads to a prolonged bleeding time. This can be treated with DDAVP.

Chapter 2

Further reading
Allman, K.G. and Wilson, I.H. *Oxford Handbook of Anaesthesia*, 2nd edn. Chapter 6: Renal disease, pp. 123–30. Oxford: Oxford University Press, 2006.

Physics and clinical measurements: Anaesthesia circuits

1. How can you classify breathing circuits?
The breathing circuits can be classified as Open, Closed, Semi-open, and Semi-closed.

2. Please draw the Mapleson circuits.
FGF = fresh gas flow; RB = reservoir bag.

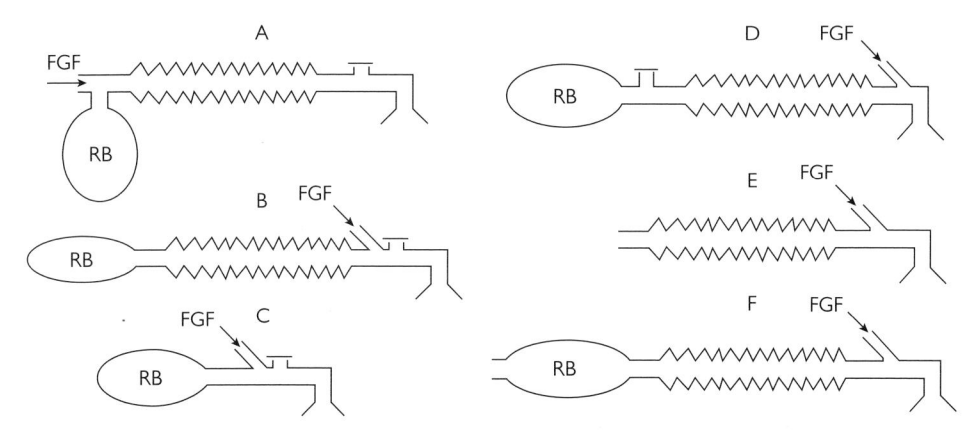

Figure 2.5a Mapleson circuits.

Figure 2.5b Mapleson circuits.

3. You have a 1-year-old patient for repair of hernia who weighs 12 kg. What breathing circuit you would use?
I would use Ayre's T-piece with Jackson–Rees modification.

4. Tell me more about the Mapleson E (Ayres T-piece).
The Ayres T-piece is a very compact breathing circuit with the following features:
- The circuit has low resistance as it is valveless.
- It is lightweight and semi-closed.
- It can be used both with spontaneous and controlled respiration.
- It is ideal for paediatric usage:
  - Expiratory limb must exceed tidal volume to prevent rebreathing of CO_2.
  - Used in children up to 25–30 kg as spontaneous or controlled ventilation.

5. In order to maintain the respiration what fresh gas flow is required?

The fresh gas flow (FGF) depends on the kind of ventilation:
- For spontaneous ventilation FGF must be 2–3 times minute volume.
- For IPPV, FGF must be 70 ml/kg/min.

6. What is the Jackson–Rees modification?

- This is also known as the Mapleson F circuit.
- It includes a 500-ml open ended bag.
- Allows for visual monitoring of respiratory effort of controlled ventilation.
- Suitable for children up to 20 kg.
- Scavenging is not possible.
- Requires high FGF.

Further reading

Allman, K.G. and Wilson, I.H. *Oxford Handbook of Anaesthesia*, 2nd edn. Anaesthesia breathing systems, pp. 768–9. Oxford: Oxford University Press, 2006.

Mapleson, W.W. Anaesthetic breathing systems-semi-closed systems. *Continuing Education in Anaesthesia Critical Care & Pain* 2001; **1**:3–7.

Chapter 3

Clinical anaesthesia

Long case: A case for elective colectomy   49
Short cases   54
   Questions   54
   Answers   56
      Short case 1: Guillain–Barré syndrome   56
      Short case 2: Squint correction   57
      Short case 3: Patient with an abnormal ECG   58

Clinical science

Questions   60
Answers   61
   Anatomy: Bone   61
   Physiology: Post-herpatic neuralgia   62
   Pharmacology: Bilirubin metabolism   63
   Physics and clinical measurements: Hyperbaric oxygen   64

Clinical anaesthesia

Long case: A case for elective colectomy

A 58-year-old coal miner is posted for sigmoid colectomy for carcinoma. He has a non-productive cough and is on nebulizers at home for asthma. He feels breathless on walking 50 metres. He is currently taking 2.5 mg prednisolone.

Clinical examination	Temperature: 38.2°C; weight: 85 kg; height: 160 cm			
	Pulse: 90/min, regular; BP: 140/82 mmHg; respiratory rate: 30/min; SpO_2: 93% on air			
	Chest: bilateral decreased air entry at bases, bilateral rhonchi			
	Cardiovascular system: normal heart sound with no murmurs			
	Central nervous system: no neurological deficit apart from visual field defects			
Laboratory investigations	Hb	12.0 g/dL	Na	137 mEq/L
	MCV	94 fL	K	4.8 mEq/L
	WBC	5.2×10^9/L	Urea	5.8 mmol/L
	Platelets	343×10^9/L	Creatinine	130 µmol/L
	INR	1.1	PO_2	10.3 kPa
			PCO_2	4.5 kPa
Pulmonary function tests		Predicted values	Measured values	% predicted
	FEV_1	4.2 L	1.8 L	40 %
	FVC	5.00 L	3.4 L	68 %
	FEV_1/FVC	84 %	55 %	60 %
	PEFR	500 L/min	200 L/min	40%

QUESTIONS

1. Summarize this case.
2. What are the main issues in this case?
3. Comment on the blood investigations.
4. What does the chest X-ray show?
5. Comment on the ECG. Why does this patient have right ventricular hypertrophy (RVH)?
6. Interpret the pulmonary function tests (PFTs).
7. What is the significance of measuring PFTs before and after bronchodilator administration?
8. What further investigations would you like?
9. How would you optimize this patient preoperatively?
10. What is the likely cause of his chronic obstructive pulmonary disease (COPD)?
11. How would you anaesthetize this man?

Structured Oral Examination Practice for the Final FRCA

12. What are the benefits of epidural analgesia? Does it improve outcome?
13. How would you manage him postoperatively?

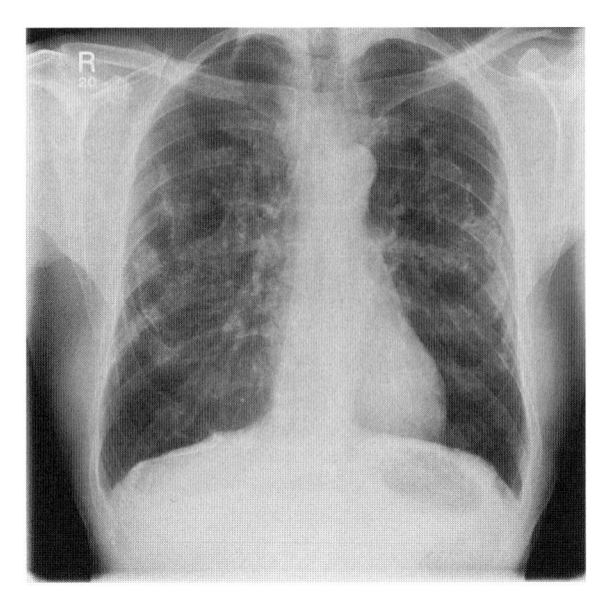

Figure 3.1 Chest-X-ray.

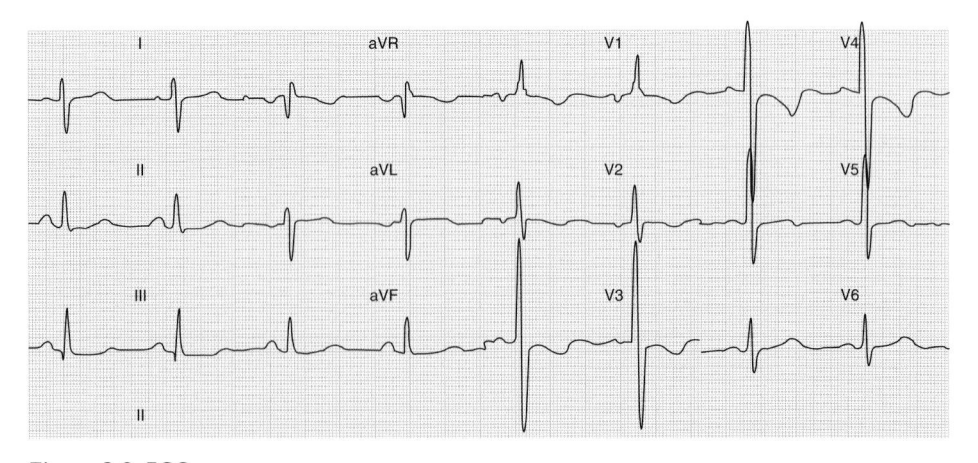

Figure 3.2 ECG.

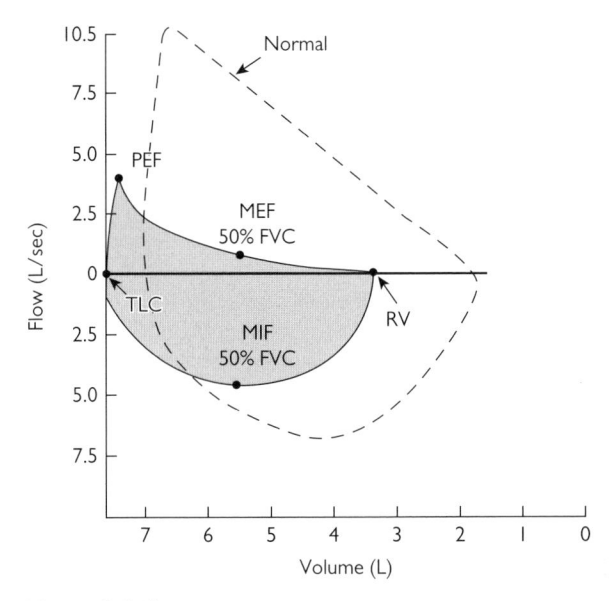

Figure 3.3 Spirometry.

ANSWERS

1. Summarize this case.

This is a middle-aged man with significant and non-optimized respiratory disease. He is listed for abdominal cancer surgery that is semi-urgent but allows time for optimization. I would not be happy to anaesthetize him today but would like to improve his respiratory status.

2. What are the main issues in this case?

- Cancer surgery: allows some time for optimization but there is not time for unnecessary delay.
- Abdominal surgery:
  - Need to consider the effects of laparotomy on postoperative respiratory function.
  - Need to consider options for pain relief.
- Respiratory status: patient is tachypnoeic, hypoxic, and has obstructive PFTs.

3. Comment on the blood investigations.

- Full blood count: mild anaemia—probably due to bowel carcinoma. Might expect polycythaemia with this respiratory history.
- Clotting: INR is normal, as are platelets—neuraxial anaesthesia is not contraindicated.
- Arterial blood gases: hypoxic-type I respiratory failure.
- Given a RR of 30 you might expect a lower $PaCO_2$.

4. What does the chest X-ray show?

The lungs are hyperexpanded and there are bilateral calcified pleural plaques. The heart size is normal.

5. Comment on the ECG. Why does this patient have right ventricular hypertrophy (RVH)?

- ECG: sinus rhythm 100 bpm
- Criteria for RVH:
  - R in V1 >7 mm or >S wave
  - T in V1 inverted
  - Right axis deviation
  - S waves in V5–V6

Longstanding hypoxia leads to hypoxic pulmonary vasoconstriction. This causes an increase in pulmonary vascular resistance and leads to pulmonary hypertension and eventually cor pulmonale or right ventricular failure. The right ventricle undergoes hypertrophy in an attempt to compensate for this.

6. Interpret the pulmonary function tests (PFTs).

The values are globally reduced and fit with a pattern of obstructive lung disease.

7. What is the significance of measuring PFTs before and after bronchodilator administration?

This allows assessment of the degree of reversibility. If there is improvement after administration of bronchodilators at least part of the respiratory disease is reversible and can be treated preoperatively.

8. What further investigations would you like?

- Echocardiogram: to allow assessment of ventricular function.
- CRP: may be elevated if concurrent infection as a cause for tachypnoea.
- Cardiopulmonary exercise testing: to allow risk stratification on basis of VO_2 max etc.

9. How would you optimize this patient preoperatively?

- Treat any reversible element of his respiratory disease.
- Cardiology review to optimize heart failure treatment.
- Preoperative nebulizers.
- Physiotherapy and antibiotics if any suggestion of superimposed chest infection.
- Nutritional support if cachexia/weight loss due to carcinoma.

10. What is the likely cause of his chronic obstructive pulmonary disease (COPD)?

- Smoking
- Coal miner-occupational exposure to dusts and pollutants

11. How would you anaesthetize this man?

- Preoperatively:
  - Nebulized bronchodilators
  - Consider risks and benefits of an epidural
- Intraoperatively:
  - Preoxygenation
  - Consider choice of muscle relaxant—atracurium may cause histamine release

- Tracheal intubation
- Pressure controlled ventilation—avoid barotrauma

12. What are the benefits of epidural analgesia? Does it improve outcome?

- Benefits:
  - Analgesia
  - Decreased thromboembolism
- Disadvantages:
  - Cardiovascular changes
  - Risk of nerve damage/haematoma

Right hemi-colectomy is usually performed via a lower midline incision—this is unlikely to have a significant effect on postoperative respiratory function.

Epidurals do not improve outcome.

13. How would you manage him postoperatively?

- Elective HDU admission
- Physiotherapy and early mobilization
- Early antibiotic therapy if increased temperature or sputum production
- Nebulized bronchodilators until fully mobile
- Humidified oxygen
- Deep vein thrombosis (DVT) prophylaxis: high risk as carcinoma

Further reading

Allman, K.G. and Wilson, I.H. *Oxford Handbook of Anaesthesia*, 2nd edn. Chapter 5: Respiratory disease, pp. 93–122. Oxford: Oxford University Press, 2006.

Wong, D.H., Weber, E.C., and Schell, M.J. Factors associated with postoperative pulmonary complications in patients with severe chronic obstructive pulmonary disease. *Anesthesia & Analgesia* 1995; **80**:276–84.

Short cases

QUESTIONS

Short case 1: Guillain–Barré syndrome

A 13-year-old boy presents with a 10-day history of malaise and generalized weakness. He complains of pins-and-needles in his toes and pain in his calves. He has now developed difficulty in swallowing and coughing. His HR is 120/min and irregular, BP is 95/60 mmHg but labile, and RR 26 breaths/min on oxygen by facemask at 6 L/min. Examination of his chest reveals bilateral air entry, harsh vesicular breath sounds, and crepitations at the right lower lung base. You have been asked to assess this patient for ICU admission.

1. What is the differential diagnosis?
2. What is the most likely diagnosis?
3. What is Guillain–Barré syndrome?
4. Can cranial nerves be affected?
5. What could be the reason for the irregularity in HR and labile BP?
6. What is your management plan?
7. After achieving control of ABC, what are the priorities in ITU management?

Short case 2: Squint correction

You are anaesthetizing for a day-case ophthalmic list. One of the cases is a 4-year-old child for strabismus surgery.

1. What is your anaesthetic plan?
2. The case is underway and the child becomes bradycardic at 40 bpm. What will you do?
3. What is the mechanism involved in the oculocardiac reflex?
4. How can you prevent this occurring?
5. Which muscle is most often involved?

Short case 3: Patient with an abnormal ECG

One of the pre-assessment nurses asks you to review an ECG for them. The patient is a healthy 29-year-old male who is listed for day-case knee arthroscopy.

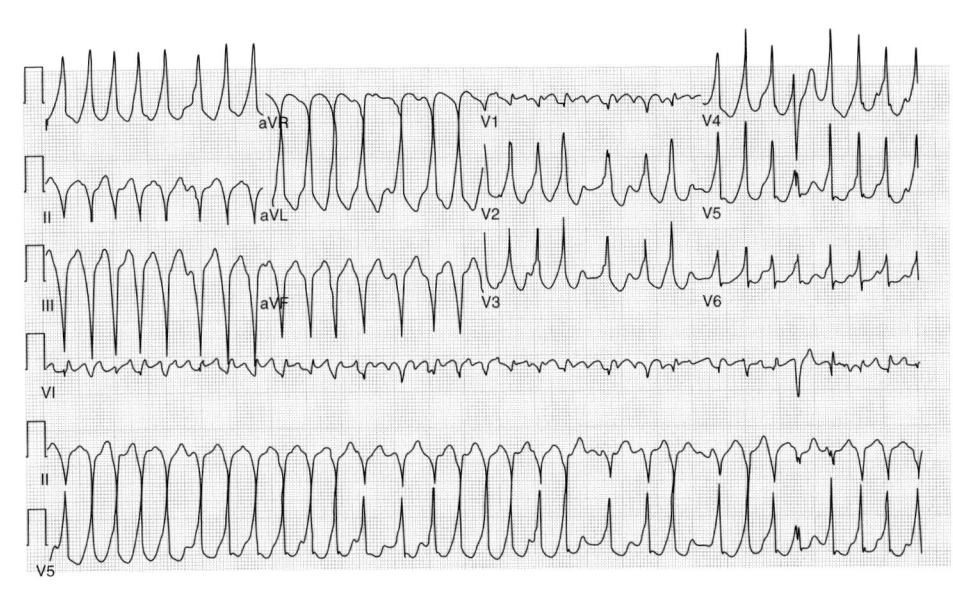

Figure 3.4 ECG.

1. Talk me through this ECG.
2. What is Wolff–Parkinson–White syndrome (WPW)?
3. What is the anaesthetic management of a patient with WPW?
4. How would you manage a perioperative supraventricular tachycardia (SVT)?
5. What else may cause SVT?
6. Do you think this patient is suitable for surgery?

ANSWERS

Short case 1: Guillain–Barré syndrome

1. What is the differential diagnosis?

- Guillain–Barré syndrome
- Poliomyelitis
- Diphtheria
- Porphyria
- Diabetes mellitus with sensorimotor neuropathy
- Lead and solvent poisoning
- Motor neuron disease
- Myasthenia gravis
- Botulism

2. What is the most likely diagnosis?

Guillain–Barré syndrome, an acute demyelinating polyneuropathy is the most likely diagnosis.

3. What is Guillain–Barré syndrome?

Guillain–Barré syndrome is an acute, ascending, immune-mediated demyelinating polyneuropathy and, in the post-polio era, is the most common cause of generalized paralysis. 50% of cases follow a viral illness.

- Incidence: 1–2 per 100,000.
- Male-to-female ratio is 1.5:1.
- Bimodal distribution, with peaks in age ranges of 15–35 years and 50–75 years.

The major symptom is rapidly progressive paralysis, which, unlike polio, is symmetrical. Paralysis of the lower extremities is followed by paralysis of the upper extremities, and both proximal and distal muscle groups are involved. Deep tendon reflexes are initially reduced and later are absent. A mild sensory disturbance or paraesthesia occurs.

One-third of patients require mechanical ventilation.

4. Can cranial nerves be affected?

Yes, the cranial nerves are involved in 45–75% of cases. Patients may present with facial weakness, dysphasia, or dysarthrias. A variation known as the *Miller–Fisher variant* is unusual in that neuropathy begins with cranial nerve deficits.

5. What could be the reason for the irregularity in HR and labile BP?

Markedly labile vital signs reflect *autonomic dysfunction*. Bradycardia or tachycardia, hypotension or hypertension, and hypothermia or hyperthermia can occur. In addition, patients may exhibit anhidrosis, paralytic ileus and urinary hesitancy.

6. What is your management plan?

The ABC approach: this patient requires airway protection (intubation) and respiratory support. Tracheostomy should be considered earlier rather than late because prolonged respiratory support is likely. He is likely to need IV fluids, inotropes, and invasive haemodynamic monitoring. After initial management, an attempt should be made to reach a definitive diagnosis (since the initial diagnosis of Guillain–Barré syndrome is clinical). Lumbar puncture and CSF analysis often shows increased CSF protein levels. A neurologist should be consulted if any uncertainty exists as to the diagnosis.

7. After achieving control of ABC, what are the priorities in ITU management?

- Specific treatment: IV immunoglobulins or exchange plasmaphoresis.
- Other measures are mainly supportive:
  - Physiotherapy.
  - Prophylaxis against DVT—extremely important as patient is likely to have limited mobility for a long time.
  - Pressure area care.
  - Nutritional support (preferably enteral).
  - Treatment of infections depending on culture and sensitivity reports.

Further reading

Vucic, S. Guillain–Barré syndrome: an update. *Journal of Clinical Neuroscience* 2009; **16**:733–41.

Short case 2: Squint correction

1. What is your anaesthetic plan?

- Preoperative:
  - EMLA/Ametop
  - Oral paracetamol 20 mg/kg
  - Some give oral atropine premed
- Induction:
  - Parent present
  - IV/gas induction as appropriate
- Airway:
  - Patients need to be paralysed, therefore south-facing RAE, armoured ETT or armoured LMA as local preference
  - Avoid suxamethonium as it increases the tone of the eye muscles
- Maintenance:
  - Usually volatile anaesthetic
  - Give PR analgesia if appropriate
  - Avoid opiates as they increase PONV
  - Give an antiemetic—high-risk surgery for PONV
  - Have atropine 20 mcg/kg available

2. The case is underway and the child becomes bradycardic at 40 bpm. What will you do?

Ask the surgeon to stop the surgery and then operate with reduce traction on the eye muscles. Give atropine IV 20 mcg/kg or glycopyrrolate 0.01 mg/kg.

This is called oculocardiac reflex (OCR) which is particularly common in children and adolescents undergoing correction of strabismus. It is characterized by a marked slowing of the HR or the occurrence of dysrhythmias in response to traction on the extraocular muscles or pressure on the globe. It may even result in cardiac arrest in extreme circumstances.

3. What is the mechanism involved in the oculocardiac reflex?

This reflex is mediated by the trigeminal–vagal reflex arc. It tends to be more marked with sudden and sustained traction compared to slow, gentle, progressive traction.
- Afferent: fibres run with the long and short ciliary nerves, via the ciliary ganglion to the trigeminal ganglion.
- Efferent: vagus nerve.

4. How can you prevent this occurring?

- I will be vigilant and consider prophylactic atropine 0.02 mg/kg or glycopyrrolate 0.01 mg/kg IV at induction.
- Inject local anaesthetic into the intraocular muscles.
- Avoid hypocarbia.

5. Which muscle is most often involved?

Medial rectus is the muscle most commonly involved.

Further reading

Allman, K.G. and Wilson, I.H. *Oxford Handbook of Anaesthesia*, 2nd edn. Chapter 27 Ophthalmic surgery, pp. 645–62. Oxford: Oxford University Press, 2006.

Short case 3: Patient with an abnormal ECG

1. Talk me through this ECG

- Irregular rhythm.
- HR around 150 bpm.
- Difficult to make out any p waves.
- δ waves are present-likely to be Wolff–Parkinson–White syndrome.

2. What is Wolff–Parkinson–White syndrome (WPW)?

- It is a congenital abnormality involving the presence of an accessory pathway between the atria and ventricles which bypasses the atrioventricular (AV) node.
- This allows more rapid conduction than the usual pathway via the AV node.
- Allows circular conduction.
- Prone to SVT and AF.

3. What is the anaesthetic management of a patient with WPW?

- Preoperative review and investigation by a cardiologist.
- Avoid sympathetic activity:
  - Avoid anxiety
  - Continue antiarrhythmics
  - Avoid tachycardia—pain/drugs/dehydration

4. How would you manage a perioperative supraventricular tachycardia (SVT)?

- Have a high index of suspicion.
- If hypotension—DC cardioversion.
- Adenosine.
- Beta-blocker such as esmolol.
- Do not give digoxin—may increase accessory conduction and lead to VF.

5. What else may cause SVT?

- Idiopathic.
- Lown–Ganong–Levine syndrome: presence of an accessory pathway bypassing the AV node.
- Hyperthyroidism.
- Caffeine.
- Nicotine.
- Alcohol.

6. Do you think this patient is suitable for surgery?

No I do not think so. This is a new diagnosis of WPW and the patient needs to be referred to a cardiologist. The tachycardia needs to be addressed before he is considered safe for surgery.

Further reading

Allman, K.G. and Wilson, I.H. *Oxford Handbook of Anaesthesia*, 2nd edn. Chapter 4 Perioperative arrhythmias, pp. 77–92. Oxford: Oxford University Press, 2006.

Yentis, S.M., Hirsch, N.P., and Smith, G.S. *Anaesthesia and Intensive Care A–Z: An Encyclopaedia of Principles and Practice* 4th edn. Edinburgh: Churchill Livingstone, 2009.

Clinical science

QUESTIONS

Anatomy: Bone

1. What layers does your needle pass through when inserting an intraosseous (IO) needle?
2. What are the indications for IO needle insertion?
3. Describe your landmarks for insertion of an IO needle into the tibia.
4. How do you know that the needle is in the correct place?
5. How does resuscitation via an IO needle work?
6. What can you give via an IO needle?
7. What are the complications of IO access?
8. What are the contraindications to using an IO needle?

Physiology: Post-herpatic neuralgia

1. What is post-herpatic neuralgia?
2. What is the pathophysiological process underlying post-herpatic neuralgia?
3. Are there any predisposing factors?
4. How do you treat it?
5. How does TENS work?
6. When is TENS not suitable?

Pharmacology: Bilirubin metabolism

1. What do you know about drug metabolism?
2. What is the pharmacological effect of liver failure?
3. What is hepatorenal syndrome?
4. Would you modify your anaesthetic for a patient with liver failure?
5. What drugs may cause jaundice?

Physics and clinical measurements: Hyperbaric oxygen

1. What is hyperbaric oxygen?
2. What are its applications?
3. Is oxygen harmless?
4. How do you know how much oxygen you are giving to your patient?
5. How do the fuel cell/Clark electrode/paramagnetic analyser work?

ANSWERS

Anatomy: Bone

1. What layers does your needle pass through when inserting an intraosseous (IO) needle?

The layers through which an IO needle pass are:
- Skin
- Epidermis
- Dermis
- Subcutaneous tissue
- Periosteum
- Compact bone (cortex)
- Marrow cavity

2. What are the indications for IO needle insertion?

The current guidelines of the European Resuscitation Council (ERC) stipulate that IO access should be used if establishing a peripheral venous access for cardiopulmonary resuscitation (CPR) would involve delays.
- Guidelines state that, during CPR in children younger than 6 years, IO access should be obtained if there is inability to achieve reliable venous access after three attempts or 90 sec.
- It can be considered where there is circulatory collapse, as in severe dehydration and diabetic ketoacidosis.
- It also gives access for rapid delivery of fluids in children with burns.

3. Describe your landmarks for insertion of an IO needle into the tibia.

The anatomical landmarks for insertion of the IO cannula to these bones are:
- Tibia: 2–3 cm below the tibial tuberosity.
- Femur: 3 cm above the lateral condyle.

The needle should be kept perpendicular to the skin in all directions.

4. How do you know that the needle is in the correct place?

Correct placement is further confirmed by:
- A sudden loss of resistance on entering the marrow cavity. This is less obvious in infants as they have soft bones.
- The needle remains upright without support. Because infants have softer bones, the needle will not stand as firmly upright as in older children.
- Fluid flows freely through the needle without swelling of the subcutaneous tissue.

5. How does resuscitation via an IO needle work?

- Fluid enters the marrow cavity.
- The cavity is filled with non-collapsible veins.
- Fluid then enters the general circulation.
- It is sometimes possible to aspirate some marrow—this can be used for blood tests.

6. What can you give via an IO needle?

- IV fluids—under pressure to overcome venous resistance.
- Nearly all drugs—follow with a 5-ml saline flush.

- It can be used to administer blood.
- It is possible to give an anaesthetic via an IO needle.
- It is possible to give all resuscitation fluids and drugs except bretylium.

7. What are the complications of IO access?

- **Immediate**: fracture, extravasation, subperiosteal infusion, embolism, compartment syndrome.
- **Late**: infection, osteomyelitis, and skin necrosis.

8. What are the contraindications to using an IO needle?

- Infection at the site of entry.
- Fracture of the bone you wish to use.

Further reading

Alawi, K.A., Morrison, G.C., Fraser, D.D., et al. Insulin infusion via an intraosseous needle in diabetic ketoacidosis. *Anaesthesia and Intensive Care* 2008; **36**:110–12.

Chatterjee, D.J., Bukunola, B., Samuels, T.L., et al. Resuscitation in massive obstetric haemorrhage using an intraosseous needle. *Anaesthesia* 2011, **66**:306–10.

European Resuscitation Council Guidelines. Available at: https://www.erc.edu/index.php/mainpage/en/

Fiser, D.H. Intraosseous infusion. *New England Journal of Medicine* 1990; **322**:1579–81.

Leidel, B.A., Kirchhoff, C., Braunstein, V., et al. Comparison of two intraosseous access devices in adult patients under resuscitation in the emergency department: A prospective, randomized study. *Resuscitation* 2010; **81**: 994–9.

Physiology: Post-herpatic neuralgia

1. What is post-herpatic neuralgia?

- Neuropathic pain following 'shingles' (herpes zoster).
- Pain must be present for longer than 1 month.
- The initial pain precedes the emergence of vesicles.
- In 10% of patients, pain and scarring persists after the initial infection.
- Pain can be triggered by contact or draughts.

2. What is the pathophysiological process underlying post-herpatic neuralgia?

- The pain originates in the peripheral nervous system.
- Activation of A-δ and C fibres occurs in the dorsal root ganglion.
- There are nerve changes in response to injury, with sensitization of nociceptors in the periphery.

3. Are there any predisposing factors?

The predisposing factors are old age and immunodeficiency.

4. How do you treat it?

The treatment options are:

- Medical drugs: tricyclic antidepressants, anticonvulsants, and local anaesthetic cream/gel
- Transcutaneous nerve stimulation (TENS)

- Acupuncture
- Sympathetic nerve block

5. How does TENS work?
- Conventional TENS is used in this setting.
- It decreases sensitization in the central nervous system, decreases nociceptive cell activity, and induces A-δ activity; this depresses central nociceptive cell activity.
- TENS also activates descending inhibitory pathways in the periaqueductal grey.
- TENS brings about the release of a variety of neurotransmitters.

6. When is TENS not suitable?
- Patients with pacemakers.
- Pregnancy—do not place TENS over pelvis or abdomen.
- Epilepsy—do not place electrodes on head or neck.
- Malignancy—do not place electrodes over area of active malignancy.

Further reading
Callin, S. and Bennett, M.I. Assessment of neuropathic pain. *Continuing Education in Anaesthesia, Critical Care & Pain* 2008; **8**:210–13.

Jones, I. and Johnson, M.I. Transcutaneous electrical nerve stimulation. *Continuing Education in Anaesthesia, Critical Care & Pain* 2009; **9**:130–5.

Pharmacology: Bilirubin metabolism

1. What do you know about drug metabolism?
Drug metabolism usually makes a substance more water soluble so that it is easier to excrete.
- Phase I:
  - Oxidation, reduction, or hydrolysis.
  - Often occurs in the liver.
  - May involve cytochrome P450 system.
- Phase II: often occurs in the liver but other tissues may be involved.
- Plasma: Hofmann degradation and ester hydrolysis.

2. What is the pharmacological effect of liver failure?
- Decreased protein synthesis affects the amount of plasma proteins and reduces protein binding.
- Decreased drug metabolism—liver failure affects phase I processes first.
- Ascites increases the volume of distribution of many drugs.
- Portocaval shunts may reduce hepatic clearance and thereby increase bioavailability.
- Encephalopathy makes patient more susceptible to the sedating effects of benzodiazepines and opioids.

3. What is hepatorenal syndrome?
- Renal failure in patients with liver failure, particularly in obstructive jaundice.
- Kidney is histologically normal.

- Diagnosis:
  - Urinary sodium <10 mmol/L.
  - Normal CVP—no renal response to central filling.
  - Ascites.

4. Would you modify your anaesthetic for a patient with liver failure?

- Propofol and thiopentone are safe.
- Isoflurane, sevoflurane, and desflurane are safe.
- Atracurium metabolism is independent of liver function.
- Remifentanil metabolism is independent of liver function.
- Paracetamol is safe.
- Caution with opioids—use reduced doses.
- Regional anaesthesia is safe if coagulation is normal.

5. What drugs may cause jaundice?

- Impaired conjugation of bilirubin: paracetamol, methyldopa.
- Obstruction of bile drainage: OCP.
- Hepatitis: halothane.

Further reading

Allman, K.G. and Wilson, I.H. *Oxford Handbook of Anaesthesia*, 2nd edn. Chapter 7: Hepatic disease, pp. 133–48. Oxford: Oxford University Press, 2006.

Peck, T.E., Hill, S.A., and Williams, M. (eds.) *Pharmacology for Anaesthesia and Intensive Care*, 2nd edn. London: Greenwich Medical Media Ltd, 2003.

Physics and clinical measurements: Hyperbaric oxygen

1. What is hyperbaric oxygen?

- Oxygen given at above atmospheric pressure.
- Administered in single- or multiperson chambers.
- Increases the amount of oxygen dissolved in blood.
- O_2 content of blood = $(10 \times Hb \times SaO_2 \times 1.34) + (10 \times PaO_2 \times 0.0225)$.
- In 100% O_2 and at 3 atm there will be 5.7 ml of oxygen per 100 ml of blood.

2. What are its applications?

The applications of hyperbaric oxygen are:

- Carbon monoxide poisoning
- Decompression sickness
- Air embolism
- Osteoradionecrosis
- To aid tissue healing (e.g. diabetic ulcers)

3. Is oxygen harmless?

- 100% O_2 may cause atelectasis.
- There are adverse effects in healthy volunteers after 12 hours of 100% O_2.
- Convulsions if 100% O_2 administered above 2–3 atm.
- Retinopathy of prematurity.

4. How do you know how much oxygen you are giving to your patient?

Oxygen content of gases can be analysed by several methods:

- Chemical: Haldane apparatus
- Physical:
    - Oxygen/Clark polarographic electrode
    - Fuel cell
    - Paramagnetic cell
    - Mass spectrometer

5. How does the fuel cell work?

- Lead anode/gold mesh cathode.
- Potassium hydroxide solution.
- Hydroxide ions produced at the cathode will react with lead at anode.
- Creates a current flow proportional to oxygen molecules.
- No external power source.
- Limited lifespan—because it acts like a battery.
- Affected by N_2O—reacts with lead to form nitrogen, alters pressure inside the cell.
- Bulky.
- Affected by temperature—overcome by a thermistor.
- Response time 30 sec.

Further reading

Lumb, A.B. Just a little oxygen to breathe as you go off to sleep...is it always a good idea? *British Journal of Anaesthesiology* 2007; **99**:769–71.

Yentis, S.M., Hirsch, N.P., and Smith, G.S. *Anaesthesia and Intensive Care A–Z: An Encyclopaedia of Principles and Practice* 4th edn. Edinburgh: Churchill Livingstone, 2009.

Chapter 4

Clinical anaesthesia

Long case: A patient with carcinoma of the sigmoid colon   *69*
Short cases   *73*
   Questions   *73*
   Answers   *75*
      Short case 1: General anaesthesia for Caesarean section   *75*
      Short case 2: Patient with an abnormal ECG   *76*
      Short case 3: Apnoeic child   *78*

Clinical science

Questions   *80*
Answers   *81*
   Anatomy: Brainstem death   *81*
   Physiology: Thyroid   *82*
   Pharmacology: Clinical trials   *83*
   Physics and clinical measurements: Carbon dioxide measurement   *84*

Clinical anaesthesia

Long case: A patient with carcinoma of the sigmoid colon

A 77-year-old-male with a history of respiratory illness is scheduled for a resection of carcinoma of the sigmoid colon. He is known to have longstanding COPD with worsening breathlessness and is unable to tolerate lying flat. He uses three pillows while sleeping and currently has a productive cough. He manages to walk 50 metres on level ground. He takes prednisolone 5 mg once a day, and uses salmeterol and budesonide inhalers. He had a partial gastrectomy 10 years previously.

Clinical examination	Temperature: 37.4°C; weight: 60 kg; height: 170 cm				
	Pulse: 95/min, regular; BP: 135/95 mmHg; respiratory rate: 12/min				
	Chest: few crepitations and rhonchi in right infraclavicular region no crepitations/ rhonchi				
	Cardiovascular system: the apex beat is not palpable, and heart sounds are soft with no murmurs				
	Central nervous system: no neurological deficit apart from visual field defects				
Laboratory investigations	Hb	15.0 g/dL	Na	135 mEq/L	
	MCV	89 fL	K	3.6 mEq/L	
	WBC	16.4 × 10^9/L	Urea	6.6 mmol/L	
	Platelets	271 × 10^9/L	Creatinine	148 μmol/L	
			Albumin	20 g/L	
			ALT/AST	Normal	
ABG: room air	pH: 7.34	PaCO$_2$: 6 kPa	PaO$_2$: 9 kPa	HCO$_3$: 29 mmol	BE: 7 mmol
Pulmonary function tests		Predicted values	Measured values	% predicted	
	FEV$_1$	4.2 L	1.8 L	40 %	
	FVC	5.00 L	3.4 L	68 %	
	FEV$_1$/FVC	84 %	55 %	60 %	
	PEFR	500 L/min	200 L/min	40%	

QUESTIONS

1. Summarize the case
2. Comment on the blood investigations. What are the common causes of hypoalbuminaemia?
3. What is the relationship between serum creatinine levels and glomerular filtration rate (GFR)? Are there any other indices of renal function that correlate more accurately with GFR?
4. Comment on the chest X-ray.
5. Comment on the ECG findings.
6. Why does this patient have RVH?
7. Interpret the PFTs.
8. What is the significance of measuring PFTs before and after bronchodilator administration?
9. What further investigations would you like to have for this patient?

Structured Oral Examination Practice for the Final FRCA

10. Does this patient need perioperative steroid cover?
11. What is your anaesthetic plan for this patient?
12. What are the benefits of epidural analgesia? Does it improve outcome?

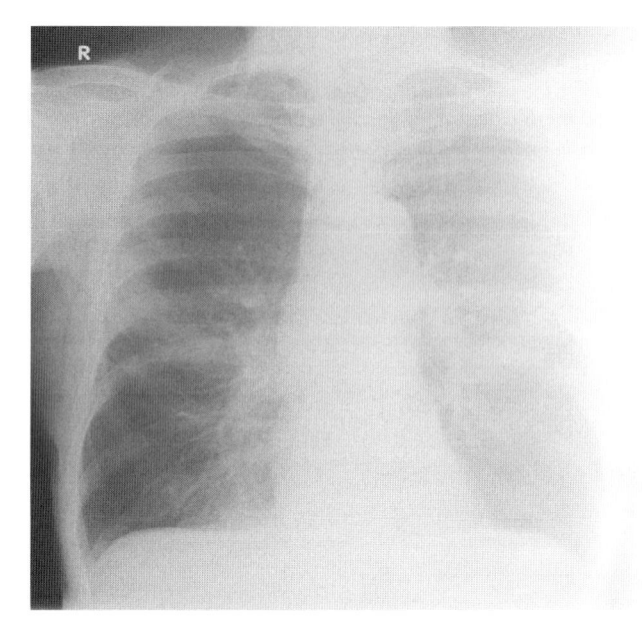

Figure 4.1 Chest X-ray.

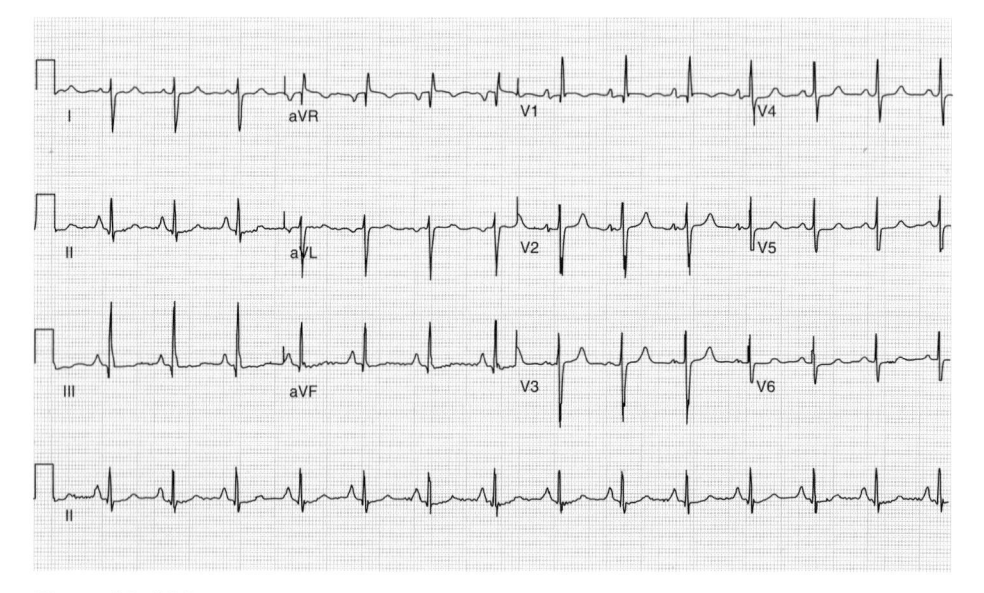

Figure 4.2 ECG.

Chapter 4

ANSWERS

1. Summarize the case

An elderly male patient is scheduled for elective bowel resection. He has severe obstructive pulmonary disease with a possible chest infection. He will need preoperative respiratory and metabolic optimization.

2. Comment on the blood investigations. What are the common causes of hypoalbuminaemia?

Low albumin; moderately elevated creatinine.

Hypoalbuminaemia indicates poor nutritional status either due to inadequate protein intake/synthesis or excessive protein loss/destruction.

The common causes of low albumin are: liver disease, nephrotic syndrome, burns, malabsorption, malnutrition, protein-losing enteropathy, and malignancy.

3. What is the relationship between serum creatinine levels and glomerular filtration rate (GFR)? Are there any other indices of renal function that correlate more accurately with GFR?

The serum creatinine begins to increase only after the GFR has decreased by more than 50%.

24-hour creatinine clearance is a more sensitive indicator of GFR.

4. Comment on the chest X-ray.

Posterior–anterior chest-X-ray. The lungs are hyperexpanded with flattening of the hemidiaphragms. There are disorganized vascular markings and paucity of lung markings and small bullae in the right upper lobe. No focal collapse or consolidation. The appearances are in keeping with COPD. Normal cardiomediastinal contour with cardiac shadow normal.

5. Comment on the ECG findings.

Right axis deviation (RAD) with RVH. The tall right precordial R waves (with a qR complex in lead V1) and the RAD are essentially diagnostic of RVH.

6. Why does this patient have RVH?

This patient has COPD where RVH occurs over time in response to pressure or volume overload. RVH is seen in primary pulmonary hypertension, obstructive pulmonary disease, pulmonic stenosis, and atrial septal defect.

7. Interpret the PFTs.

Reduction in FEV_1/FVC and PEFR suggest moderate to severe COPD.

8. What is the significance of measuring PFTs before and after bronchodilator administration?

Patients are tested without bronchodilators and then tested following the bronchodilator. This is to evaluate the amount of bronchoconstriction that was present and how responsive the patient is to a bronchodilator medication. This assesses the degree of reversibility of the airway obstruction. After the drug has been administered, the PFT is repeated. If two out of three measurements (FVC, FEV_1, and $FEF_{25-75\%}$) improve, then it can be said that the patient has a reversible airway obstruction that is responsive to medication. The amount of improvement is variable between clinics but some standards are presented below:

- FVC: an increase of 10% or more.
- FEV_1: an increase of 200 ml or 15% of the baseline FEV_1.
- $FEF_{25-75\%}$: an increase of 20% or more.

9. What further investigations would you like to have for this patient?

I would like to know about the infective state of the patient by checking CRP and will consider sputum culture. If the temperature is raised then I would do blood cultures as well.

10. Does this patient need perioperative steroid cover?

Yes, the patient requires the steroid cover preoperatively and I would prescribe hydrocortisone 25 mg four times a day for 3 days. This is because endogenous cortisol production is normally 25–30 mg/24 hours which increases to 75–100 mg/24 hours under stress response. There is increased secretion of adrenocorticotropic hormone (ACTH) and cortisol as a normal response to illness or surgery. Low-dose steroid treatment carries little danger of suppressed hypothalamo–pituitary–adrenal (HPA) axis. But the treatment with above 10 mg has a risk of HPA suppression and at risk of developing hypoadrenal crisis (e.g. circulatory collapse and shock).

11. What is your anaesthetic plan for this patient?

- Preoperative stage:
    - Further history, examination, investigations, and continue the treatment
- Pre-optimization:
    - Admit at least 3 days before surgery to treat the chest infection prior to surgery
    - Optimizing bronchodilators—add ipratropium
    - Physiotherapy; deep breathing and incentive spirometry
    - Consider oxygen therapy
    - Antibiotics to treat the infection
    - Consider systemic steroids
- Conduct of anaesthesia:
    - General anaesthesia with thoracic epidural analgesia
    - Invasive monitoring: arterial line, CVP catheter, and urinary catheter
    - Temperature monitoring, warm fluids, warming blanket, low fresh gas flows
- Postoperative:
    - High dependency or critical care management
    - Continue the physiotherapy

12. What are the benefits of epidural analgesia? Does it improve outcome?

Benefits of the epidural: less respiratory compromise from abdominal pain, less postoperative morbidity from pneumonia, DVT, PE, etc.

MASTER trial showed decreased:

- Respiratory failure and postoperative pneumonia
- Lower pain scores
- Transfusion requirements
- DVT/PE

Further reading

Allman, K.G. and Wilson, I.H. *Oxford Handbook of Anaesthesia*, 2nd edn. Chapter 8: Endocrine and metabolic disease, pp. 166–7. Oxford: Oxford University Press, 2006.

Peyton, P.J., Myles, P.S., Silbert, B.S., et al. Perioperative epidural analgesia and outcome after major abdominal surgery in high-risk patients. *Anesthesia & Analgesia* 2003; **96**:548–54.

Peyton, P.J., Rigg, J.A., Jamrozik, K., et al. The MASTER trial has successfully addressed requirements of protocols for large trials. *Anesthesia & Analgesia* 2003; **97**:922–3.

Salem, M., Tainsh, R.E. Jr, Bromberg, J.S., et al. Perioperative glucocorticoid coverage: A reassessment 42 years after emergence of a problem. *Annals of Surgery* 1994; **219**:416–25.

Symreng, T., Karlberg, B.E., Kdgedal, B., et al. Physiological cortisol substitution of long-term steroid treated patients undergoing major surgery. *British Journal of Anaesthesia* 1981; **53**:949–53.

Chapter 4

Short cases

QUESTIONS

Short case 1: General anaesthesia for Caesarean section

You are the on-call anaesthetist for maternity services. A 'category 1' Caesarean section is required for a sustained fetal bradycardia.

1. What initial steps will you take before commencing anaesthesia?
2. You decide to give a general anaesthetic. At laryngoscopy you are unable to see the vocal cords. What will be your priority?
3. How will you proceed?
4. How would your anaesthetic management differ if the indication for operative delivery was placental abruption rather than fetal distress?

Short case 2: Patient with an abnormal ECG

A 70-year-old gentleman is admitted to the ICU following abdominal aortic aneurysm (AAA) repair. Admission ECG (12-lead and rhythm strip); his BP is 98/55 mmHg.

1. What do you see on the ECG (diagnosis)?
2. Classify heart block.
3. What are the features of complete heart block?
4. What are the causes?
5. What is the management of new onset 3rd-degree AV block?
6. What are the indications for temporary pacing?
7. What are the indications for permanent pacing?

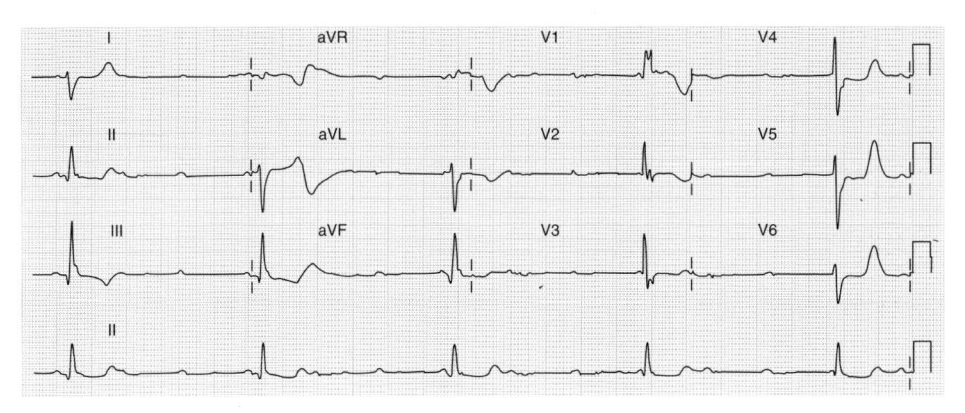

Figure 4.3 ECG.

Short case 3: Apnoeic child

A 10-year-old child who you have anaesthetized for an appendicectomy fails to breath at the end of the operation.

1. What is the differential diagnosis?
2. What is suxamethonium apnoea?
3. What would you see if you use a nerve stimulator in a patient with suxamethonium apnoea?
4. How would you manage a case of suxamethonium apnoea?

Chapter 4

ANSWERS

Short case 1: General anaesthesia for Caesarean section

1. What initial steps will you take before commencing anaesthesia?

A category 1 Caesarean section is required where there is imminent threat to maternal or fetal life. It is recommended that the baby be delivered within 30 min from the time of decision for operative delivery. However, the evidence behind this timescale is limited and in some instances an even more rapid delivery will be required. A multidisciplinary approach is essential if this is to be achieved.

Attempts should be made at fetal resuscitation. Simple techniques include placing the mother in the left-lateral position, oxygen administration, discontinuing any Syntocinon infusion, and optimizing placental perfusion with IV fluids.

A rapid, focused, anaesthetic history should be obtained. In particular, evidence of maternal compromise should be sought. Informed consent for the chosen anaesthetic technique must be obtained if possible. Additional help should be obtained early if anaesthetic difficulties are foreseen.

Close communication with the obstetric team will be required to determine the most appropriate action. A general anaesthetic would be a common approach but a regional technique may still be appropriate if the operator is confident that adequate anaesthesia is achievable in the available time.

2. At laryngoscopy you are unable to see the vocal cords. What will be your priority?

Maternal well-being is always the priority and the mother should not be placed at undue risk. It is therefore essential to ensure maternal oxygenation, which will be rapidly compromised if ventilation is suspended due to the reduced functional residual capacity and increased oxygen requirements of pregnancy.

3. How will you proceed?

Failed intubation is more common in obstetric anaesthesia and conditions for intubation (pre-oxygenation, head position, choice of laryngoscope, etc.) should be optimized before induction. If endotracheal intubation is not immediately possible, for example with laryngeal manipulation or use of an endotracheal introducer, re-oxygenation by mask ventilation must be commenced. A difficult intubation should be verbally declared to the team and help obtained.

If mask ventilation is effective, a repeat attempt at intubation is generally appropriate once the anaesthetist is sure that the conditions and choice of equipment is optimal. It may be necessary to relax the cricoid pressure. If intubation is again impossible, a failed intubation should be declared and mask ventilation recommenced. In the absence of maternal compromise, the mother should be woken up irrespective of any fetal compromise. A regional technique (or awake fibreoptic intubation if this is contraindicated) may then be attempted.

Where mask ventilation is difficult or impossible with the usual airway adjuncts, ventilation with a laryngeal mask may be attempted. Cricoid pressure will need to be relaxed whilst the device is inserted. If adequate ventilation still cannot be achieved, a 'can't intubate, can't ventilate' situation should be declared.

Oxygenation must be maintained by cannula cricothyrotomy and jet ventilation or surgical cricothyrotomy where this fails. Surgery must be postponed and the mother woken up.

4. How would your anaesthetic management differ if the indication for operative delivery was placental abruption rather than fetal distress?

Placental abruption may be associated with significant antepartum haemorrhage, which may be concealed. Under these circumstances, operative delivery cannot be postponed since it is essential for maternal survival. Maternal oxygenation must still be maintained as above. However, if adequate mask or laryngeal mask ventilation is achievable a spontaneous breathing technique is appropriate and minimizes the chances of gastric insufflation and subsequent regurgitation.

Further reading

Difficult Airway Society Guidelines. Available at: http://www.das.uk.com/guidelines/guidelineshome.html
Henderson, J.J., Popat, M.T., Latto, I.P., *et al*. Difficult airway society guidelines for management of the difficult airway. *Anaesthesia* 2004; **59**:675–94.

Short case 2: Patient with an abnormal ECG

1. What do you see on the ECG?

- There are regular non-conducted P waves with a broad complex QRS escape rhythm. There is no association between the atrial and the ventricular rates.
- Complete heart block with broad complex bradycardia.

2. Classify heart block.

Heart block (or atrioventricular conduction block, AVB) is typically classed as:
- 1st-degree AVB (PR interval prolongation > 0.2 ms).
- 2nd-degree AVB:
  - Mobitz type I (progressive increase in PR interval until ventricular beat not conducted).
  - Mobitz type II (periodic failure of ventricular activity either with regular period e.g. 2:1, 3:1 or variable degree).
- 3rd-degree AVB/complete heart block (CHB):
  - Complete atrioventricular dissociation.
  - Escape rhythm may be narrow or broad complex indicating further degrees of atrioventricular conduction path dysfunction.

3. What are the features of complete heart block?

Primary AVB is most commonly a benign finding in young, fit individuals or a result of high vagal tone. It may also occur as a result of hyperkalaemia or hypercalcaemia. Mobitz type I AVB is also usually a benign finding. However, either may also occur as a result of:
- Beta-blockers, calcium channel antagonists, and cholinesterase inhibitors
- After myocardial infarction
- Myocarditis

Mobitz type II AVB is usually a consequence of myocardial infarction.

Extensive anterior myocardial infarction may lead to 3rd-degree AVB with a broad ventricular escape rhythm due to destruction of the septal conduction system. Inferior myocardial infarction is also associated with 3rd-degree block although this is usually a narrow complex bradycardia due to dysfunction of the AV node, which may recover in time. Congenital CHB is also seen.

4. What are the causes?

1st-degree and Mobitz type I block are stable conduction defects and intervention is not usually required. Treatment for Mobitz type II and CHB is necessary if the patient is haemodynamically compromised or in the presence of adverse feature suggesting an increased risk of asystole:

- Increased risk of asystole:
  - Previous asystole
  - Ventricular pauses > 3 sec
  - Mobitz type II block
  - CHB with broad complex ventricular rhythm
- Adverse signs from bradycardia:
  - Hypotension.
  - Inadequate cardiac output
  - Heart rate sustained below 40 min^{-1}
  - Ventricular escape beats requiring suppression

5. What is the management of new-onset 3rd-degree AV block?

- Initial treatment for non-benign bradycardias should be with atropine 500 micrograms to 3 mg IV.
- If this fails, temporary pacing should be instituted.
- Transcutaneous pacing (with appropriate sedation) or percussion pacing may be useful temporizing manoeuvres while transvenous pacing is arranged.
- Transvenous pacing is both more reliable and effective and relatively easy. A Swan–Ganz sheath of adequate size to pass the wire is inserted into the internal jugular or subclavian vein.
- An infusion of a chronotrope such as isoprenaline may also be considered although this runs the risk of precipitating other arrhythmias.

6. What are the indications for temporary pacing?

Temporary pacing is required as a treatment of acute cardiovascular compromise probably related to cardiac arrhythmia. It is repetitive, extrinsic electrical stimulation of cardiac activity.

Emergency pacing may be required if symptomatic and requiring resuscitation. This is just a temporary situation and external pacing is replaced by transvenous insertion of a pacing wire.

The following conditions are indications if contributing to low BP or cardiac output:
- Ventricular asystole with atrial ECG activity
- Sinus bradycardia
- Complete (3rd-degree) heart block
- Möbitz type II 2nd-degree AV block (high risk of progression to CHB)
- Ventricular tachyarrhythmias requiring overdrive pacing

7. What are the indications for permanent pacing?

Permanent pacing is usually appropriate for CHB or Mobitz type II AVB. It may be appropriate for symptomatic cases of Mobitz type I AVB. It is very rarely employed in severe primary AVB where atrial filling is compromised.

Further reading

Allman, K.G. and Wilson, I.H. *Oxford Handbook of Anaesthesia*, 2nd edn. Chapter 4: Perioperative arrhythmias, pp. 77–92. Oxford: Oxford University Press, 2006.

Short case 3: Apnoeic child

1. What is the differential diagnosis?
- Residual anaesthetic and/or opioid
- Residual neuromuscular block/inadequate reversal
- Suxamethonium apnoea
- Hypocapnia
- Sub-clinical fits
- Intraoperative cerebral catastrophe

2. What is suxamethonium apnoea?
Reduced plasma cholinesterase function leading to a prolonged neuromuscular blockade after suxamethonium.

Inherited
- Rare, autosomal condition
- Usual genotype E1U
- Originally described in terms of *in vitro* resistance to inhibition by dibucaine or fluoride
- Atypical form E1A (approx 5% of Caucasian population):
    - Heterozygous (E1U/E1A)—block prolonged (30 min)
    - Homozygous (E1A/E1A)—rarer but greatly prolonged block (2 hours)
- Other rarer forms:
    - 'Fluoride resistant' (E1F)
    - Silent (E1S):
        - Mixed qualitative/qualitative
        - (E1S/E1S) virtually no plasma cholinesterase function: greatly prolonged block >2 hours
    - Quantitative variants: Kallow (K), James (J), and Hammersmith (H)

Acquired
- Degree of block prolongation is not usually a clinical problem:
    - Pregnancy
    - Liver failure
    - Renal failure

Awareness may occur at emergence—sweating, papillary dilatation.

Mivacurium metabolism also by plasma cholinesterase and therefore also affected.

3. What would you see if you use a nerve stimulator in a patient with suxamethonium apnoea?
Train-of-four stimulation may give a mixed picture: prolonged exposure to suxamethonium typically results in a 'non-depolarizing' picture (presence of fade).

4. How would you manage a case of suxamethonium apnoea?
Initial management
- Re-anaesthetize and ventilate.
- Arrange for ventilation until train-of-four restored without fade (e.g. on ITU) and no residual block evident (e.g. with double-burst stimulation).
- Wake patient.

- Extubate only when full muscle functions clinically apparent—replacement of cholinesterase with blood products (FFP) possible, but carries risks of immunological reaction and blood-borne-viruses.
- Explain/counsel patient and family—may need to counsel patient for awareness at emergence.

Subsequent management

- Send serum samples for suxamethonium apnoea screen:
  - Test involves: total cholinesterase, dibucaine number (DN), fluoride number (FN), and Roche number (RN).
  - Not before 24 hours after suxamethonium administration.
  - Need to wait 3 weeks if FFP given.
- Need to screen 1st-degree relatives.
- Clear documentation in patient notes, 'allergies' section.
- Counsel patient/family regarding significance of test results and explain actions in the event of an anaesthetic being required in the future—written documentation to patient/family and GP.

Further reading

Allman, K.G. and Wilson, I.H. *Oxford Handbook of Anaesthesia*, 2nd edn. Chapter 37: Practical anaesthesia; Neuromuscular blockers, reversal, and monitoring, pp. 953–1000. Oxford: Oxford University Press, 2006.

Lenz, A., Hill, G., and White, P.F. Emergency use of sugammadex after failure of standard reversal drugs. *Anesthesia & Analgesia* 2007; **104**(3):585–6.

Clinical science

QUESTIONS

Anatomy: Brainstem death

1. Who is allowed to perform brainstem testing?
2. How many tests are performed?
3. Under what circumstances can brainstem testing be performed?
4. Anatomically, which parts of the brainstem and cranial nerves are tested?
5. How is the apnoea test performed?
6. What time of death is recorded?

Physiology: Thyroid

1. Describe the synthesis, transport, and control of thyroid hormones.
2. What are the functions of the thyroid hormones?
3. What are the clinical features of hyperthyroidism?
4. What are the anaesthetic implications of hyperthyroidism?
5. What investigations are performed prior to thyroidectomy?
6. What drugs are used in the treatment of hyperthyroidism and how do they work?

Pharmacology: Clinical trials

1. What is the principal aim of drug trials?
2. How are drugs tested?
3. What is a 'null hypothesis'?
4. What is a power calculation? Why is it important?

Physics and clinical measurements: Carbon dioxide measurement

1. List the methods of measuring carbon dioxide.
2. Describe a common method for measuring the carbon dioxide content of a gas.
3. What are the advantages and disadvantages of infrared spectrometry?
4. What are the advantages of capnography?
5. Draw, label, and discuss the normal capnogram.

Chapter 4

ANSWERS

Anatomy: Brainstem death

1. Who is allowed to perform brainstem testing?
Two doctors:
- Either together or independently.
- May not be part of a transplant team.
- Both must have held full General Medical Council registration for at least 5 years.
- At least one must be a consultant.

2. How many tests are performed?
Two sets of tests are performed—time interval between tests is not defined.

3. Under what circumstances can brainstem testing be performed?
- Patient must have an identified pathology causing irreversible brainstem death.
- The patient must be unconscious, apnoeic, and requiring mechanical ventilation.
- Where unconsciousness/unresponsiveness is not due to:
    - Hypothermia <34°C (core).
    - CNS depressant drugs or muscle relaxants.
    - Potentially reversible metabolic, endocrine, or circulatory dysfunction.
- The patient is over 2 months old.

4. Anatomically, which parts of the brainstem and cranial nerves are tested?
- Cranial nerve (CN) II, III: pupils fixed and dilated.
- CN V, VII: absent corneal reflex.
- CN VIII, III: absent vestibulo-ocular reflexes.
- CN V, VII, and sensory/motor pathways through brainstem: absent motor response in the CN distribution in response to somatic stimulation. No peripheral response to supraorbital pressure.
- CN IX: absence of gag reflex.
- CN X: absent cough reflex in response to endobronchial suctioning.

5. How is the apnoea test performed?
- The patient is disconnected from the ventilator and observed for respiratory efforts until a CO_2 tension of 6.65 kPa is achieved (on arterial blood gas sampling).
- Desaturation is prevented by pre-oxygenation/insufflation of O_2 via a tracheal catheter.

6. What time of death is recorded?
The time of death is that of the first time brainstem death testing criteria were satisfied.

Further reading
Academy of Medical Royal Colleges. *A Code of Practice for the Diagnosis and Confirmation of Death*. London: Academy of Medical Royal Colleges, 2008.
Conference of Medical Royal Colleges and their Faculties in the UK. Criteria for the diagnosis of brainstem death. *Journal of the Royal College of Physicians of London* 1995; **29**:381–2.
Eelco, F. and Widjdicks, M. Determining brain death in adults. *Neurology* 1995; **45**:1003–11.
Eelco, F. and Widjdicks, M. The diagnosis of brain death. *New England Journal of Medicine* 2001; **344**:1215–21.

Physiology: Thyroid

1. Describe the synthesis, transport, and control of thyroid hormones.
- The thyroid secretes thyroxine (T_4) and triiodothyronine (T_3).
- Regulated by thyroid-stimulating hormone (TSH) from thyrotrophs in the posterior pituitary in response to thyrotropin-releasing hormone (TRH) from the hypothalamus.
- TSH release is inhibited by high blood T_3/T_4 forming a negative feedback loop.
- T_3 and T_4 synthesized in follicular cells by successive iodination of tyrosine bound to thyroglobulin by the enzyme thyroperoxidase.
- The iodide required for this reaction is sequestered by a sodium-dependent iodide transporter.
- Ultimately thyroglobulin is cleaved to release hormones.
- Almost all of the circulating T_3 and T_4 is protein bound (mainly to thyroid binding protein). <1% free hormone.
- Additionally T_4 is converted peripherally to the more active T_3 (or the inactive reverse-T_3) depending on the metabolic state of the peripheral tissues.

2. What are the functions of the thyroid hormones?
T_3 and T_4 bind to G protein-coupled receptors present in nearly every cell in the body. Functions include:
- Increasing basal metabolic rate and regulating carbohydrate, fat, and protein metabolism. Consequently increase cardiac output, CO_2 production, and respiratory rate.
- Increasing catecholamine sensitivity.
- Regulation of anabolic processes, e.g. protein synthesis, growth.
- Increase in thermogenesis.
- Potentiation of neural development.
- Increasing endometrial thickness.

3. What are the clinical features of hyperthyroidism?
- Tachycardia, tachyarrhythmias, palpitations, hypertension, cardiac failure if severe.
- Tremor.
- Anxiety, irritability, hyperactivity, poor sleep.
- Heat intolerance, sweating, warm peripheries, facial flushing.
- Weight loss.
- Proptosis (with Graves disease).

4. What are the anaesthetic implications of hyperthyroidism?
- Increased anaesthetic requirement.
- Hyperdynamic circulation.
- Danger of 'thyroid storm': uncontrolled hypermetabolic crisis.

5. What investigations are performed prior to thyroidectomy?
- BP, ECG.
- CT to evaluate retrosternal extension or tracheal involvement.
- Nasendoscopy to confirm laryngeal nerve function.
- Routine bloods including serum calcium (as baseline, in case parathyroids also accidentally removed) and thyroid function test.

6. What drugs are used in the treatment of hyperthyroidism and how do they work?

Antithyroid drugs:
- Carbimazole:
  - Pro-drug.
  - Inhibits thyroid peroxidase.
- Propylthiouracil:
  - Inhibits thyroid peroxidase.
  - Inhibits peripheral conversion of T_4 to T_3.
- Beta-blockers (e.g. propranolol): for catecholaminergic control.

Further reading

Farling, P.A. Thyroid disease. *British Journal of Anaesthesia* 2000; **85**:15–28.
Malhotra, S. and Sodhi, V. Anaesthesia for thyroid and parathyroid surgery. *Continuing Education in Anaesthesia Critical Care & Pain* 2007; **7**:55–8.

Pharmacology: Clinical trials

1. What is the principal aim of drug trials?
To assess the safety and efficacy of a new drug.

2. How are drugs tested?

- Pre-clinical testing: *in vitro* and *in vivo* (animal) testing to gain information on likely toxicity and pharmacokinetics. Estimation of likely doses for human subjects.
- Phase 0 clinical studies:
  - Sub-therapeutic studies to estimate preliminary pharmacokinetic/pharmacodynamic properties.
- Phase I clinical studies:
  - Small groups of healthy volunteers.
  - Verification of safety and tolerability.
  - Measurement of pharmacokinetic properties.
- Phase II clinical studies:
  - Larger groups including patients, usually randomized control studies.
  - To determine the effectiveness and safety of the drug in patients.
  - Establish optimal dosing.
- Phase III clinical studies:
  - Large groups of patients.
  - Randomized, controlled, blinded studies to determine the safety and effectiveness of the drug in treating the condition.
  - Comparison with existing treatment.
- Licensing.

- Phase IV:
  - Post-marketing surveillance.
  - Ongoing vigilance/reporting for adverse effects.

3. What is a 'null hypothesis'?
- The hypothesis that an intervention has no effect.
- Statistical analysis tests the observed effect against the null hypothesis. If the observed effect is greater than that expected by chance, the null hypothesis is rejected.

4. What is a power calculation? Why is it important?
- Power calculations use pilot data to estimate the minimum sample size likely to be required to be able to observe a statistically and clinically significant difference if it exists.
- It is unethical to conduct a study without an estimate of the number of subjects which will be needed:
  - If too few are recruited, these subjects have potentially been exposed to risk in a study which could never show a significant result.
  - If too many are recruited, more subjects are exposed to a potential risk than is necessary.

Physics and clinical measurements: Carbon dioxide measurement

1. List the methods of measuring carbon dioxide.
CO_2 can be measured by the following methods:
- Infrared spectrometry
- Mass spectrometry
- Raman spectrometry
- Photo-acoustic spectrometry

2. Describe a common method for measuring the carbon dioxide content of a gas.
Infrared absorption is by far the most common method:
- CO_2 absorbs in the far infrared.
- Pulsed infrared source.
- Measure transmitted infrared intensity with detector.
- Light source is pulsed using mechanical 'shutter'—allows discrimination against ambient infrared light.
- Beer–Lambert law gives concentration of CO_2, $[CO_2] = -\log(I/I0)/\varepsilon\, l$ (where ε = molar absorption, l = optical path length).
- Calibrated against sample gases with known CO_2 concentration.

3. What are the advantages and disadvantages of infrared spectrometry?
Advantages
- Relatively low cost/simple.
- Robust.
- Easily adapted to sidestream or mainstream use.

Disadvantages
- Needs to warm up.
- Does not work at low ambient temperatures.
- Vulnerable to condensation on optical cell.
- Needs correction for nitrous oxide, which has similar infrared absorption properties.

4. What are the advantages of capnography?

Routine monitoring of CO_2
- Operating theatre
- ICU
- Transport of critically ill patient
- Sedation
- Recovery

Detection of airway, respiratory, and circulatory problems
- Correct ETT placement (it does not exclude endobronchial intubation)
- Disconnection
- Airway obstruction
- Pulmonary embolism
- Rebreathing
- Falls in cardiac output
- Malignant hyperpyrexia
- Cardiopulmonary resuscitation (adequacy of chest compressions, correct ETT placement).

5. Draw, label, and discuss the normal capnogram.

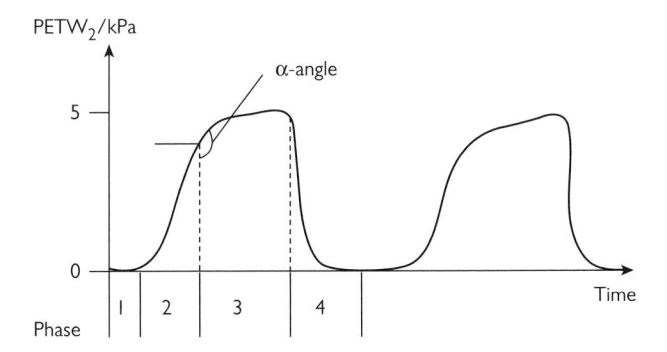

Figure 4.4 Normal capnogram trace.

Normal $ETCO_2$ trace

Phase 1: dead-space phase. As the patient breathes out, the first part represents anatomical dead-space gas, which contains no CO_2.

Phase 2: mixture of anatomical and alveolar dead-space phase. Gas from the alveoli, which has been involved in gas exchange, is mixed with dead-space gas and the CO_2 concentration rises until pure alveolar gas is detected.

Phase 3: alveolar plateau phase. This is practically all alveolar gas. It usually has a positive up-slope since CO_2 is being continuously excreted into the alveoli. In addition, alveoli with low V/Qs tend to empty late.

Phase 4: inspiratory phase. The CO_2 falls to zero as fresh gas is inhaled.

The A *angle* is the angle between phase 2 and phase 3, and is supposed to represent the V/Q status of the lungs.

Increased ETCO$_2$	Decreased ETCO$_2$
Decreased alveolar ventilation: • Reduced respiratory rate • Increased respiratory rate • Increased equipment dead space Increased CO_2 production: • Fever • Hypercatabolic state Increased inspired CO_2: • Rebreathing space • CO_2 absorber exhausted • External CO_2	Increased alveolar ventilation: • Increased respiratory rate • Increased tidal volume Reduced CO_2 production: • Hypothermia • Hypocatabolic state Increased alveolar dead: • Reduced cardiac output • PE • High PEEP during IPPV Sampling error: • Inadequate tidal volume • Water blocking sampling line • Air entrainment into sampling line

Further reading

Bhavani Shankar, K., Moseley, H., Kumar, Y., et al. Capnometry and anaesthesia. A Review Article. *Canadian Journal of Anaesthesia* 1992; **39**:617–32.

Chapter 5

Clinical anaesthesia

Long case: A patient for total hip replacement   *89*

Short cases   *95*

    Questions   *95*

    Answers   *97*

        Short case 1: Emergency case with Colles' fracture   *97*

        Short case 2: A patient with acute pain   *98*

        Short case 3: Major obstetric haemorrhage   *100*

Clinical science

Questions   *103*

Answers   *104*

    Anatomy: Anatomical features of the eye   *104*

    Physiology: Neuromuscular junction   *106*

    Pharmacology: Sedation   *107*

    Physics and clinical measurements: Temperature   *108*

Clinical anaesthesia

Long case: A patient for total hip replacement

You are conducting a preoperative assessment of a 76-year-old woman who is scheduled for a right total hip replacement on a routine orthopaedic list. You are seeing her for the first time on the morning of her surgery.

Reading her surgical care pathway, you obtain the following information:

Past medical/surgical history

- Osteoarthritis.
- Age 30: appendicectomy, uncomplicated.
- 5 years ago: myocardial infarction, angioplasty/stenting.
- 1 year ago: cardiological investigation for multiple syncopal episodes. Asymptomatic since a permanent 'pacemaker' was fitted.

Social history

The patient lives with her husband in a bungalow and describes herself as independent. Her exercise tolerance is limited by pain from her hip although she is sometimes short of breath in the mornings. She ceased smoking 5 years ago after her myocardial infarction.

Drug history

- Perindopril 4mg twice a day.
- Furosemide 20mg twice a day.
- Aspirin 75mg once a day.
- Clopidogrel 75mg once a day.
- Atorvastatin 20mg once a day.
- No recorded drug allergies or adverse reactions.

Clinical examination	Temperature: 38.2°C; weight: 90 kg; height: 170 cm
	Pulse: 80/min, regular; BP: 150/90 mmHg; respiratory rate: 20/min; SpO$_2$: 93% on air
	Chest: breath sounds and air entry equal on both sides. Fine crackles at both lung bases
	Cardiovascular system: normal heart sound with no murmurs
	Central nervous system: no neurological deficit apart from visual field defects
Laboratory investigations	Hb 13.0 g/dL Na 135 mEq/L
	MCV 89 fL K 3.5 mEq/L
	WBC 7.1 × 10^9/L Urea 7.6 mmol/L
	Platelets 271 × 10^9/L Creatinine 187 μmol/L
	PT 13 sec Glucose 11.2 mmol/L
	APTT 26 sec Alkaline phos. 400 IU/L

Structured Oral Examination Practice for the Final FRCA

QUESTIONS

1. Summarize the case.
2. What does the ECG show?
3. What is your observation from the chest X-ray?
4. List some common indications for insertion of a permanent pacemaker.
5. Do you require further information or investigation?
6. What perioperative risks would you anticipate/discuss with this patient?
7. In what ways can surgical diathermy affect pacemakers?
8. What precautions should be taken when diathermy is being used?
9. What would be your anaesthetic technique for this patient?
10. What will be your postoperative care plan?

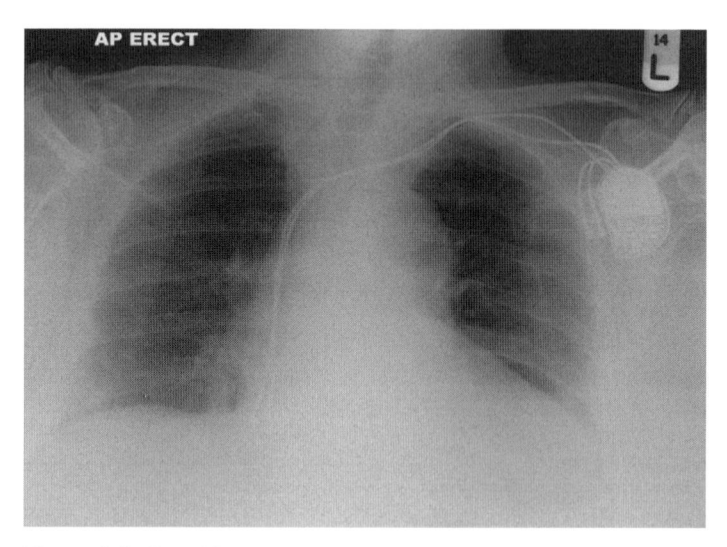

Figure 5.1 Chest X-ray.

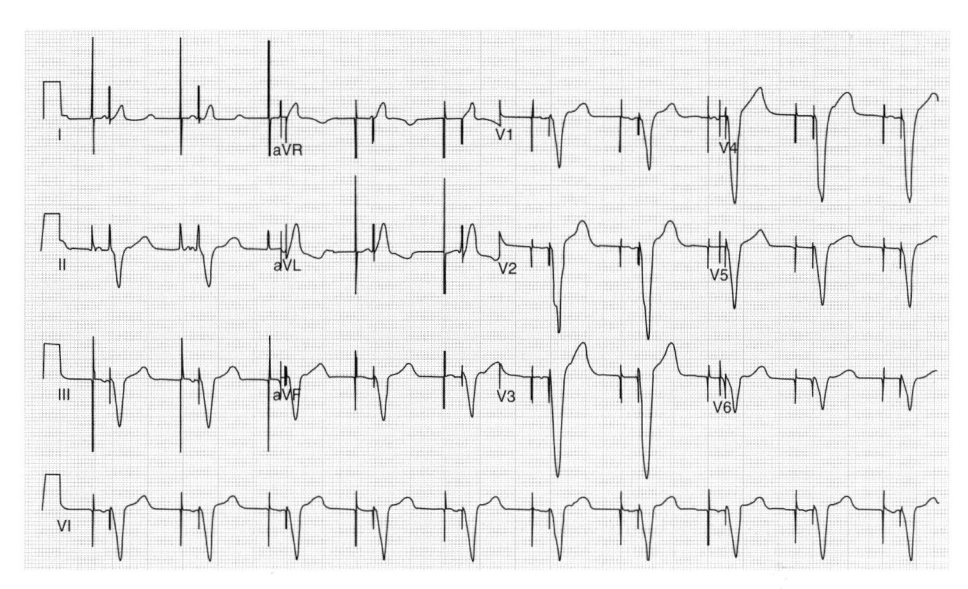

Figure 5.2 ECG.

ANSWERS

1. Summarize the case.

This is a 76-year-old woman with a background history of ischaemic heart disease for which coronary stenting has taken place and a recent permanent pacemaker, presenting for elective hip total arthroplasty for osteoarthritis. From the information we also note her obesity and possibly a degree of heart failure as evidenced by her dyspnoea and chest findings, which are in keeping with the diuretic therapy in her drug history. Her functional status is likely to be difficult to assess due to immobility from her hip pain.

Also of particular note from an anaesthetic point of view is her ongoing long-term use of clopidogrel. The nature of her coronary stent and pacemaker are unknown.

2. What does the ECG show?

The 12-lead ECG provided shows a paced broad ventricular rate of approximately 80 min^{-1}. There are pacing spikes preceding each atrial and ventricular complex signifying that there is a dual chamber pacemaker.

3. What is your observation from the chest X-ray?

Anterior–posterior chest X-ray with poor inspiratory effort. Dual chamber pacemaker *in situ* with apparently intact leads. The left hemidiaphragm is obscured with the tissue being pulled inferiorly giving a straight edge to the heart border. The appearances are in keeping with a left lower lobe collapse. The right lung is clear.

4. List some common indications for insertion of a permanent pacemaker.

There are numerous indications for consideration of a permanent pacemaker devices including:

- Heart block:
  - Complete heart block
  - Symptomatic 2nd-degree heart block
  - Symptomatic bifascicular or trifascicular block
  - Symptomatic bradycardia
- After myocardial infarction:
  - Persistent 2nd/3rd-degree heart block as above
  - Infranodal AV block with left bundle branch block
- Sinus node dysfunction:
  - Sick-sinus syndrome/tachy-brady syndrome

Additionally, pacemakers with cardioversion/defibrillation (ICD) function may be used in the treatment of tachyarrhythmias. Finally, biventricular pacing is used in the treatment of heart failure.

5. Do you require further information or investigation?

A full anaesthetic evaluation is mandatory. Particular attention will need to be paid to any symptoms suggestive of ongoing ischaemia, syncope, or heart failure. Additionally a cardiology opinion would be prudent in this patient. Specific questions include:

- Nature of coronary stent (bare metal vs. drug eluting). Require assessment of risk of stent thrombosis if clopidogrel omitted. This needs to be balanced against the risks of intra/postoperative bleeding.
- Original indication for and nature of implanted 'pacemaker':
  - Interrogation of device and evaluation of remaining battery life.
  - Rate responsive function?
  - ICD functions?
  - Confirm response of unit to an applied magnet.
  - Availability of pacemaker technician to disable anti-tachyarrhythmia/rate responsiveness.
- Echocardiographic evaluation of ventricular function to guide intraoperative technique and risk stratification.
- Chest x-ray is not essential but may be helpful in identifying the type of pacemaker, broken leads, or signs of heart failure/cardiomegaly.

Additionally the patient should be cross-matched.

6. What perioperative risks would you anticipate/discuss with the patient?

The combination of stable ischaemic heart disease and moderate surgery places the patient at a risk of perioperative cardiac event of ≤5%. This risk would be increased significantly in the presence of ongoing ischaemia or decompensated left ventricular failure. Death might be expected in half of these cases.

Additionally, risks of pulmonary and thromboembolic complications are increased in this patient due to her obesity.

The risk of arrhythmia due to pacemaker malfunction will depend on the original indication for the device.

7. In what ways does surgical diathermy affect pacemakers?

Surgical diathermy may affect pacemakers in three ways:

- It may lead to inhibition of the unit, resulting in no output and potentially asystole or severe bradycardia.

- It may induce eddy currents in the pacing lead, resulting in ventricular arrhythmias including ventricular fibrillation.
- The software programming in some DDD units may be erased by diathermy, resulting in potentially unsuitable pacing parameters.

8. What precautions will you think of when diathermy is being used?
- Diathermy must be used in short bursts.
- Bipolar diathermy is preferable to unipolar.
- If unipolar diathermy is being used for the procedure: place the diathermy plate well away from pacemaker, pacemaker may need to be converted in the asynchronous mode.

9. What would be your anaesthetic technique for this patient?
- If clopidogrel can be safely discontinued, then there is merit in delaying the procedure for a week whilst platelet function recovers. Otherwise, and once appropriate cardiological evaluation has been obtained, a careful general anaesthetic balanced with opioid analgesia and muscle relaxation with endotracheal intubation and positive pressure ventilation would appear to be a reasonable technique.
- Standard intraoperative monitoring should be adequate but additional invasive monitoring or 5-lead ECG may be warranted depending on the results of the cardiological evaluation (e.g. in the presence of severely impaired ventricular function). However, placement of central lines should be done with particular care so as not to damage the pacemaker leads.
- A stable anaesthetic from the point of view of BP and HR are highly desirable to optimize coronary perfusion and minimize the risk of arrhythmias.
- Total hip replacement may be associated with moderate blood loss, particularly given the clopidogrel treatment. Large-bore IV access should be obtained.
- Monopolar diathermy is highly desirable from a surgical point of view. The increased risk of electromagnetic interference may be offset by: the distance of the surgical site from the heart; positioning the diathermy current return plate away from the heart; and minimizing diathermy use to short bursts as much as possible. Selection of a non-rate responsive mode by reprogramming may not be required.
- With pacemakers, application of a magnet over an implanted pacemaker will activate a fixed rate mode, typically around 80min^{-1}. Whilst this may not be necessary, a magnet should be available in case diathermy leads to inappropriate triggering of the pacemaker.
- However, a magnet should not routinely be used with pacemakers with cardioversion/defibrillation functions since the resulting mode is unpredictable and depends on the device. Anti-tachyarrhythmia functions should, instead, be deactivated by reprogramming preoperatively given the elective nature of this case.
- In the event of a life-threatening arrhythmia, sources of electromagnetic interference should be removed (e.g. diathermy).
- Anti-tachyarrhythmia functions should be re-activated where appropriate and if there is time. If external pacing, cardioversion or defibrillation is required, the pads should be positioned away from the pacemaker pulse generator/leads, as far as is possible (anterior/posterior position).
- Careful intraoperative fluid balance is essential and catheterization is probably justifiable if there is concern regarding ventricular function. Acidosis and hypoxia are particularly undesirable in this case as they may alter pacemaker threshold.

10. What will be your postoperative care plan?

The implanted device should be interrogated so that any disabled functions can be reactivated in the post-anaesthetic recovery unit. The HR should be measured continuously in the immediate recovery period and cardioversion/defibrillation equipment should be immediately to hand.

Postoperative analgesia is particularly important if the stress-response is to be obtunded.
- A patient-controlled analgesia system would seem to be a reasonable approach.
- The patient may return to the ward if the operation is otherwise uneventful and if blood loss has not been too great.
- Careful attention to postoperative detail including fluid balance is important.
- Oxygen should be administered by nasal cannulae at least for the first 3 postoperative nights.
- Some degree of postoperative bleeding is common after hip replacement and haemoglobin levels should be monitored.
- Electrolytes, including magnesium, should be checked daily and appropriate potassium replacement is essential.
- Antithrombotic therapy is essential in this obese patient.
- If this level of care cannot be delivered on the standard ward, consideration should be given to admitting the patient to an intermediate level of care postoperatively. Clearly, adverse cardiological evaluation may mandate elective critical care admission.

Further reading

Allman, K.G. and Wilson, I.H. *Oxford Handbook of Anaesthesia*, 2nd edn. Chapter 4: Perioperative arrhythmias, pp. 77–92. Oxford: Oxford University Press, 2006.

Atlee, J.L. and Bernstein, A.D. Cardiac rhythm management devices. (Part I) Indications, device selection and function. *Anesthesiology* 2001; **95**:1265–80.

Diprose, P. and Pierce, J.M.T. Anaesthesia for patients with pacemakers and similar devices. *Continuing Education in Anaesthesia Critical Care & Pain* 2001; **1**:166–70.

Levine, P.A., Balady, G.J., Lazar, H.L., et al. Electrocautery and pacemakers: Management of the paced patient subject to electrocautery. *Annals of Thoracic Surgery* 1986; **41**:313–17.

Saluke, T.V., Dob, D., and Sutton, R. Pacemakers and defibrillators: Anaesthetic implications. *British Journal of Anaesthesia* 2004; **93**:95–104.

Chapter 5

Short cases

QUESTIONS

Short case 1: Emergency case with Colles' fracture

A 65-year-old gentleman, obese, heavy smoker, heavy drinker has a Colles' fracture. He is booked for manipulation under anaesthetic and the surgeon tells you this will be a 'quick pull'. He tells you he has a productive cough.

1. Would you anaesthetize now or defer?
2. What do you see on the chest X-ray?
3. How would you anaesthetize him?
4. What regional techniques would be appropriate?
5. Describe the intravenous Bier block procedure.

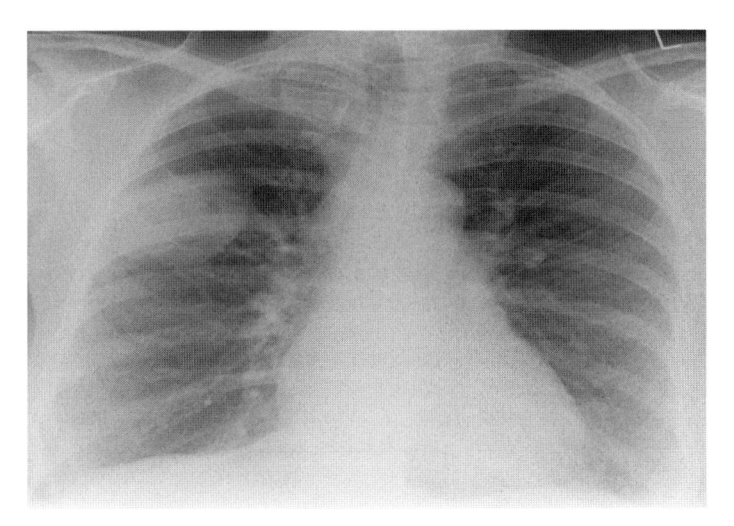

Figure 5.3 Chest X-ray.

Short case 2: A patient with acute pain

A 44-year-old man is referred to you by the acute pain team in your pain clinic for evaluation and management. He was recently diagnosed with adenocarcinoma of the pancreas with retroperitoneal lymph nodes in the para-aortic region. He has pain in the epigastric region which is worst in the night and decreases during the day. He is taking sustained-release morphine 100 mg orally every 8 hours and also takes 30 mg for rescue pain. He wishes to know what the other options available for him are.

1. Why is the patient in extreme pain?
2. Why do you say this is neuropathic pain?
3. How are you going to screen the neuropathic pain patient?

4. What are the modalities of treatment available for him?
5. What are the indications for a coeliac plexus block?
6. Briefly describe the applied anatomy for coeliac plexus.
7. Briefly describe the technique for coeliac plexus block.
8. What drugs are used to perform the block?
9. What complications can occur during and following this block?

Short case 3: Major obstetric haemorrhage

A patient in late pregnancy at 38 weeks' of gestation is brought in to hospital from home by ambulance with a major antepartum haemorrhage. She has, up to this point, concealed her pregnancy and is not known to obstetric services.

1. What do you think is happening?
2. What is the differential diagnosis?
3. What will be your initial management?
4. The midwife estimates a blood loss of 1500 ml. How would you proceed?
5. An emergency Caesarean section is planned. What anaesthetic technique will you choose?
6. The baby is successfully delivered but the estimated blood loss is >3.5 L. What will you do?

Chapter 5

ANSWERS

Short case 1: Emergency case with Colles' fracture

1. Would you anaesthetize now or defer?

General anaesthesia for this quick procedure may be acceptable but is likely to be associated with increased hazards: risk of hypoxia secondary to atelectasis, aspiration, and possibly a difficult airway. Rapid desaturation is likely, due to shunt and limited functional residual capacity. There is a need to consider possible paraneoplastic implications. A regional technique would seem to be a safer option.

2. What do you see on the chest X-ray?

Anterior–posterior chest X-ray. At the right apex is a mass. There is no bone destruction identified. There is a further mass at the right mid zone. The left lung is clear. Even allowing for projection the heart is enlarged. The appearances are suggestive of a primary bronchial carcinoma (Pancoast tumour) with lung metastases. A full staging CT is suggested.

3. How would you anaesthetize him?

Little margin for further optimization and further investigation of likely chest neoplasm can be deferred until after the orthopaedic procedure so delay is inappropriate although the patient should be fasted unless neurovascular compromise present.

4. What regional techniques would be appropriate?

If a regional technique is selected choices include:
- Brachial plexus block:
  - An axillary approach is likely to be the most appropriate for this distal procedure.
  - May be supplemented by individual distal nerve blocks.
- Intravenous regional anaesthesia (IVRA, 'Bier block').
  - Needs discussion with surgeon as limited duration of action if manipulation unsuccessful or prolonged.
  - Need to ensure double-cuff is appropriately sized for the arm.

5. Describe the intravenous Bier block procedure.

IVRA is indicated for any procedure on the arm below the elbow or leg below the knee that will be completed within 40–60 min.

Onset of anaesthesia is rapid and reasonable muscle relaxation can be obtained.

Mechanisms of action

The local anaesthetic injected diffuses into the small veins surrounding the nerves and then into the vasa nervorum and capillary plexus of the nerves, leading to conduction block in the nerves in the limb. Further, there is conduction block in the skin nerves. The tourniquet produces ischaemia, which contributes to the analgesic action of the local anaesthetic by blocking nerve conduction and motor endplate function. 20 min after tourniquet application alone there will be analgesia to pinprick without the injection of any local anaesthetic. The use is limited to procedures lasting less than an hour because of increasing discomfort from the tourniquet.

Contraindications
- The technique should not be employed if a tourniquet cannot safely be used, for example, in patients with severe Reynaud's or homozygous sickle cell disease.

- Caution should be employed in patients who have sustained crush injuries of the relevant limb as potentially viable tissue will be subjected to a further period of hypoxia.

Equipment and procedure
- The procedure is conducted in the operating theatre with full resuscitation equipment available.
- Tourniquet which is tested for leak and can be inflated to a pressure at least 50 mmHg above the patient's systolic BP.
- IV cannula inserted in a distal vein.
- IV cannula in the other arm for resuscitation.

Before the procedure the patient should be:
- Starved for 6 hours.
- Monitored closely (standard monitoring applied).
- Placed on a tipping trolley.
- Adequately informed about the procedure and have consented to it.

The equipment required for IVRA includes:
- Pneumatic tourniquet (checked for leaks before the procedure) and a pressure gauge.
- Esmarch bandage or Rhys-Davies exsanguinator.
- Local anaesthetic solution.
- Resuscitation equipment and drugs.

Drugs

The drug of choice for IVRA is prilocaine as it is the least toxic local anaesthetic and has the largest therapeutic index. If prilocaine is not available, lignocaine is an acceptable alternative. It is essential that plain and not adrenaline-containing solutions are used.

A suitable dose to use in an arm is 40 ml of 0.5% prilocaine (or 0.5% lignocaine). This can be increased to 50 ml in muscular individuals or decreased to 30 ml in small or frail patients. Larger volumes are necessary in the leg, e.g. 50–60 ml. Maximum recommended volumes for a 60–70-kg patient are 400 mg prilocaine (80 ml 0.5% solution) or 250 mg lignocaine (50 ml 0.5% solution).

Further reading

Brown, E.M., McGriff, J.T., and Malinowski, R.W. Intravenous regional anaesthesia (Bier block): review of 20 years' experience. *Canadian Journal of Anaesthesia* 1989; **36**:307–10.

Casale, R., Glynn, C., and Buonocore, M. The role of ischaemia in the analgesia which follows Bier's block technique. *Pain* 1992; **50**:169–75.

Short case 2: A patient in acute pain

1. Why is the patient in extreme pain?

In view of the symptoms and maximal dose of morphine this is a typical example of neuropathic pain.

2. Why do you say this is neuropathic pain?

Neuropathic pain is defined as 'pain initiated or caused by a primary lesion or dysfunction of the nervous system'.

This patient has history of pancreatic tumour and pain could be due to presence and progression of tumour itself leading to nerve injury or indirect effect of tumour, i.e. metabolic imbalance etc., unrelated mechanisms such as migraine and myofascial pain.

3. How are you going to screen the neuropathic pain patient?

There are some screening tools which are not designed as diagnostic tools as such but which highlight the need for a more detailed clinical assessment. These are: the neuropathic pain scale, Leeds assessment of neuropathic symptoms and signs (LANSS), neuropathic pain questionnaire, painDETECT, ID-pain, and the Douleur neuropathique (DN4).

The LANSS has shown good validity and reliability as it is suitable for assessing neuropathic pain in a range of clinical contexts, including chronic pain populations, and comprises five symptom and two examination items (allodynia and pin-prick testing).

4. What are the modalities of treatment available for him?

- Pharmacotherapy is a key component in the multimodal treatment of chronic pain. The options are:
  - Switching the opioids to oxycodone or fentanyl patch or buprenorphine.
  - Non-opioid non-analgesic: antidepressant, antiepileptic, and antiarrhythmic drugs.
- Interventional management: coeliac plexus block.

5. What are the indications for coeliac plexus block?

The indications are for relief of pain from non-pelvic intra-abdominal organs.

- **Acute pain:** may be performed during surgery for postoperative pain relief.
- **Chronic pain:** useful for any condition that causes chronic severe upper abdominal visceral pain, e.g. chronic pancreatitis (local anaesthetic blocks only).
- **Cancer pain:** useful for upper abdominal organ cancer pain, and is frequently used for carcinoma of the pancreas—initial diagnostic local anaesthetic block, followed by neurolytic block.

6. Briefly describe the applied anatomy for the coeliac plexus.

The coeliac ganglia lie either side of the L1 vertebral body. The coeliac ganglia and interconnecting fibres are involved in autonomic supply of the upper abdominal organs and first two-thrids of the large bowel (mid-gut). The coeliac plexus block is therefore useful in controlling autonomically-mediated chronic pain, for example from chronic pancreatitis or from upper abdominal malignancy. It is formed from:

- Greater splanchnic nerve (T5/6 to T9/10).
- Lesser splanchnic nerve (T10/11).
- Least splanchnic nerve (T11/12).
- The upper abdominal organs receive their parasympathetic supply from the left and right vagal trunks, which pass through the coeliac plexus but do not connect there.

7. Briefly describe the technique for coeliac plexus block.

The procedure is explained to the patient and consent obtained. The block is usually performed under fluoroscopic guidance. The patient is positioned in the prone position and may be lightly sedated. IV access must be obtained. Superficial local anaesthetic infiltration is used at the needle insertion point below the tip of the 12th rib. The needle tip is angled anteromedially aiming at the L1 vertebral body. The needle is re-directed past the vertebral body and passes forwards into the plexus taking care to avoid the inferior vena cava and aorta. Correct needle placement is confirmed by injection of X-ray contrast before injection of the local anaesthetic and/or neurolytic solution (e.g. aqueous phenol). A second injection on the other side is typically required unless convincing contralateral contrast spread is seen.

8. What drugs are used to perform the block?

- For non-malignant pain: 10 ml 0.5% levobupivacaine on each side
- For malignant pain: 5 ml 6% aqueous phenol + 5 ml 0.5% levobupivacaine on each side

9. What complications can occur during and following this block?

The patient must be warned and consented for the following side effects:

- Discomfort.
- Failure either to perform the technique or due to non-autonomically transmitted pain.
- Infection.
- Hypotension secondary to venous pooling due to splanchnic sympathectomy. This may be particularly severe in dehydrated patients. IV fluid preloading may offset this.
- Haemorrhage from aortic or inferior vena caval injury. The block is contraindicated in pathological or iatrogenic coagulopathy or in the presence of an abdominal aortic aneurysm.
- Perforation of upper abdominal viscera.
- Inadvertent intravascular injection. Injection of neurolytic into the spinal arterial supply may lead to permanent paraplegia.
- Sexual dysfunction.

Further reading

Bennett, M.I., Attal, N., Backonja, M.M., et al. Using screening tools to identify neuropathic pain. *Pain* 2007; **127**:199–203.

Cherny, N.I. The management of cancer pain. *CA: A Cancer Journal for Clinicians* 2000; **50**:70–116.

Kaplan, R., Schiff-Keren, B., and Alt, E. Aortic dissection as a complication of celiac plexus block. *Anesthesiology* 1995; **83**:632–5.

Rykowski, J.J. and Hilgier, M. Continuous celiac plexus block in acute pancreatitis. *Regional Anesthesia* 1995; **20**:528–32.

Short case 3: Major obstetric haemorrhage

1. What do you think is happening?

This is a case of antepartum haemorrhage (APH) which is bleeding from the genital tract after 24 weeks of gestation. According to the triennial Confidential Enquiry into Maternal Deaths (2003–2005) 14 women died from haemorrhage. The incidence of APH is about 3% of all pregnancy—a significant cause of maternal mortality.

2. What is the differential diagnosis?

Most APHs are benign ('show'). Pathological causes include placental abruption, placenta (or vasa) previa, uterine rupture, and bleeding from the genital tract.

3. What will be your initial management?

A multidisciplinary approach including the obstetric and midwifery teams as well as obstetric anaesthetist is essential in cases of life-threatening haemorrhage. The usual ABCDE approach must be adapted. Use of a wedge prevents aortocaval compression. Reliable large-bore IV access is essential. Significant haemorrhage may be concealed and haemodynamic compromise may initially be absent

Chapter 5

due to the compensatory reserves of young, otherwise fit women. The fetal heartbeat should be assessed although maternal resuscitation is paramount if either mother or baby is to survive.

4. The midwife estimates a blood loss of 1500 ml. How would you proceed?

My management plan would be along the lines of:
- Call for help—senior staff midwife, obstetric/anaesthetic.
- A multidisciplinary approach.
- Resuscitation ABCDE approach with 15°, left lateral tilt:
    - Assess, high oxygen.
    - IV access, blood samples.
    - Replace volume with colloid to start, followed by packed cells.
- Monitor appropriately.
- Stop bleeding, move in to theatre by:
    - Medical
    - Surgical
    - Radiological
    - Anaesthetic intervention

5. An emergency Caesarean section is planned. What anaesthetic technique will you choose?

For emergency Caesarean section, a general anaesthetic with appropriate aspiration precautions is generally the most appropriate technique since regional techniques may cause significant hypotension in the presence of hypovolaemia and general anaesthesia gives the greatest physiological control.

In cases of life-threatening haemorrhage, packed red cells and FFP should be given from the outset in a ratio approaching 1:1. Cryoprecipitate and platelets should be considered early. Hypothermia must be carefully avoided. Invasive monitoring is helpful but should not delay haemorrhage control.

6. The baby is successfully delivered but the estimated blood loss is >3.5 L. What will you do?

This is a major haemorrhage and I will initiate major haemorrhage protocol—this involves the haematologist and gynaecologist.
- Continue resuscitation with:
    - Cross-match blood 4 units with FFP and a bag of platelets.
    - Warm fluids crystalloids (2 L max), colloids (1.5 L max).
    - Consider O −ve blood.
- Blood component management:
    - Red blood cells.
    - Correction of defective blood coagulation:
        - Clotting factors.
        - Platelets, and
        - Cryoprecitate.
    - Use of Haemostatic agents:
        - Aprotinin (Trasylol).
        - Vitamin K.
        - Tranexamic acid.
        - Recombinant Factor VIIa (NovoSeven).
    - Cell salvage procedures.

- Surgical management:
  - Delivery for placental and uterine pathology.
  - B-Lynch suture (brace suture).
  - Uterine tamponade, e.g. Rusch urological balloon or Sengstaken–Blakemore tube.
  - Surgical ligation of uterine and internal iliac arteries.
  - Hysterectomy.
  - Compression/clamping aorta to buy time.
  - Uterine replacement if uterine inversion.
- Interventional radiological techniques:
  - Bilateral iliac artery balloons may be placed electively and inflated at Caesarean section or should bleeding occur.
  - Selective uterine artery embolization can be performed.
- Continue monitoring:
  - FBC and electrolytes.
  - Coagulation studies to guide the use of further blood products:
    - APTT ratio/INR; aim for <1.5.
    - Platelet count; aim for $>50 \times 10^9$/L.
    - Fibrinogen >1 g/L.
  - CVP and arterial line.
  - Temperature.
- HDU care :
  - Transfer to a high dependency unit or intensive care facility.
  - Anticipate coagulopathy and treat clinically until coagulation results available.

Further reading

Banks, A. and Norris, S. Massive haemorrhage in pregnancy. *Continuing Education in Anaesthesia Critical Care & Pain* 2005; **5**:195–8.

Welsh, A., McLintock, C., Gatt, S., *et al*. Guidelines for the use of recombinant activated factor VII in massive obstetric haemorrhage. *Australian and New Zealand Journal of Obstetrics and Gynaecology* 2008; **48**:12–16.

Clinical science

QUESTIONS

Anatomy: Anatomical features of the eye

1. Describe the muscles of the eye, their nerve supply, and their relation to the orbit.
2. What is the nerve supply to the eye? Where do the nerves originate?
3. What is the autonomic supply to the eye?
4. What anatomical features of the orbit and eye should you be aware of before performing regional anaesthesia on the eye?
5. What eye blocks can be performed to provide anaesthesia for ophthalmic surgery?
6. What are the risks of the peribulbar and sub-Tenon's blocks?

Physiology: Neuromuscular junction

1. Describe the structure of the neuromuscular junction.
2. Describe the structure of the neuromuscular acetylcholine receptor.
3. How does neuromuscular transmission take place?
4. What are the implications in myasthenia and myasthenic syndromes?

Pharmacology: Sedation

1. What is meant by the term 'context sensitive' half-life? How does it arise?
2. What pharmacological strategies are available for the sedation of patients in intensive care?
3. What factors influence the choice of agent?
4. What problems are associated with sedation on the intensive care unit?

Physics and clinical measurements: Temperature

1. What are the methods of measuring temperature?
2. What techniques are used to measure temperature in anaesthesia and how do they work?
3. Why does core temperature drop under anaesthesia? How may this be prevented?
4. What are the consequences of hypothermia?
5. How can you prevent peroperative hypothermia?

ANSWERS

Anatomy: Anatomical features of the eye

1. Describe the muscles of the eye, their nerve supply and their relation to the orbit.

Muscle	Movement produced	Cranial nerve
Superior rectus	Up	Oculomotor (III)
Inferior rectus	Down	Oculomotor (III)
Medial rectus	In towards nose	Oculomotor (III)
Lateral rectus	Away from nose	Abducens (VI)
Superior oblique	Down and in (intortion)	Trochlear (IV)
Inferior oblique	Up and out (extortion)	Oculomotor (III)
Levator palpebrae superioris	Lifts upper eyelid	Oculomotor (III)

- Superior, medial, lateral, and inferior rectus muscles arise from tendinous ring surrounding optic foramen (superior rectus inserts by means of a fibro-cartilaginous pulley system).
- Superior oblique arises from orbital surface of sphenoid bone.
- Inferior oblique arises from orbital surface of maxilla.

2. What is the nerve supply to the eye? Where do the nerves originate?

The sensory supply is mainly from the ophthalmic division of the 5th (trigeminal) cranial nerve. The lacrimal branch innervates the conjunctiva and the nasociliary branch the cornea, sclera, iris, and ciliary body. The 2nd cranial nerve (optic) conveys vision.

3. What is the autonomic supply to the eye?

The parasympathetic supply is from the Edinger Westphal nucleus accompanying the 3rd cranial nerve to synapse with the short ciliary nerves in the ciliary ganglion. The sympathetic fibres are from T1 (the first thoracic sympathetic outflow) and synapse in the superior cervical ganglion before joining the long and short ciliary nerves.

4. What anatomical features of the orbit and eye should you be aware of before performing regional anaesthesia on the eye?

Each orbit is in the shape of an irregular pyramid with its base at the front of the skull and its axis pointing posteromedially towards the apex. The angle between the lateral walls of the two orbits is approximately 90° (and the angle between the lateral and medial walls of each orbit is nearly 45°). Thus the medial walls of the orbit are almost parallel to the sagittal plane.

The orbital fat is divided into central (retrobulbar, intracone) and peripheral (peribulbar, pericone) compartments by the cone of the recti muscles. The central space contains the optic, oculomotor, abducens, and nasociliary nerves. The peripheral space contains the trochlear, lacrimal, frontal, and infraorbital nerves. All the motor and sensory nerves can be blocked by an injection into the orbital fat.

The depth of the orbit measured from the rear surface of the eyeball to the apex is about 25 mm (range 12–35 mm). The axial length (AL) of the globe (eyeball) is the distance from the corneal surface to the retina and is often measured preoperatively. An AL of 26 mm or more denotes a large eye, indicating that great caution is necessary as globes longer than this are easier to perforate during regional anaesthesia.

5. What eye blocks can be performed to provide anaesthesia for ophthalmic surgery?

The common blocks are peribulbar and sub-Tenon's, and also surface anaesthesia.

6. What are the risks of the peribulbar and sub-Tenon's blocks?

Complications of regional blocks for ophthalmic surgery may result either from the agents used or the block technique itself:

Common complications of peribulbar block

Complication of agent:
- Intravascular injection and systemic toxicity.

Complication of technique:
- Subconjunctival oedema and chemosis.
- Bruising.
- Haemorrhage:
  - Retrobulbar haemorrhage incidence of 0.1–1.7% and is characterized by a sudden rise of IOP and usually requires postponing of surgery. It is very rare with shallow retrobulbar or peribulbar injections.
  - Subconjunctival haemorrhage is less significant as it will eventually be absorbed. Surgery need not be postponed.
- Globe penetration:
  - Incidence of 1 in 12,000.
  - Common in:
    - Myopic eyes which are longer but also thinner than normal (>26 mm AL), enophthalmos, staphyloma.
    - Previous extraocular surgery, e.g. for strabismus.
    - Sharp needles vs. blunt needles. Sharp needles are more likely to perforate sclera but blunt needles that do perforate are likely to cause more intraocular trauma.
  - Perforation may be avoided by carefully inserting the needle tangentially and by not going 'up and in' until the needle tip is clearly past the equator of the globe.
- Central spread of local anaesthetic:
  - This is due to either direct injection into the dural cuff which accompanies the optic nerve to the sclera or to retrograde arterial spread.
- Oculocardiac reflex is the bradycardia which may follow traction on the eye.
- Myotoxicity: extra-ocular nerve palsies.
- Optic nerve atrophy:
  - Optic nerve damage and retinal vascular occlusion may be caused by direct damage to the optic nerve or central retinal artery, injection into the optic nerve sheath or haemorrhage within the nerve sheath. These complications may lead to partial or complete visual loss.

Complications of sub-Tenon's block

- Conjunctival haemorrhage.
- Conjunctival chemosis can be a problem.
- Case reports of scleral perforation.

Further reading

Bellucci, R. Anesthesia for cataract surgery. *Current Opinion in Ophthalmology* 1999; **101**:36–41.
Rubin, A.P. Complications of local anaesthesia for ophthalmic surgery. *British Journal of Anaesthesia* 1995; **75**:93–6.
Thind, G.S. and Rubin, A.P. Local anaesthesia for eye surgery – no room for complacency. *British Journal of Anaesthesia* 2001; **86**:473–6.

Physiology: Neuromuscular junction

1. Describe the structure of the neuromuscular junction.
- Motor neuron terminal.
- Membrane voltage gated Ca^{2+} channels.
- Acetylcholine (ACh) vesicles.
- Synaptic cleft.
- Post-synaptic membrane convoluted to increase surface area with ligand gated acetylcholine receptors (AChR).

2. Describe the structure of the neuromuscular acetylcholine receptor.
- Type of nicotinic receptor.
- Five transmembrane domains.
- Ligand gated ion channel.
- Binding of two ACh leads to channel opening and non-specific increase in Na/K permeability.

3. How does neuromuscular transmission take place?
- Action potentials transmitted from motor neuron to end plate.
- Action potentials trigger Ca^{2+} influx into motor neuron terminal.
- ACh vesicle exocytosis via Ca^{2+} mediated SNARE protein mechanism.
- ACh released into synaptic cleft and diffuse to post-synaptic membrane.
- Binding to AChR leads to channel opening:
    - Partial depolarization of myocyte membrane—miniature end plate potentials (MEPPS).
    - MEPPS summate to raise myocyte membrane threshold reached leading to myocyte action potential.
- Synaptic ACh removed by acetylcholinesterase attached to post-synaptic membrane.

4. What are the implications in myasthenia and myasthenic syndromes?
Myasthenia gravis is characterized by muscle weakness and fatigability. It is caused by autoimmune disruption of postsynaptic acetylcholine receptors at the neuromuscular junction, with up to 80% of functional receptors lost. The disease may occur at any age but is most common in young adult women. It may be associated with thymus hyperplasia with 15% of affected patients having thymomas.

Conduct of anaesthesia
- Continue the anticholinesterase therapy up to the time of induction.
- Premedication is to continue the drug treatment.
- Intubation/ventilation is often achievable using non-paralysing techniques.
- Use of non-depolarizing drugs should be used cautiously along with the monitoring of neuromuscular junction. If the muscle relaxants are required then the reduced dosage should be used; initial doses of 10–20% of normal are usually adequate.
- Short and intermediate duration non-depolarizing drugs such as atracurium, is preferred but mivacurium, or rocuronium can also be used.
- Reversal of neuromuscular blocking drugs should be achievable with standard doses of neostigmine if preoperative symptom control has been good. Avoidance of reversal is preferred since further doses of anticholinesterase may introduce the risk of overdose (cholinergic crisis). Drugs with spontaneous reversal such as atracurium are optimal.

Myasthenic syndromes

Eaton–Lambert myasthenic syndrome (ELMS) is a paraneoplastic syndrome associated with small-cell carcinoma of the lung. It presents as proximal muscle weakness affecting lower limbs. There is a prejunctional defect in release of ACh due to antibodies against calcium channels. Anticholinesterases do not cause an improvement. ELMS patients are sensitive to both depolarizing and non-depolarizing relaxants whereas myasthenia gravis patients are often resistant to depolarizing relaxants.

Reduced doses should be used if the disease is suspected. Maintain a high index of suspicion in those undergoing procedures related to diagnosis and management of carcinoma of the lung.

Further reading

Allman, K.G. and Wilson, I.H. *Oxford Handbook of Anaesthesia*, 2nd edn. Chapter 11: Neurological and muscular disorders, pp. 229–66. Oxford: Oxford University Press, 2006.

Pharmacology: Sedation

1. What is meant by the term 'context sensitive' half-life? How does it arise?

- A drug is said to have a context sensitive half-life when the elimination or redistribution half-life is increased with prolonged exposure to the drug (i.e. with the duration of the infusion).
- It is due to gradual accumulation of the drug in 'slow' compartments.

2. What pharmacological strategies are available for the sedation of patients in intensive care?

Sedation can be either by infusion (more common) or by boluses.

Two classes of agents in use:

- Hypnotics:
    - E.g. propofol, midazolam, clonidine.
    - Neuroleptics (e.g. haloperidol).
    - Alpha-2 agonists (e.g. clonidine, dexmedetomidine).
- Analgesics:
    - E.g. morphine, fentanyl, remifentanil.
- Usually use combinations but pure hypnotic or analgesic regimens possible.

3. What factors influence the choice of agent?

Most drugs (except remifentanil) have context sensitive half-life after prolonged infusion.

- Makes sedation breaks difficult.
- Short periods of sedation: propofol/remifentanil useful:
    - Propofol—danger of lipaemia and propofol infusion syndrome (especially children) after longer periods.
    - Propofol may contribute to hypotension and increase inotropic requirements.
    - Remifentanil—expensive (although may shorten intensive care unit stay).
- Morphine/midazolam—accumulation in hepatic failure.
- Morphine—also very significant accumulation of active metabolite in renal failure (morphine-6-glucuronide).

- Analgesia-based sedation may lead to withdrawal.
- Neuroleptics more appropriate if the patient experiences hallucinations.

For painful procedures or conditions analgesia-based sedation is particularly important.

4. What problems are associated with sedation on the intensive care unit?

- Inadequate techniques may adversely affect morbidity, length of stay, and mortality.
- Increased risk of infection (especially pulmonary).
- Cardiovascular disturbances:
  - Propofol: hypotension, increased inotrope requirements.
  - Clonidine: bradycardia/hypotension.
  - Neuroleptics: QT interval prolongation.
- Abnormal sleep or circadian rhythm—dexmedetomidine may be advantageous.
- Strategies:
  - Move from deep to lighter sedation.
  - Avoidance of oversedation:
    - Daily sedation breaks.
    - Patient-oriented sedation scoring.
  - Analgesia scoring.
  - Tracheostomy/sedation avoidance.
  - Use of shorter-acting agents as patients wean.

Further reading

Murdoch, S. and Cohen, A. Intensive care sedation: a review of current British practice. *Intensive Care Medicine* 2000, **26**:922–8.

NICE. *Sedation for children and young people* (Clinical Guideline 112). London: NICE, 2010. Available at: http://www.nice.org.uk/CG112.

Physics and clinical measurements: Temperature

1. What are the methods of measuring temperature?

- Electrical: resistance thermometer, thermistor, thermocouple.
- Non-electrical: alcohol, mercury, Bourdon gauge.

2. What techniques are used to measure temperature in anaesthesia and how do they work?

- Thermocouples:
  - Junction formed between two dissimilar metals.
  - Small voltage generated as temperature increases—small size, low-cost technology.
- Thermistors:
  - Semiconducting material.
  - Resistance is a function of temperature.
- Infrared:
  - Infrared detector detects radiated heat.
  - Non-contact applications (e.g. tympanic thermometer).

Chapter 5

3. Why does core temperature drop under anaesthesia? How may this be prevented?

- Initial temperature drop due to vasodilation/relative vasoplegia:
  - Causes mixing of cooler peripheral blood with core.
  - May be prevented by ensuring patients are kept warm before anaesthesia.
- Ongoing heat loss increased as vasodilation leads to increased thermal losses from skin:
  - Radiation (60% of total heat loss):
    - Increases as fourth power of temperature difference between body and surroundings.
    - Reduced by forced air warming and maintaining a warm theatre environment.
  - Convection (25% of total heat loss):
    - Reduced by preventing passive air movements around patient.
    - E.g. blanketing, forced air warming.
  - Respiration (10% of total heat loss)
    - Due to warming and humidification (latent heat of evaporation of water lost).
    - Reduced by use of heat and moisture exchange filter.
  - Conduction (1–2% total losses):
    - Reduced by warming mattress, forced air warming (forms insulating layer of air).
  - Evaporation (normally small contribution, may be significant is patient wet).
  - Thermodilution:
    - Due to infusion of cold fluid.
    - Prevented by fluid warming.
- Hypothalamic temperature set-point for shivering reduced.
  - Use of muscle relaxants prevents shivering/thermogenesis.

4. What are the consequences of hypothermia?

- Mild hypothermia:
  - Postoperative patient discomfort.
  - Impaired coagulation and platelet function, increased blood loss.
  - Increased postoperative sepsis.
  - Poor wound healing.
  - Prolonged anaesthetic recovery.
- Moderate hypothermia:
  - Increased catecholamine secretion.
  - Hypertension and myocardial irritability.
  - Impaired immune function.
  - Reduced drug metabolism.
  - Shivering increases myocardial oxygen consumption.
  - Reduction in cerebral metabolic rate, potential cerebral protection.
- Severe hypothermia:
  - Myocardial depression, bradycardia, circulatory collapse.

5. How can you prevent peroperative hypothermia?

The prevention of hypothermia can be divided in the following phases

Perioperative care

- Patients should be informed staying warm before surgery will lower the risk of postoperative complications. The hospital environment may be colder than their own home.

- The staff should be trained in taking temperature and document appropriately if required act as well.

Preoperative phase

Each patient should be assessed for their risk of inadvertent perioperative hypothermia and potential adverse consequences before transfer to the theatre suite. Patients should be managed as higher risk if any two of the following apply:

- ASA grade II to V (the higher the grade, the greater the risk).
- Preoperative temperature below 36.0°C (and preoperative warming is not possible because of clinical urgency).
- Undergoing combined general and regional anaesthesia.
- Undergoing major or intermediate surgery.
- At risk of cardiovascular complications.

If the patient's temperature is below 36.0°C:

- Forced air warming should be started preoperatively on the ward or in the emergency department (unless there is a need to expedite surgery because of clinical urgency, for example bleeding or critical limb ischaemia).
- Forced air warming should be maintained throughout the intraoperative phase.

Intraoperative phase

- The patient's temperature should be measured and documented before induction of anaesthesia and then every 30 min until the end of surgery.
- Induction of anaesthesia should not begin unless the patient's temperature is 36.0°C or above (unless there is a need to expedite surgery because of clinical urgency, for example bleeding or critical limb ischaemia).
- IV fluids (500 ml or more) and blood products should be warmed to 37°C using a fluid warming device.
- Patients who are at higher risk of inadvertent perioperative hypothermia and who are having anaesthesia for less than 30 min should be warmed intraoperatively from induction of anaesthesia using a forced air warming device.
- All patients who are having anaesthesia for longer than 30 min should be warmed intraoperatively from induction of anaesthesia using a forced air warming device.

Postoperative phase

- The patient's temperature should be measured and documented on admission to the recovery room and then every 15 min.
- Ward transfer should not be arranged unless the patient's temperature is 36.0°C or above.
- If the patient's temperature is below 36.0°C, they should be actively warmed using forced air warming until they are discharged from the recovery room or until they are comfortably warm.

Further reading

NICE. *Perioperative hypothermia (inadvertent)*(Clinical Guideline 65). London; NICE, 2008. Available at: http://www.nice.org.uk/CG65.
Sessler, D.I. Temperature monitoring and perioperative thermoregulation. *Anesthesiology* 2008; **109**:318–38.
Torossian, A. Thermal management during anaesthesia and thermoregulation standards for the prevention of inadvertent perioperative hypothermia. *Best Practice & Research Clinical Anaesthesiology* 2008; **22**:659–68.

Chapter 6

Clinical anaesthesia

Long case: A patient with spinal stenosis   *113*
Short cases   *119*
   Questions   *119*
   Answers   *121*
      Short case 1: Pneumothorax   *121*
      Short case 2: Critical illness neuropathy   *123*
      Short case 3: Intrapleural block   *124*

Clinical science

Questions   *126*
Answers   *127*
   Anatomy: Larynx   *127*
   Physiology: Parathyroid glands   *129*
   Pharmacology: Lungs and bronchomotor tone   *131*
   Physics and clinical measurements: Ultrasound   *133*

Clinical anaesthesia

Long case: A patient with spinal stenosis

An 85-year-old female presents for elective decompression of C3–C5 for spinal stenosis. There is subluxation of C3 on C4. MRI showed spinal cord compression at C3–C4 level. She has advanced rheumatoid arthritis. The patient complains of pain and paraesthesia in both arms. She can walk 15 metres and feels short of breath.

Drug history: sulphasalazine, prednisolone, diclofenac, and lansoprazole.

Clinical examination	Temperature: 37.1°C; weight: 85 kg; height: 160 cm			
	Pulse: 78/min, regular; BP: 138/70 mmHg; respiratory rate: 12/min			
	Chest: decreased air entry bilateral bases, vesicular breath sound, few crepitations at right base			
	Cardiovascular system: normal heart sound with no murmurs			
	Central nervous system: pain and paraesthesia in both arms			
Laboratory investigations	Hb	9.7 g/dL	Na	142 mEq/L
	MCV	105 fL	K	3.7 mEq/L
	WBC	17.0×10^9/L	Urea	8.7 mmol/L
	Platelets	351×10^9/L	Creatinine	100 μmol/L
Pulmonary function tests		Predicted values	Measured values	% predicted
	FEV_1	4.90 L	3.52 L	72%
	FVC	5.68 L	4.43 L	78%
	FEV_1/FVC	84%	79%	94%

QUESTIONS

1. Summarize the case.
2. What are the important issues in this case?
3. What are the causes of a high WBC count?
4. Why is she anaemic? What type of anaemia could she have?
5. Would you consider transfusing her preoperatively?
6. Describe the chest X-ray and ECG.
7. Discuss her pulmonary function test results. How do they fit with her history?
8. What are the side effects of sulphasalazine and prednisolone?
9. What other examinations and investigations would you like to do before you proceed?
10. How would you assess and manage her airway? What other techniques are there for managing her airway?
11. How would you plan to anaesthetize this patient?
12. How do you know if someone is safe to extubate?

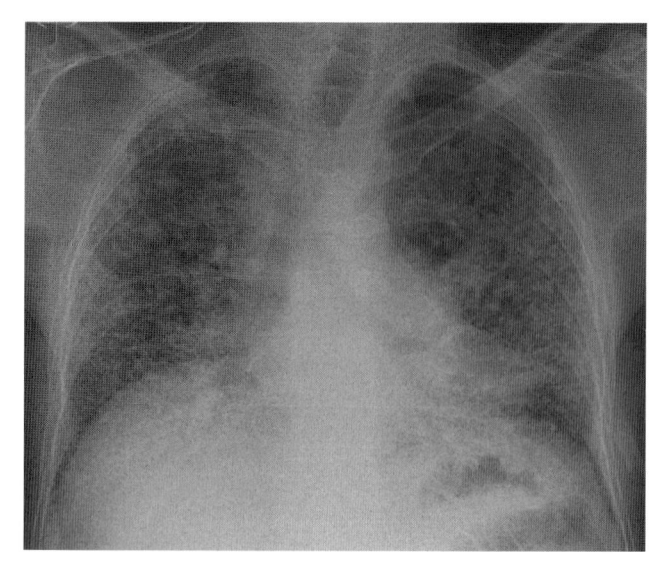

Structured Oral Examination Practice for the Final FRCA

Figure 6.1 Chest X-ray.

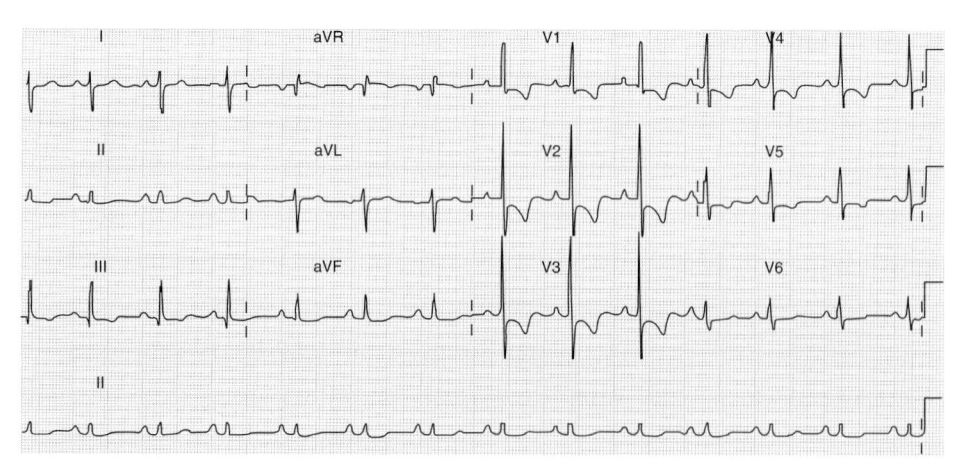

Figure 6.2 ECG.

Chapter 6

ANSWERS

1. Summarize the case
We have an elderly lady for elective decompression of C3–C5 for spinal stenosis. She is anaemic with high white blood cells, her chest X-ray shows fibrosis and collapse. PFTs show a restrictive picture.

2. What are the important issues in this case?
Important issues which needs addressing in the preoperative assessment include:
- She suffers from short of breath and limited exercise tolerance:
  - May require high-dependency postoperative care.
  - Analgesia: PCA with the traditional handset could be difficult for the patient if she has severe hand joint involvement.
  - Explore other forms of pain relief in this patient.
- She has advanced rheumatoid arthritis:
  - Difficult airway.
  - Unstable neck.
  - Care of joints and skin during positioning.
  - Poor venous access.
  - Prone positioning and its problems.
  - Steroid supplementation if already on steroids.
  - DVT prophylaxis.

3. What are the causes of a high WBC count?
- Infection: bacterial infection, viral infection, fungal infection, acute inflammation.
- Physiological; pregnancy.
- Others: lymphoma, leukaemia (chronic myelomonocytic leukaemia):
  - Raised neutrophils: infection, cold.
  - Raised eosinophils: allergic.
  - Raised monocyte: mononucleosis.
  - Raised lymphocyte: parasitic.
  - Raised basophil: parasitic.
  - When WBC raised manyfold then suspect leukaemia or lymphoma is considered.

4. Why is she anaemic? What type of anaemia could she have?
The patient could be anaemic due to:
- Anaemia of chronic disease.
- NSAID-associated blood loss.
- Drug-associated bone depression.
- Felty's syndrome—a combination of splenomegaly and neutropenia, and may be associated with anaemia and thrombocytopenia.

Causes of anaemia
- Inadequate dietary intake of iron; decreased MCV.
- Chronic blood loss; haematemesis, NSAIDs; normochromic microcytic anaemia.
- Renal failure; raised urea and creatinine.
- Haematopoietic disease; blood picture and blood film.
- Malignancy.
- Dilutional; pregnancy.

5. Would you consider transfusing her preoperatively?

This patient does not have a history of ischaemic heart disease and I would be comfortable with blood group and save as long as haemoglobin is between 9 and 10.

6. Describe the chest-X-ray and ECG.

Chest-ray: bilateral reticular shadowing predominantly in the mid and lower zones. Normal heart size. The chest X-ray appearances are in keeping with bilateral established fibrosis.

ECG shows right ventricular hypertrophy, demonstrated by right axis deviation, large R waves with T-wave inversion in leads V1–V3 and a prominent p wave (p pulmonale).

7. Discuss her pulmonary function test results. How do they fit with her history?

Restrictive lung disease:
- FEV_1 is reduced
- FVC is reduced
- FEV_1/FVC ratio is increased

8. What are the side effects of sulphasalazine and prednisolone?

The side effects of sulphasalazine are:

- Loss of appetite
- Blood disorders: megaloblastic anaemia
- Kidney: proteinuria, crystalluria
- Ataxia, vertigo, tinnitus.

The side effects of prednisolone include:

- GIT: dyspepsia, peptic ulceration, oesophageal ulceration, pancreatitis
- Musculoskeletal: osteoporosis, proximal myopathy, vertebral and long bone fracture
- Endocrine: adrenal suppression, Cushing syndrome
- Hirsutism
- Negative nitrogen and calcium balance
- Increased susceptibility to infection
- Neuropsychiatric disorder
- Impaired healing
- Skin atrophy
- Fluid and electrolyte disturbance

9. What are other examinations and investigations you would like to do before you proceed?

Examinations

Airway assessment, extent of disability, document neurological deficit.

Investigations

- U&Es.
- Blood gas (restrictive lung disease).
- Depending on systemic manifestations, CRP, LFTs may be indicated.
- ECG.
- Echocardiogram: valvular or pericardial involvement.
- Neck X-ray: cervical spine radiographs flexion/extension views, MRI, and CT scan.
- Fibreoptic nasendoscopy if indicated.

10. How would you assess and manage her airway? What other techniques are there for managing her airway?

Airway assessment
- Range of neck flexion/extension
- TMJ mobility
- Mouth opening
- Mallampati score
- Thyromental distance

Investigations
- Cervical spine X-rays (flexion/extension)
- MRI scan
- Fibreoptic nasopharyngoscopy (ENT consultation)

Airway management
- Awake fibreoptic intubation would be the safest method which I will use.
- Manual in-line stabilization when doing direct laryngoscopy.

11. How would you plan to anaesthetize this patient?

Pre-optimize patient accordingly in view of restrictive airway disease and shortness of breath.

Preoperatively
- Full routine anaesthetic assessment:
  - Assess airway.
  - Extent of disability.
  - Document neurological deficit.
- Check results of investigations.

Intraoperatively
- Routine monitoring with intra-arterial and CVP monitoring.
- Full aseptic technique for establishing IV access.
- Maintain normothermia.
- Endotracheal intubation—awake fibreoptic technique with reinforced ETT size 7.0.
- Pressure-controlled ventilation with high rate and low tidal volume.
- Movement and positioning of the patient should be meticulous and all pressure areas padded to avoid pressure sores.
- Methylcellulose eye drops should be applied as up to 15% of patients with RA suffer from kerato-conjunctivitis sicca and are at risk of corneal ulceration.
- Patients taking an equivalent dose greater than prednisolone 10 mg daily require steroid cover.
- Blood glucose concentrations should be monitored closely and controlled with insulin if necessary.
- Patients taking steroids and NSAIDs are at risk of developing gastrointestinal tract bleeding and should receive gastric acid prophylaxis.
- Analgesia:
- Paracetamol.
  - Morphine.

Postoperatively
- Careful positioning and neck movement at emergence from anaesthesia.
- Extubate in sitting position.
- Cricoarytenoid inflammation may occur, necessitating tracheostomy.
- Transferring patient from the operating table to a bed should be as gentle as possible.
- Patient may need ITU/HDU.
- Supplemental oxygen, maintain sats >92%.
- Good physiotherapy and analgesia (PCA morphine).
- Mobilize early.
- Ensure steroid cover.

12. How do you know if someone is safe to extubate?

Patient can be extubated while deeply anaesthetized if:
- No residual neuromuscular block using neuromuscular monitor.
- Easy mask ventilation.
- Easy intubation.
- Not at increased risk of aspiration.
- Normothermic.

If does not meet criteria for deep extubation, then extubate if:
- Awake.
- Following commands.
- Breathing spontaneously:
    - Well oxygenated.
    - Not excessively hypercarbic.
- Fully recovered from neuromuscular blockade:
    - Sustained head lift.
    - Strong hand grip.
    - Strong tongue protrusion.
    - Evidence of recovery on nerve stimulation.

Further reading

Allman, K.G. and Wilson, I.H. *Oxford Handbook of Anaesthesia*, 2nd edn. Chapter 5: Respiratory disease, pp. 93–122. Oxford: Oxford University Press, 2006.

Henzler, D., Rossaint, R., and Kuhlen, R. Anaesthetic considerations in patients with chronic pulmonary disease. *Current Opinion in Anaesthesiology* 2003; **16**:323–30.

Wong, D.H., Weber, E.C., Schell, M.J., *et al*. Factors associated with postoperative pulmonary complications in patients with severe chronic obstructive pulmonary disease. *Anesthesia & Analgesia* 1995; **80**:276–84.

Chapter 6

Short cases

QUESTIONS

Short case 1: Pneumothorax

A 35-year-old cyclist had a road traffic accident and presented to accident and emergency with an open radial fracture. Just before induction he had acute onset of dyspnoea. A chest X-ray shows tension.

1. What is going through your mind?
2. What do you see in the X-ray?
3. What are the clinical presentations you would see?
4. What would you treat this situation?
5. How would you proceed?

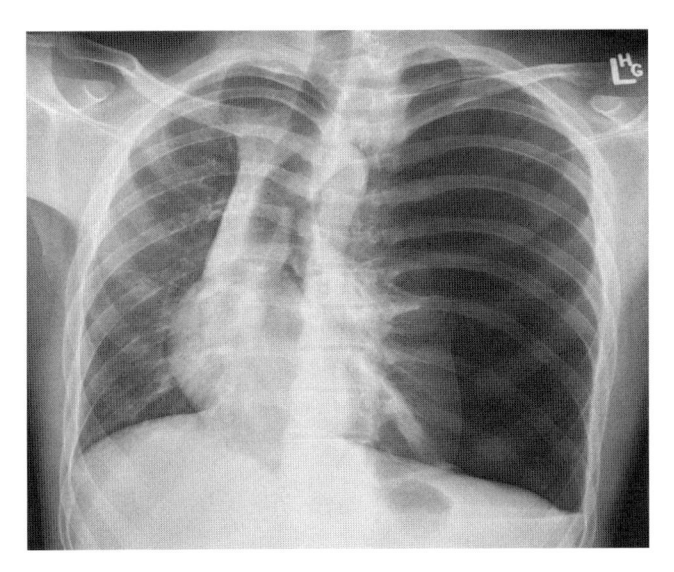

Figure 6.3 Chest X-ray.

Short case 2: Critical illness neuropathy

1. In a critically ill patient what neuromuscular problems have you come across?
2. What are the causes of muscle weakness in an intensive care unit?
3. What is critical illness neuropathy? How is it diagnosed? What is the incidence?
4. What investigations can be performed to diagnose critical illness neuropathy?
5. What is the prognosis?
6. What are its implications for perioperative management?

Short case 3: Intrapleural block

The acute pain team would like you to assess a patient in the ward who was admitted with left-side chest injury with few broken ribs on the left side. The right side is ok and there is no pneumothorax.

1. What are the indications for intrapleural block?
2. What is the mechanism of action?
3. Describe the procedure you would perform, in terms of the site, position, and type of needle, and the catheter used.
4. What would be your choice of anaesthetic?
5. What complications might you encounter?

Chapter 6

ANSWERS

Short case 1: Pneumothorax

1. What is going through your mind?

The patient had a recent road traffic accident with acute onset of dyspnoea. The patient is feeling unwell, is tachycardic and hypotensive. This could be pneumothorax and this is an emergency condition. I would get a chest X-ray if the patient is stable.

2. What do you see in this X-ray?

The chest X-ray shows a left-sided pneumothorax with a shift of the mediastinum to the right side.

Tension peumothorax: this causes shortness of breath that quickly becomes more and more severe. This occurs when the 'tear' on the lung acts like a one way valve. In effect, each breath in (inspiration) 'pumps' more air out of the lung, but the valve action stops air coming back into the lung to equal the air pressure. The volume and pressure of the pneumothorax increases which puts pressure on the lungs and heart.

Emergency treatment is needed to release the trapped air.

3. What are the clinical presentations you would see?

Pneumothorax occurs when gas enters the pleural cavity progressively but is unable to leave.

Features include:

- Respiratory distress.
- Tracheal deviation to the opposite side.
- Absent breath sounds on the affected site.
- Hyper-resonance over the affected site.
- Distended neck veins, hypotension, and loss of consciousness.
- If the patient is on IPPV—distended inflation pressures.

Diagnosis is entirely clinical. Do not waste time on getting an X-ray.

4. How would you would treat this situation?

This is an acute, life-threatening emergency. My aim is to:

- Oxygenate by facemask and call for help.
- Give circulatory support.
- Decompress the pneumothorax by inserting a wide-bore cannula in the mid clavicular line in the second intercostal space.
- Insert a chest drain on the affected site and then remove the cannula and get an X-ray.

5. How would you proceed?

Chest tube insertion

- Supine patient with the left arm behind the patient's head to expose and identify the 5th intercostal space anterior to the mid-axillary line.
- Make a 2–3-cm incision along the rib in the intercostal space.
- Blunt dissection with an artery forceps up to the pleural space.

- Puncture the pleura with artery forceps.
- Put a finger into the space to ensure safe passage and determine the presence of adhesions. Insert the chest drain to about 10–15 cm in adults and aim towards the apex.
- Connect the drain to an underwater seal and keep the bottle below the level of the patient. The fluid column should swing with respiration.

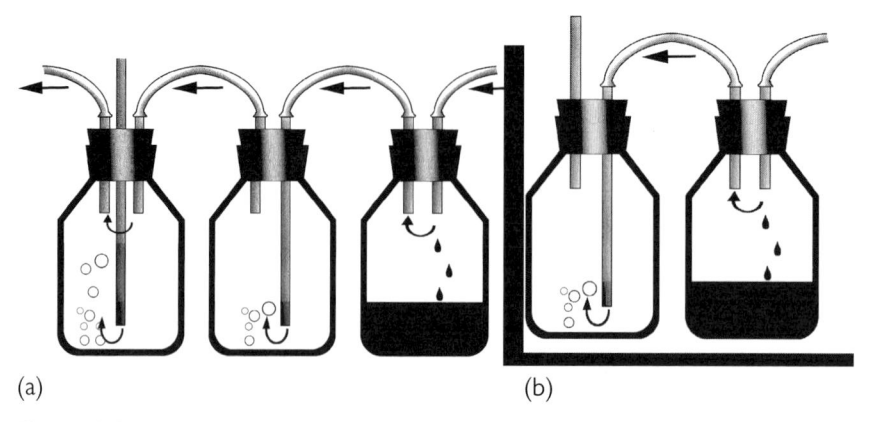

(a)   (b)

Figure 6.4 Underwater seal.

An underwater seal is used to allow air to escape through the drain but not to re-enter the thoracic cavity. The drainage bottle should always be kept below the level of the patient, otherwise its contents will siphon back into the chest cavity.

Persistent bubbling of air through the water indicates an air leak from the lung. Chest tubes should **never** be clamped for any reason, to avoid the development of a tension pneumothorax.

The air outlet of the underwater seal may be connected to moderate suction (-20 cm H_2O) to assist in lung re-expansion. This is more important in the presence of an air leak.

Chest tube removal

Chest drains may be removed when they are no longer draining any fluid and any air leak has resolved. Removal is ideally performed with two people—one to remove the tube and one to occlude the drain site. The tube should be removed either at the end of expiration or at peak inspiration, to avoid further air being entrained into the pleural cavity.

Further reading

British Thoracic Society. *Guidelines for the Management of Spontaneous Pneumothorax*. London: British Thoracic Society, 2003.

Tschopp, J.M., Rami-Porta, R., Noppen, M., et al. Management of spontaneous pneumothorax: state of the art. *European Respiratory Journal* 2006; **28**:637–50.

Chapter 6

Short case 2: Critical illness neuropathy

1. In a critically ill patient, what neuromuscular problems have you come across?
- **Peripheral neuropathy:**
  - Critical illness polyneuropathy
  - Acute motor neuropathy
- **Neuromuscular junction dysfunction:**
  - Transient neuromuscular blockade (pharmacological)
- **Myopathy:**
  - Disuse muscle fibre atrophy
  - Necrotizing myopathy

2. What are the causes of muscle weakness in an intensive care unit?
- **Pre-existing medical conditions**: Guillain–Barré syndrome, myasthenia, poliomyelitis, botulism, trauma, motor neuron disease.
- **Drug related**: aminoglycoside, muscle relaxants, steroids.
- **Metabolic and nutritional**: hypokalaemia, hypophosphataemia, magnesium deficiency.
- **Myopathy secondary to**: ARDS, liver and lung transplantation, hepatocellular failure, acidosis, malnutrition, disuse atrophy.

3. What is critical illness neuropathy? How is it diagnosed? What is the incidence?
It is polyneuropthy due to distal axonopathy involving both sensory and motor neurons without inflammation. This is associated with multiorgan failure and sepsis (60–70% of patients). Usually diagnosed when there is difficulty in weaning from mechanical ventilator or limb weakness. Occurs in up to 70% of patients who are in ICU for >5 days. Its severity is associated with length of stay in ICU.

4. What investigations can be performed to diagnose critical illness neuropathy?
- **EMG and nerve conduction**: relative preservation of conduction velocities and latencies (as myelination preserved; primary axonal degeneration). Reduction of amplitude of muscle and sensory compound action potentials.
- **Muscle biopsy**: denervation atrophy.
- **CPK**: near normal or mildly elevated.
- **CSF**: at most mildly raised protein.

5. What is the prognosis?
Most patients who survive their underlying illness will recover nerve function. Clinical recovery may take weeks in mild cases and months in severe cases. Nerve conduction studies may remain abnormal for several years.

6. What are its implications for perioperative management?
Critical illness neuropathy has been implicated in cases of severe hyperkalaemia following suxamethonium administration.

Further reading
Fletcher, S.N., Kennedy, D.D., Ghosh, I.R., et al. Persistent neuromuscular and neurophysiologic abnormalities in long term survivors of prolonged critical illness. *Critical Care Medicine* 2003; **31**:1012–16.

Mohr, M., Englisch, L., Roth, A., et al. Effects of early treatment with immunoglobulins on critical illness polyneuropathy following multiple organ failure and gram negative sepsis. *Intensive Care Medicine* 1997; **23**:1144–9.

Short case 3: Intrapleural block

1. What are the indications for intrapleural block?

Intrapleural analgesia is an established technique for providing hemithoracic analgesia and sympathetic block and offers some advantage in the management of widespread chest wall pain by minimizing the number of injections required compared with intercostal block.

Indications

- **Acute pain relief:**
  - Postoperative analgesia: mastectomy, cholecystectomy, renal operations, thoracic procedures.
  - Rib fractures, pancreatitis.
  - Acute exacerbations of pain in advanced stages of various cancers.
- **Chronic pain states:**
  - Pancreatic pain due to chronic pancreatitis or cancer of the pancreas.
  - Post-thoracotomy pain syndrome.

2. What is the mechanism of action?

Analgesia is thought to occur as a result of:
- Diffusion of local anaesthetic through the parietal pleura and the innermost intercostal muscles to reach the intercostal nerves where blockage occurs.
- Blockage of the intrathoracic sympathetic chain.
- Direct action of local anaesthetic on nerve endings within the pleura.
- Diffusion of local anaesthetic into the brachial plexus and cervical sympathetic ganglion can relieve upper extremity pain while also producing Horner's syndrome. The success of this block depends on the correct positioning of the patient such that the solution gravitates to the appropriate paravertebral area.

3. Describe the procedure you would perform, in terms of the site, position, and type of needle, and the catheter used.

- **Site**: the 6th or 7th intercostal space is identified.
- **Positioning**: performed with the patient in a lateral (and slightly oblique) or sitting position.
- **Surface anatomy**: needle insertion is performed about at a level between T6 and T8, a point anywhere between 8 cm lateral to the posterior midline and posterior axillary line.

Technique

- An epidural needle tip is advanced until it rests on the cephalad edge of the rib below the intercostal space to be entered. A syringe filled with saline or air is then attached to the needle, and the unit is advanced slowly over the superior edge of the rib.
- When the tip of the needle enters the parietal pleura, the solution in the syringe is drawn into the chest cavity because of the negative intrathoracic pressure. This effect can be observed in mechanically- and in spontaneously-ventilating patients, but it is accentuated in the latter group.

The patient's breath is held at end inspiration if spontaneously breathing, or at end expiration if ventilated, to maintain maximal negative pressure during needle insertion.
- The catheter is then inserted approximately 5–8 cm into the interpleural space and is secured on the chest wall.

4. What would be your choice of anaesthetic?

Bupivacaine in concentrations ranging from 0.25–0.5%, with or without epinephrine, is the local anaesthetic that has been studied most often. 20–25 ml of local anaesthetic (usually 0.25% bupivacaine) is usually injected. The reported mean duration of analgesia is 2–18 hours (mean 7 hours). Continuous infusion dose is at a rate of 0.125 ml/kg/hour (0.125% bupivacaine at the rate of 10 ml/hour). Interpleural administration of phenol has also been successful in the long-term relief of cancer pain.

5. What complications might you encounter?

- Pneumothorax: during needle positioning and catheter placement, care must be taken to minimize entrainment of air through the needle.
- Tension pneumothorax.
- Lung parenchymal damage can occur with loss-of-resistance techniques or insertion of excessive lengths of catheter.
- Pleural infection.
- Local anaesthetic systemic toxicity from rapid tissue absorption can also occur.
- Intravascular injection.

Further reading

Dravid, R.M. and Paul, R.E. Interpleural block – part 1. *Anaesthesia* 2007; **62**:1039–49.
Dravid, R.M. and Paul, R.E. Interpleural block – part 2. *Anaesthesia* 2007; **62**:1143–53.

Clinical science

QUESTIONS

Anatomy: Larynx

1. Draw a functional diagram to demonstrate the anatomy of the larynx.
2. What is the blood supply of the larynx?
3. What bones, cartilages, and membranes are present in the larynx?
4. What are the laryngeal muscles? What are their functions?
5. What is the nerve supply of the larynx?
6. What are the effects of partial and complete nerve damage (e.g. during thyroid surgery) on functioning of the larynx?

Physiology: Parathyroid glands

1. What do you know about the parathyroid glands?
2. What do they synthesize and what are its main effects?
3. What are the anaesthetic implications for parathyroidectomy?
4. How is calcium homeostasis maintained?
5. When would you suspect a patient has hypocalcaemia and how would you manage the condition?
6. When would you consider a patient has hypercalcaemia and how would you manage the condition?

Pharmacology: Lungs and bronchomotor tone

1. What is the nerve supply of lungs and pleura?
2. What are the receptors in the respiratory tract?
3. What are the ganglionic neurotransmitters in the sympathetic and parasympathetic systems?
4. What are the mediators of bronchoconstriction?
5. What are G proteins?
6. Classify the drugs acting as bronchodilators with their mechanism of action.
7. How do beta-2 agonists act on the bronchial smooth muscle?
8. You have intubated a patient and transferred onto the operating table and the ventilator alarm goes off with high pressure and the tidal volume reduces. How would you proceed?

Physics and clinical measurements: Ultrasound

1. Discuss the physics of ultrasound—how is it generated, what is the frequency used?
2. How does the system know the depth of the reflection?
3. What is the piezoelectric effect?

Chapter 6

4. What is the Doppler effect?
5. How is the Doppler principle used in clinical ultrasound?
6. Describe some uses of ultrasound in anaesthesia and intensive care.
7. Describe the various types of echocardiography.

ANSWERS

Anatomy: Larynx

1. Draw a functional diagram to demonstrate anatomy of the larynx.

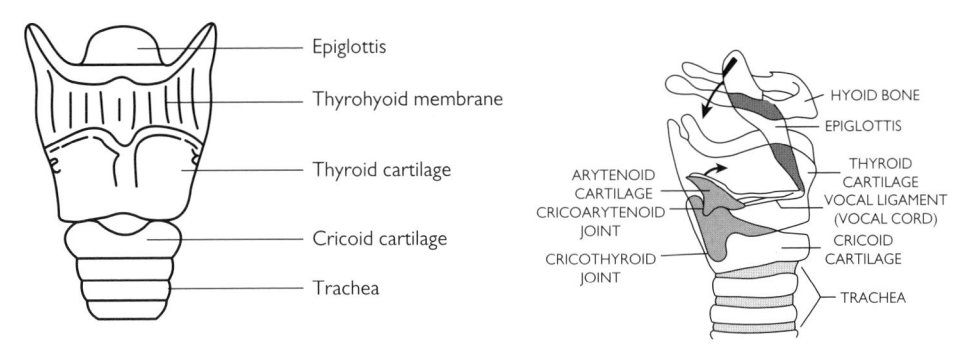

Figure 6.5 Anatomy of the larynx.

2. What is the blood supply of the larynx?
The blood supply to larynx comes from the branches of the superior and inferior thyroid arteries.

3. What bones, cartilages, and membranes are present in the larynx?
The larynx extends from root of the tongue to cricoid cartilage (C3–C6). It is composed of:
- **Bone:**
  - Hyoid bone (level with C3, attached superiorly to mandible and tongue (by hypoglossus, mylohyoid, geniohyoid, and digastric muscles) and styloid process, attached inferiorly to thyroid cartilage, sternum).
- **Cartilages**—3 unpaired, 6 paired:
  - Epiglottis (leaf shaped, vallecula = depression on either side of the midline glossoepiglottic fold, attached to thyroid cartilage by thyro-epiglottic ligament, attached to arytenoids laterally by aryepiglottic membrane).
  - Thyroid cartilage (largest cartilage, borders carry cornua posteriorly, inferior cornu has a facet for articulation with the cricoid cartilage).
  - Cricoid (signet ring shaped, level with C6, articulates with thyroid cornua and with arytenoids cartilages).
  - Arytenoids (pyramid shaped, vocal cord pass from vocal processes anteriorly to back of thyroid cartilage).
  - Corniculate (paired) and cuneiform (paired) cartilages (provide attachment for some intrinsic laryngeal muscles and are both found within the aryepiglottic folds).
  - Joined by several muscles and ligaments.

- **Membranes:**
  - Aryepiglottic membrane
  - Cricothyroid membrane
  - Thyrohyoid membrane

4. What are the laryngeal muscles? What are their functions?

- **Three extrinsic muscles:**
  - Sternothyroid—depresses larynx.
  - Thyrohyoid—elevates larynx.
  - Inferior constrictor—constricts pharynx.
- **Six intrinsic muscles:**
  - Cricothyroid are the tensor of cords.
  - Thyroarytenoid and vocalis relax the cords.
  - Posterior cricoarytenoids abduct the cords.
  - Adductor of the cords lateral cricoarytenoids and transverse arytenoids.
  - Larynx elevated by muscles of the pharynx, depressed by sternohyoid.

5. What is the nerve supply of the larynx?

The nerve supply of larynx is derived from **vagus** nerve and the nerves are:

- **Superior laryngeal nerve:** arises from the middle of the ganglion nodosum and in its course receives a branch from the superior cervical ganglion of the sympathetic. It descends, by the side of the pharynx, behind the internal carotid artery, and below and anterior to greater cornua of hyoid bone divides into two branches:
  - **Internal laryngeal nerve** supplies mucous membrane down to vocal cords.
  - **External laryngeal nerve** supplies cricothyroid muscle and inferior constrictor muscle of the pharynx.
- **Recurrent laryngeal nerve:**
  - Supplies all intrinsic laryngeal muscles except cricothyroid, and mucous membrane of the larynx below vocal cords, which is innervated by the external branch of the superior laryngeal nerve.
  - Motor to all intrinsic muscles; sensory below cords.

6. What are the effects of partial and complete recurrent laryngeal nerve damage (e.g. during thyroid surgery) on functioning of the larynx?

- **Superior laryngeal** : slack cord and weak voice.
- **Recurrent laryngeal (partial)**: cord held in midline because *abductors are affected more than the adductors*, hoarse voice, if bilateral severe airway obstruction possible.
- **Recurrent laryngeal (complete)**: cord held midway between midline and abducted position, if bilateral cords may be snapped during inspiration, causing stridor. Voice is lost.
- If one side only is affected, the contralateral cord may move across and restore the voice.
- The right recurrent laryngeal nerve is more susceptible to damage during thyroid surgery due to its relatively medial location.

Further reading

Jeannon, J.P., Orabi, A.A., Bruch, G.A., *et al*. Diagnosis of recurrent laryngeal nerve palsy after thyroidectomy: a systematic review. *International Journal of Clinical Practice* 2009; **63**(4):624–9.

Physiology: Parathyroid glands

1. What do you know about the parathyroid glands?
There are usually four parathyroid glands embedded in, but separate from, the thyroid gland. The glands consist of densely packed cells arranged in nests around abundant capillaries. These cells produce parathyroid hormone (PTH) and contain calcium-sensing receptors that regulate blood calcium levels.

2. What do they synthesize and what are its main effects?
Parathyroid hormone; PTH is synthesized in the parathyroid cells and then packaged in vesicles and secreted into the blood by exocytosis in response to low calcium levels. It is a protein consisting of 84 amino acids. It acts to raise blood calcium and lower phosphate levels. This is achieved by three mechanisms:

- Stimulating osteoclasts which resorb bone, releasing calcium.
- Indirectly increasing calcium absorption from the small bowel via increased production of vitamin D by the kidney. This induces production of a calcium-binding protein in the gut which facilitates absorption of calcium.
- Decreasing calcium loss in the urine by stimulating reabsorption.

3. What are anaesthetic implications for parathyroidectomy?
Surgery involves a full neck dissection with removal of either a single gland or, in the case of generalized hypertrophy, removal of three glands. Anaesthesia is as for thyroid surgery, but the airway is less likely to be compromised preoperatively. If the patient is markedly hypercalcaemic, dehydration should be considered and corrected.

Postoperative issues

- Airway complications can occur due to bleeding.
- Bilateral recurrent laryngeal nerve damage.
- Hypocalcaemia is commonly seen at 24–72 hour postoperatively.
- Tetany and laryngospasm may occur.
- Calcium levels should be measured twice daily until stable.

4. How is calcium homeostasis maintained?
Calcium is the most abundant mineral in the body, accounting for about 1 kg of body weight. Blood calcium levels are closely controlled in the range of 2.20–2.55 mmol/L. Approximately half is free in the blood—the rest is bound to albumin. If blood albumin levels are abnormal, a corrected calcium level should be used. This is calculated as follows:

$$\text{Corrected calcium} = \text{uncorrected calcium (mmol/L)} + 0.02(40 - \text{albumin})$$

There are three main regulatory mechanisms:

- **PTH** is very important in raising calcium levels.
- **Calcitriol** is formed in the kidney from vitamin D. It increases intestinal absorption of calcium and hence raises blood levels.
- **Calcitonin** is a 32-amino acid hormone s formed by the parafollicular cells of the thyroid gland. It counteracts the effects of PTH, lowering calcium and raising phosphate levels. It is thought to be of little importance in calcium homeostasis in humans and is not essential for life.

5. When would you suspect a patient has hypocalcaemia and how would you manage the condition?

This is defined as a calcium level <2.2 mmol/L (or ionized calcium <1.1 mmol/L). The most common causes are:

- Primary hypoparathyroidism
- Vitamin D deficiency
- Acute or chronic renal failure
- Pancreatitis

Clinical features include:

- Paraesthesia and perioral tingling.
- Tetany and carpopedal spasm occur:
    - Trousseau sign describes carpopedal spasm on sustained inflation of BPcuff, and tendon reflexes are depressed.
    - Chovstek's sign (twitching of facial muscles on repeat tapping over zygoma) may be seen.
    - In severe cases, laryngospasm and arrhythmias are seen.

Management involves replacing calcium as either IV calcium gluconate or chloride. Oral calcium and calcitriol supplements may be necessary long term. Treatment should be reserved for symptomatic patients or for those with calcium <1.5 mmol/L.

6. When would you consider a patient has hypercalcaemia and how would you manage the condition?

Hypercalcaemia is described as blood calcium >2.6 mmol/L, but is not usually symptomatic until the calcium level is >3 mmol/L.

- Symptoms: fatigue, mood change, confusion, diarrhoea, and polyuria. Renal stones can develop.
- ECG changes include shortened QT interval and arrhythmias.
- If levels rise above 3.7 mmol/L, coma and cardiac arrest occur.

Causes of hypercalcaemia

- Primary hyperparathyroidism—adenoma, hyperplasia, carcinoma.
- Malignancy—breast, lung, kidney, phaeochromocytoma.
- Vitamin D intoxication.
- Rhabdomyolysis.
- High bone turnover—Paget's disease, immobilization.
- Drugs—thiazide diuretics, lithium.
- Renal failure (secondary hyperparathyroidism).
- Milk alkali syndrome.

Together, malignancy and primary hyperparathyroidism account for 90% of cases.

Treatment of hypercalcaemia

- Rehydration to replace renal or gut fluid losses.
- Furosemide to decrease renal calcium reabsorption and allow further IV rehydration. Bisphosphonates (e.g. pamidronate) to inhibit osteoclast activity and bone resorption.

Further reading

Aguilera, M. and Vaughan, R.S. Calcium and the anaesthetist. *Anaesthesia* 2000; **55**:779–90.
Bushinsky, D.A. and Monk, R.D. Calcium. *Lancet* 1998; **352**:306–11.

Guyton AC. Parathyroid hormone, calcitonin, calcium and phosphate metabolism, vitamin D, bone and teeth. In Guyton, A.C. and Hall, J.E. (eds.) *Textbook of Medical Physiology* 12th edn., pp. 955–71. Philadelphia, PA: Saunders, 2010.

Pharmacology: Lungs and bronchomotor tone

1. What is the nerve supply of lungs and pleura?
- Tracheobronchial tree and lung:
  - Sensory: vagus nerve (X), recurrent laryngeal nerve.
  - Motor: vagus (X) (bronchoconstriction) and sympathetic fibres from T2 and T4 (bronchodilation and minor vasoconstriction).
- Pleura:
  - Parietal sensory: phrenic and intercostals nerves.
  - Visceral sensory: autonomic supply.

2. What are the receptors in the respiratory tract?
- B_2 adrenergic receptor stimulation causes bronchodilation.
- Muscarinic receptor stimulation causes bronchoconstriction.
- H_1 receptor stimulation causes bronchoconstriction.
- H_2 receptors cause bronchodilation. However, the predominant effect of histamine is bronchoconstriction.

3. What are the ganglionic neurotransmitters in the sympathetic and parasympathetic systems?
- Sympathetic: preganglionic—acetylcholine; postganglionic—acetylcholine.
- Parasympathetic: preganglionic—acetylcholine; postganglionic—noradrenaline.

4. What are the mediators of bronchoconstriction?
Bronchoconstriction or dilatation is mediated by alpha and beta receptors. Their action is mediated through G proteins.

Bronchoconstriction is caused by:
- B_2 receptor blockade.
- Parasympathetic activity and acetylcholine.
- A fall in PCO_2 in alveolar gas (apparently as a result of direct action).
- Histamine.
- As a reflex stimulation of the receptors in the trachea and large bronchi by irritants.

5. What are G proteins?
Guanine nucleotide binding proteins—these are a group of heterotrimeric proteins that act as cellular transducers, involved in bringing about an intracellular change from an extracellular stimulus. Activation of a receptor by a ligand causes an alteration in the guanine binding site of the G protein, with displacement of GDP by GTP. This results in the G protein splitting into its alpha and beta subunits—the alpha unit initiates intracellular events which lead to the cell's response to stimulation.

6. Classify the drugs acting as bronchodilators with their mechanism of action.

- **Beta-2 agonists:** transmembrane receptors which stimulates adenylate cyclase in smooth muscle cells which reduces cellular calcium causing smooth muscle relaxation; also inhibit mast cell degranulation. Short-acting salbutamol and long-acting salmeterol.
- **Anticholinergics:** cause a decrease in cGMP—this results in bronchodilation as cGMP opposes cAMP action. Example: ipratropium.
- **Phosphodiesterase inhibitors:** enzyme phosphodiesterase inhibitors cause increased cAMP levels which results in bronchodilation. Example: theophylline: methyl xanthines.
- **Mast cell stabilizers:** stabilize the mast cells preventing release of inflammatory mediators such as histamine from mast cells. Example: cromoglycate.
- **Corticosteroids:** have anti-inflammatory action—reduced capillary permeability and also potentiate action of beta-2 agonists.
- **Magnesium:** smooth muscle relaxant causing bronchodilation.

7. How do beta-2 agonists act on the bronchial smooth muscle?

These drugs act by activation of G-protein coupled receptors causing activation of adenylate cyclase resulting in an increase in cAMP and hence causing relaxation of bronchial smooth muscle.

8. You have intubated a patient and transferred onto the operating table and the ventilator alarm goes off with high pressure and the tidal volume reduces. How would you proceed?

This could be severe bronchospasm which is a life threatening situation.

Diagnosis and management occur simultaneously.

Call for help; ventilate with 100% oxygen, deepen anaesthesia using the Inhalational agent.

I will rule out other causes of raised airway pressure at machine end, tubing and patient's end.

- Inform the surgeon of the situation.
- Check the following :
  - $EtCO_2$: effective ventilation/cardiac output.
  - SpO2: saturation.
  - ECG: tachycardia or arrhythmia.
  - NIBP: hypotensive (or possibly hypertensive).

Potential diagnoses are:

- Bronchospasm (secondary to histamine release due to IV drug administration?).
- Anaphylaxis.
- Light plane of anaesthesia.
- ETT in one of the main bronchi.
- Obstructed ETT (kinked, cuff herniation, secretions, etc.).
- Pneumothorax.

Rapid check for:

- Chest movement.
- Trachea shift.
- Breath sounds/wheeze/patient coughing.
- Colour of the patient.
- ETT position, blocked, kinked, etc.
- Breathing circuit kinked, stood on, etc.
- Ventilator problem.

Chapter 6

Further reading

British Thoracic Society and Scottish Intercollegiate Guidelines Network. British guideline on the management of asthma. *Thorax* 2008; **63**(Suppl 4):1–121.

Physics and clinical measurements: Ultrasound

1. Discuss the physics of ultrasound—how is it generated, what is the frequency used?

- Ultrasound imaging is based on transmission and reflection of high-frequency longitudinal, mechanical waves ('ultrasonic sound' waves) in tissues that are transmitted from, and received by, an ultrasound transducer.
- Image information is provided by the energy of these waves as they are reflected from the surfaces between different tissues. The reflections are due to differences in the mechanical properties of the tissues.
- Utilize frequencies of 2–15 MHz (human hearing operates at 1–20 kHz).
- Most transducers use artificial polycrystalline ferroelectric materials (ceramics) [e.g. lead zirconate titanate (PZT)], which have piezoelectric properties.

2. How does the system know the depth of the reflection?

The system calculates how long it takes for the echo to return to the scan head using:

$$\text{Distance} = \text{velocity}/\text{time}$$

The velocity of sound in tissue is assumed constant at 1540 m/sec.

3. What is the piezoelectric effect?

When an electric potential is applied across a crystal of quartz it causes a dimensional change of the crystal. The crystal then emits ultrasonic waves, this is known as the piezoelectric effect. It is a characteristic of transducer elements (crystals) which converts electrical to mechanical energy and vice versa.

4. What is the Doppler effect?

The Doppler effect is an increase in observed frequency of a signal when the signal source approaches the observer and a decrease when the source moves away. The Doppler effect is based on work by Austrian physicist Johann Christian Doppler.

- Source moving TOWARD receiver = HIGHER frequency.
- Source moving AWAY from receiver = LOWER frequency.

5. How is the Doppler principle used in clinical ultrasound?

The principle is used clinically to determine velocities and flow rates of moving substances, e.g. in cardiac output measurement. An ultrasound beam may be directed along the path of flow; the sound waves reflect from the surface of blood cells as they approach or move away. Analysis of the reflected frequencies allows determination of velocity of flow. Doppler probes contain both emitter and detector in the probe tip.

$$F_d = \frac{2 F_t V \cos\theta}{C}$$

where F_t is the transmitted Doppler frequency, V is the speed of blood flow, $\cos\theta$ is the cosine of the blood flow to beam angle, and C is the speed of sound in tissue.

6. Describe some uses of ultrasound in anaesthesia and intensive care.

- Imaging vessels for safe cannulation (SonoSite).
- Locate pleural effusions and to guide taps.
- Locating vessels anterior to the trachea prior to tracheotomy.
- Guidance for nerve block procedures.
- TOE may be used perioperatively to aid fluid management, detect air embolism, and monitor valvular function during cardiac surgery.
- There is research into the use of ultrasound to locate the epidural space.
- Transcranial Doppler ultrasonography to study CBF.

7. Describe the various types of echocardiography.

- **A-mode:** now obsolete in medical imaging. Wave spikes are represented when a single beam passes through objects of different consistency and hardness.
- **B-mode**: same as A-mode, but one-dimensional graphical display, with brightness corresponding to amplitude of reflected sound.
- **M-mode**: a single beam in an ultrasound scan can be used to produce an M-mode picture, where movement of a structure such as a heart valve can be depicted in a wave-like manner. Because of its high sampling frequency (up to 1000 pulses per second), this is useful in assessing rates and motion and is still used extensively in cardiac and fetal cardiac imaging.
- **Transthoracic echocardiography** (TTE) employs low-frequency transducers (2–4 MHz), which allows better penetration of the acoustic energy through the chest wall, but at the cost of reduced longitudinal resolution.
- **Transoesophageal echocardiography** (TOE) does not require such penetration and so uses higher frequency transducers (3.5–7 MHz) to produce better resolution imaging.
- **2D-real time**: Most modern ultrasound devices are 2D-real time imaging systems. Multiple crystals (linear, curved, or phased-array) or moving crystal. Sequential B-mode pulses sweeping across a plane to display the image in either a linear or 'sector' format. Displayed as real-time imaging with up to 100 images per second.

NICE guidelines summary

- 2D imaging ultrasound guidance should be the preferred method when inserting a central venous catheter into the internal jugular vein in adults and children in elective or an emergency situations.
- Everyone who uses 2-D imaging ultrasound guidance to insert central venous catheters should have appropriate training to ensure they are competent to use the technique.
- Audio-guided Doppler ultrasound guidance is not recommended for use when inserting central venous catheters.

Further reading

Carty, S. and Nicholls, B. Ultrasound-guided regional anaesthesia. *Continuing Education in Anaesthesia Critical Care & Pain* 2007; **7**:20–4.

Davis, P.D. and Kenny, G.N.C. *Basic Physics and Measurement in Anaesthesia*, 5th edn. Oxford: Butterworth-Heinemann, 2003.

Hatfield, A. and Bodenham, A. Ultrasound for central venous access. *Continuing Education in Anaesthesia Critical Care & Pain* 2005; **5**:187–90.

NICE. *Central venous catheters – ultrasound locating devices: summary* (Technology appraisals TA49). London: NICE, 2002. Available at: http://www.nice.org.uk/TA49

Roscoe, A. and Strang, T. Echocardiography in intensive care. *Continuing Education in Anaesthesia Critical Care & Pain* 2008; **8**:46–9.

Chapter 7

Clinical anaesthesia

Long case: A case of hiatus hernia   *137*
Short cases   *142*
   Questions   *142*
   Answers   *144*
      Short case 1: Myasthenia gravis   *144*
      Short case 2: Aspiration pneumonia   *145*
      Short case 3: Chronic pain   *147*

Clinical science

Questions   *150*
Answers   *151*
   Anatomy: Intercostal nerves   *151*
   Physiology: Aldosterone   *154*
   Pharmacology: Serotonin   *155*
   Physics and clinical measurements: Laminar and turbulent flow   *158*

Clinical anaesthesia

Long case: A case of hiatus hernia

An 83-year-old woman was admitted with complaints of severe nausea and vomiting and abdominal pain, which responded to GTN and Gaviscon. Within 2 days of admission, she developed atrial fibrillation and was started on digoxin. She became febrile that was treated with cefuroxime. She gives a history of similar problems 2 years ago.

She is now scheduled for laparoscopic/open repair of a hiatus hernia.

Clinical examination	Temperature: 36.9°C; weight: 85 kg; height: 160 cm			
	Pulse: 85/min, regular; BP: 138/86 mmHg; respiratory rate: 12/min			
	Chest: decreased air entry bilateral bases, vesicular breath sound, no crepitations/rhonchi			
	Cardiovascular system: normal heart sound with no murmurs			
	Central nervous system: no neurological deficit apart from visual field defects			
Laboratory investigations	Hb	9.1 g/dL	Na	139 mEq/L
	MCV	89 fL	K	3.6 mEq/L
	WBC	9.0×10^9/L	Urea	4.3 mmol/L
	Platelets	351×10^9/L	Creatinine	85 μmol/L
	CRP	50	Glucose	5.2 mmol/L
			Albumin	20 g/L
	Mg	0.55	Total Ca	1.96

QUESTIONS

1. Summarize the case.
2. What are the important issues?
3. What are the abnormal biochemical investigations?
4. In this patient what are the causes of low albumin and why?
5. Comment on the chest X-ray and ECG.
6. What features in the information provided suggest that this patient might have an infection?
7. Where is C-reactive protein (CRP) produced and what are the conditions which cause raised CRP?
8. What would you do to rule out ischaemia/infarction?
9. Would you accept this patient for surgery? If not, what further investigations would you need?
10. Would you like to transfuse this lady prior to taking up for surgery?
11. How would you optimize this lady?
12. Once the lady is optimized, what will be the induction technique?
13. Considering the lady has a laparoscopic procedure, what are the problems/complications that can arise?
14. How would you deal with postoperative pain and further management if the patient has a laparoscopic repair?

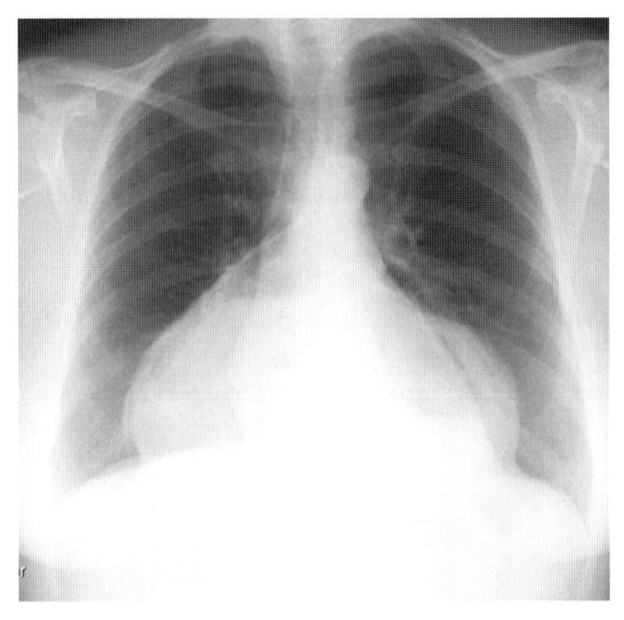

Structured Oral Examination Practice for the Final FRCA

Figure 7.1 Chest X-ray.

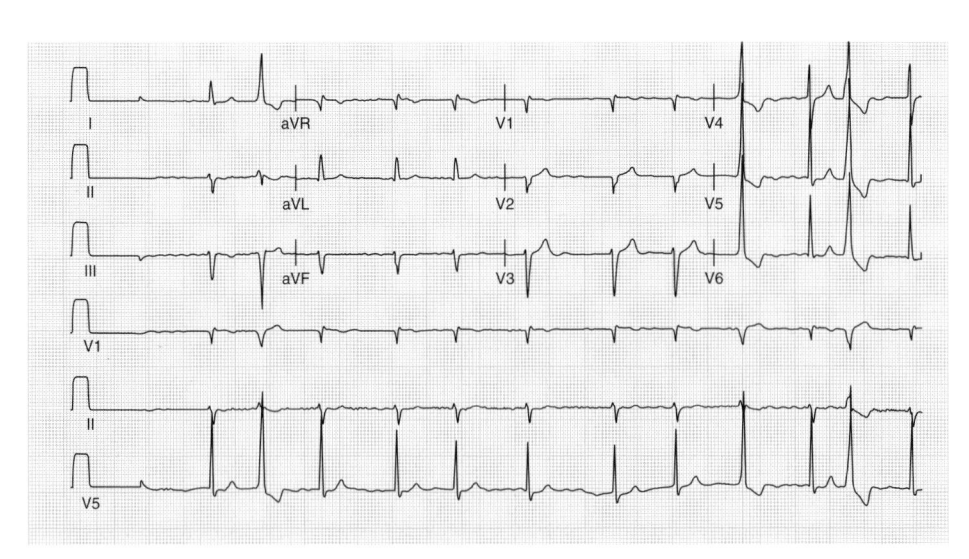

Figure 7.2 ECG.

138

Chapter 7

ANSWERS

1. Summarize the case.
We have an elderly lady with significant cardiac history with symptoms of chest infection requiring repair of hiatus hernia.

2. What are the important issues?
- Significant cardiac disease.
- Sings of chest infection.
- Problems related to the elderly: CNS, respiratory, hydration, blood loss, temperature, pressure points.

3. What are the abnormal biochemical investigations?
There is hypomagnesaemia and the patient is on digoxin. Digoxin along with hypomagnesaemia can precipitate or accentuate digoxin toxicity.

4. In this patient what are the causes of low albumin and why?
The causes of low albumin are:
- **Decreased production:** malnutrition, malabsorption, chronic liver disease (e.g. cirrhosis), or the acute phase response.
- **Increased loss:** protein-losing states (nephrotic syndrome, protein-losing enteropathy), severe burns, during operative procedures.
- **Redistribution:** during sepsis, albumin may be lost into the extravascular compartment due to increased vascular permeability, in ascites due to an exudate albumin is lost into the abdominal cavity.

5. Comment on the chest X-ray and ECG.
Chest X-ray: posterior–anterior chest X-ray. There is a large fluid filled viscus seen projected behind the heart which contains an air fluid level. The appearances are in keeping with a large hiatus hernia. The lungs are clear with no evidence of current aspiration. Heart size is within the upper limits of normal.

ECG: shows absent P waves, variable RR interval, normal QRS complexes. HR is variable, 75 bpm, the rhythm is irregular with normal QRS complexes and narrow complex tachycardia with irregular rhythm. My impression is atrial fibrillation with occasional premature ventricular contraction.

6. What features in the information provided suggest that this patient might have infection?
The patient has raised CRP, along with other signs of infection rise in temperature and currently on antibiotics.

7. Where is C-reactive protein (CRP) produced and what are the conditions which cause raised CRP?
CRP is produced in the liver.

The causes of raised CRP are:
- Inflammation/inflammatory disorders.
- Infection, tissue necrosis or injury.
- Haemolysis, malignancy.
- Pregnancy and with use of oral contraceptive pills. Recent research suggests mild CRP elevation has emerged as a valuable marker of cardiovascular risk.

8. What would you do to rule out ischaemia/infarction?

The cardiac ischaemia could be ruled out by doing troponin T test. This test is quite reliable between 6–12 hours. There are other test which can be done to rule out myocardial ischaemia are CPK MB; ECHO; thallium test if facilities available.

9. Would you accept this patient for surgery? If not, what further investigations would you need?

No, I would like to get an echocardiography to know about the left ventricular function and ejection fraction.

10. Would you like to transfuse this lady prior to taking up for surgery?

This lady has haemoglobin of 9.1 and in view of coronary artery disease I would not transfuse but would cross-match 4 units prior to surgery.

11. How would you optimize this lady?

I would first like to know her cardiac status by performing echocardiography.

Plan to optimize by:

- Continuous monitoring of BP, ECG, and saturation level.
- Central venous line and arterial line to guide the resuscitation.
- Correct magnesium, calcium.
- Resuscitate by correcting the hydration, improve nutrition, and continue antibiotics and coagulation screen.

12. Once the lady is optimized, what will be the induction technique?

This lady has hiatus hernia and there is also a high level of stress. I would pre-medicate the patient with IV rantidine and just before induction also give sodium citrate.

My technique of induction would be rapid sequence with cricoid pressure.

13. Considering the lady has a laparoscopic procedure, what are the problems/complications that can arise?

- **Injury from the instruments**: haemorrhage, perforation of intra-abdominal structures, subcutaneous emphysema.
- **Complications due to pneumoperitoneum**: increased intra-abdominal pressure, bowel ischaemia, gas embolism.
- **Systemic effect of carbon dioxide absorption**: hypercarbia, acidosis, increased sympatho-adrenal stimulation, hypertension, arrhythmias, and pain.
- **Trendelenburg position**: venous congestion of head and neck, increased ICP, increased intraocular pressure, retinal haemorrhage, etc.
- **Late complications**: bowel obstruction and injury, hernia, adhesion.

14. How would you deal with postoperative pain and further management if the patient has a laparoscopic repair?

I would manage this patient in HDU/ITU depending on course of events/surgery for full monitoring, fluid management, and normothermia.

- 100% O_2 for 48–72 hours.
- DVT prophylaxis and gastric prophylaxis.
- Simple analgesics like paracetamol, and morphine PCA.

Further reading

Conacher, I.D., Soomro, N.A., and Rix, D. Anaesthesia for laparoscopic urological surgery. *British Journal of Anaesthesia* 2004; **93**:859–64.

Póvoa, P. C-reactive protein: a valuable marker of sepsis. *Intensive Care Medicine* 2002; **28**:235–43.

Short cases

QUESTIONS

Short case 1: Myasthenia gravis

You have a 25-year-old female patient for larngopharyngoscopy with a history of increasing dysphagia and diplopia. She is on pyridostigmine and prednisolone.

1. What do you think about the case?
2. What is the pathophysiology?
3. How is it different from myasthenic syndrome?
4. How is the diagnosis made?
5. What are the treatment options for a patient with myasthenia gravis?
6. What are the main anaesthetic concerns for this patient?
7. What is the difference between a myasthenic and a cholinergic crisis?

Short case 2: Aspiration pneumonia

You have a 35-year-old male patient anaesthetized with LMA for removal of metal work from the femur. In the middle of the operation you notice copious gastric contents coming up the LMA.

1. What do you think is going on?
2. What would you do now?
3. Comment on the chest X-ray displayed. What does it show and what is the diagnosis?
4. What happens when aspiration occurs? Discuss the pathophysiology of aspiration.
5. What lobes of the lung are likely to be affected and does the position of the patient have any influence on the site of aspiration?
6. What is the likely complication following aspiration pneumonia?
7. Would you give antibiotics?

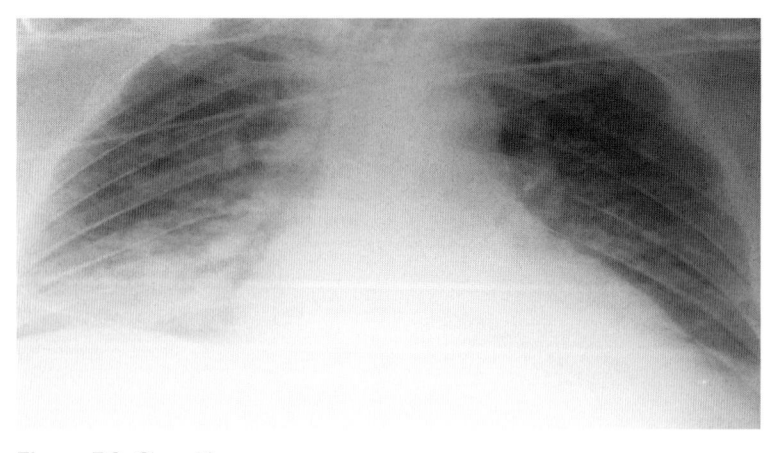

Figure 7.3 Chest-X-ray.

Chapter 7

Short case 3: Chronic pain

A woman with a history of carcinoma of the breast has presented with a tight, burning sensation in the upper arm and axilla. She had a mastectomy 4 months ago. She is on morphine sulphate tablets twice a day but complains that her pain is getting worse.

1. What are your thoughts?
2. What type of pain is this woman experiencing? What is the likely cause of this pain?
3. What are the proposed mechanisms for neuropathic pain?
4. What are the features of neuropathic pain?
5. What are allodynia, hyperalgesia, and hyperpathia?
6. What is complex regional pain syndrome (CRPS)?
7. What are the treatment modalities for neuropathic pain?

ANSWERS

Short case 1: Myasthenia gravis

1. What do you think about the case?
This is a young female patient who is suffering from a rare condition of autoimmune disorder causing weakness of muscles.

2. What is the pathophysiology?
Myasthenia gravis is an autoimmune disease caused by an antibody to and T-cell attack on nicotinic acetylcholine receptor (AChR) of motor end-plate. These reduce the number of functional receptors at the neuromuscular junction. The lowered transmission at the neuromuscular junction causes the clinical symptoms of muscle fatigue in myasthenic patients.

The clinical features are:
- Increased muscle weakness with increased activity affecting:
  - Ocular muscle causing ptosis and diplopia.
  - Bulbar muscles leading to dysarthria, dysphagia, and difficulty in chewing.
  - Proximal limbic muscles are involved as well.
- Twice as common in females, associated with thymomas, thymic hyperplasia.
- Associated with other autoimmune conditions—thyrotoxicosis, pernicious anaemia, rheumatoid arthritis.

3. How is it different from myasthenic syndrome?
- Eaton–Lambert myasthenic syndrome (ELMS) is a paraneoplastic syndrome associated with small-cell carcinoma of the lung. It presents as proximal muscle weakness affecting lower limbs.
- There is a prejunctional defect in release of ACh due to antibodies against calcium channels.
- Exercise causes improvement in weakness in ELMS but worsening in myasthenia gravis.
- Anticholinesterases do not cause an improvement.
- ELMS patients are sensitive to both depolarizing and non-depolarizing relaxants whereas myasthenia gravis patients are often resistant to depolarizing relaxants.
- Dysautonomia is more likely in ELMS patients.

4. How is the diagnosis made?
- **Edrophonium test:** injection of the edrophonium (Tensilon) may result in a sudden, although temporary, improvement in muscle strength.
- **Blood analysis:** confirms the presence of abnormal antibodies that disrupt the receptor sites.
- **Repetitive nerve stimulation:** nerve conduction study.
- **Single-fibre electromyography (EMG):** measures the electrical activity in single nerve fibre and muscle unit.
- **Imaging scans:** CT scan or an MRI to see tumours or other abnormality in the thymus.
- **Other tests:**
  - PFTs—vital capacity.
  - Blood gas (ABGs), chest-X-ray.
  - Hypokalaemia, metabolic acidosis, and hypomagnesaemia can potentiate weakness.

5. What are the treatment options for a patient with myasthenia gravis?
- Pharmacological:

Chapter 7

- ◆ Anticholinesterases (pyridostigmine).
- ◆ Steroids: prednisolone 20–60 mg/day.
- ◆ Immunosuppressants: prednisone, cyclosporine, mycophenolate mofetil, and azathioprine.
- ◆ Plasmapheresis and IV venous immunoglobulins.
- Surgical: thymectomy.

6. What are the main anaesthetic concerns for this patient?

- Increased sensitivity to non-depolarizing relaxants—decrease atracurium dose.
- Resistance to effects of depolarizing relaxants due to decreased number of ACh receptors—suxamethonium best avoided (risk of phase II block).
- Preoperative plasmapheresis decreases plasma esterase levels—possibility of prolonged action of drugs metabolized by this enzyme.
- Severity of disease—respiratory or bulbar involvement.
- Coexisting medical diseases and intercurrent medications (steroids).
- Implications of the operative technique—risk of damage to SVC, pneumothorax.
- Postoperative ventilatory support may be required depending on severity of disease. Predictors of postoperative ventilation:
  - ◆ Duration of disease >6 years
  - ◆ Coexisting respiratory disease
  - ◆ Pyridostigmine dose >750 mg/day
  - ◆ Preoperative vital capacity <2.9 L.

7. What is the difference between a myasthenic and a cholinergic crisis?

- Both present as increasing muscle weakness: edrophonium can be used to differentiate.
- Myasthenic crisis: due to inadequate treatment with anticholinesterases, improvement in muscle power with edrophonium—ability to cough or clench a fist.
- Cholinergic crisis: due to excessive administration of anticholinesterases; results in pronounced muscarinic effects. Depolarizing neuromuscular block, sweating, salivation, and miosis.

Further reading

Aitkenhead, A.R., Rowbotham, R.J., and Smith, G. *Textbook of Anaesthesia* 5th edn. Edinburgh: Churchill Livingstone Elsevier, 2006.
Allman, K.G. and Wilson, I.H. *Oxford Handbook of Anaesthesia*, 2nd edn. Oxford: Oxford University Press, 2006.
Thavasothy, M. and Hirsch, N. Myasthenia gravis. *Continuing Education in Anaesthesia Critical Care & Pain* 2002; **2**:88–90.

Short case 2: Aspiration pneumonia

1. What do you think is going on?

This is regurgitation of gastric content and as LMA does not protect the airway there is a high potential for pulmonary aspiration of gastric contents.

2. What will you do now?

- Immediately tilt the operating table to about 30° head-down position to have the larynx at a higher level than pharynx to allow drainage.
- Simultaneously call for help and ask the surgeon to stop.
- Remove LMA and suck the oropharynx. Check the pH level of the aspirate.
- Ensure oxygenation, 100% O_2, avoid ventilating gastric contents into lungs.
- Deepen the anaesthesia with IV propofol.
- The earliest and most reliable sign of aspiration is hypoxia.
- Depending on degree of contamination, consider intubation, IPPV, bronchoalveolar lavage, antibiotics, bronchodilators, rescheduling of surgery, and ITU if necessary.

3. Comment on the chest X-ray displayed. What does it show and what is the diagnosis?

Anterior–posterior chest X-ray. There is bilateral lower zone and right mid zone alveolar shadowing. Normal cardiomediastinal contour. The differential includes aspiration or infection.

4. What happens when aspiration occurs? Discuss the pathophysiology of aspiration.

The acute inflammatory-phase response (possibly to an infection) involves massive recruitment of neutrophils, with the systemic elaboration of various cytokine-mediated cascades. Some recent studies have revealed the key role played by interleukin-8 in the process.

The consequences of aspiration include bronchial obstruction, infection, and direct chemical destruction of tissues.

A hydrogen ion concentration (pH) lower than 2.5 causes considerable damage, including haemorrhagic tracheobronchitis and pulmonary oedema. Massive aspiration of acid substance such as gastric contents leads to the development of diffuse bilateral lung parenchymal opacities. Aspirated material in the lungs may lead to pneumonia, abscess, and empyema.

Large particles can cause acute airway obstruction with lobar or segmental atelectasis.

Pathophysiology: aspirated foreign material may cause obstruction. The primary sites for damage by chemical or microbial aspirates are the small airway and alveoli in which the delicate structures are particularly prone to infections and inflammation.

5. What lobes of the lung are likely to be affected and does the position of the patient have any influence on the site of aspiration?

Most commonly, the aspirated material lands in the posterior segment of upper lobes and superior segment of lower lobes, typically in supine positioned patients; therefore, these sites are most commonly the locations of aspiration pneumonia. The mechanical obstruction impedes the usual mucosal cleansing mechanism, leading to increased vulnerability to seeded pathogens.

The distribution of aspirated material in the lung depends on the person's position during the event. If aspiration occurs when a person is upright, the opacities usually are in the right lower lobe. If the individual aspirates in the supine position, the material tends to accumulate in the upper lobes.

6. What is the likely complication following aspiration pneumonia?

Acute lung injury leading to ARDS.

7. Would you give antibiotics?

The initial aspirate is usually sterile and remains for the first 24 hours. The antibiotic therapy should depend on the clinical features—chest signs, bronchospasm, pyrexia, productive cough.

Chapter 7

Further reading

Marik, P.E. Aspiration pneumonitis and aspiration pneumonia. *New England Journal of Medicine* 2001; **344**: 665–71.

Short case 3: Chronic pain

1. What are your thoughts?

This is a case of cancer pain which is taking the nature of chronic pain.

2. What type of pain is this woman experiencing? What is the likely cause of this pain?

The lady is suffering with neuropathic pain which occurs when there is abnormal activation of these pain pathways as a result of damage or dysfunction within the nervous system itself. In this case it is due to intercostobrachial nerve injury. This is commonly referred to as the post-mastectomy syndrome.

3. What are the proposed mechanisms of neuropathic pain?

The mechanisms underlying neuropathic pain are complex. It is clear that the nervous system is capable of significant plasticity with various peripheral and central changes occurring in response to injury or experience, altering both structure and function. The peripheral changes include sensitization of nociceptors resulting in reduced thresholds for activation and enhanced responses to stimuli, abnormal neuronal sprouting leading to enlargement of receptive fields and ectopic firing in A-delta and C-fibres in the dorsal root ganglion. This increased expression of abnormal sodium and calcium channels are considered to be generating the spontaneous discharges from the damaged neurons.

The central changes induced by peripheral nerve damage include sensitization of spinal cord neurons resulting in 'wind-up' with loss of central inhibitory mechanisms and enhanced nociceptive transmission, despite reduced peripheral input. Upregulation and activation of central N-methyl-D-aspartic acid (NMDA) receptors have been shown to play an important role centrally.

4. What are the features of neuropathic pain?

The International Association for the Study of Pain (IASP) defines neuropathic pain as 'pain resulting from disease or damage of the peripheral or central nervous systems, and from dysfunction of the nervous system'.

Neuropathic pain is characterized as a persistent and severe pain, often with sensory pain qualities that are described as burning, sharp and stabbing. Associated features include hyperalgesia, allodynia, sympathetic hyperfunction, and secondary myofascial pain. There is often a delay in the onset of the pain after the initial injury (days–months) and there is a lack of identifiable clinical or radiographic abnormalities.

5. What are allodynia, hyperalgesia, and hyperpathia?

Definitions:

- **Allodynia**: pain produced by a stimulus that would not normally be expected to produce pain.
- **Hyperalgesia**: increased response to a stimulus that is normally painful.

- **Hyperpathia**: altered perception such that stimuli which would normally be innocuous, if repeated or prolonged, result in severe explosive or persistent pain.

6. What is complex regional pain syndrome (CRPS)?

CRPS is characterized by pain with sudomotor or vasomotor instability. It is triggered by noxious stimuli (Type I) or by nerve injury (Type II).
- Type I: formerly known as reflex sympathetic dystrophy.
- Type II: formerly known as causalgia.

The diagnosis of CRPS can be made when there is history of trauma to the affected area associated with pain which exceed in both magnitude and duration the expected course of the inciting event plus one of the following
- Abnormal function of sympathetic nervous system
- Swelling
- Movement disorder
- Changes in tissue growth (dystrophy and atrophy)

Clinical features of CRPS
- **Inflammatory**: pain, colour change, temperature change, limitation of movement, exacerbation by exercise, oedema.
- **Neurological**: allodynia, involuntary muscle spasms, hyperpathia, paresis.
- **Dystrophic**: changes in skin, muscle, nails, bone.
- **Sympathetic**: hyperhidrosis, changed hair and nail growth, vasomotor abnormalities.

7. What are the treatment modalities for neuropathic pain?

- **Topical**: local anaesthetic, capsaicin.
- **Local**: transcutaneous electrical stimulation (TENS), acupuncture, thermal (heat, cold), vibration, massage.
- **Nerve blocks**: nerve or plexus, root block of sympathetic of ganglia, or regional guanethidine.
- **Central**: spinal cord stimulation (SCS) and deep brain stimulation (DBS).
- **Spinal drugs**: epidural or intrathecal (local anaesthetics, opioids).
- **Pharmacological drugs**: a key component in the multimodal treatment of chronic pain.
- **Antidepressant drugs**: the exact mechanism is unknown. There is generally central blockade of CNS monoamine uptake, specifically serotonin and/or norepinephrine, in addition to other neurotransmitters. They may alter nociceptive processing by prolonging synaptic activity of these monoamines, thereby enhancing descending inhibitory action in the spinal cord in addition to monoaminergic effects elsewhere in the CNS. Tricyclic antidepressants remain one of the first-line therapies for neuropathic pain.
    - Doses range of antidepressants:
        - Amitriptyline: initially 10–25 mg, increasing to 75 mg NOCTE every night.
        - Dosulepin: 25–75 mg NOCTE every night.
        - Nortriptyline: initially 10–25 mg, increasing to 75 mg NOCTE every night.
        - Venlafaxine: 37.5–75 mg NOCTE every night.
        - Fluoxetine: 20 mg NOCTE every night.
- **Antiepileptic drugs**: these reduce neuronal excitability by means of frequency-dependent blockade of sodium channels. Phenytoin is now used infrequently although given IV may have some utility in the management of acute flare-ups of neuropathic pain. Carbamazepine remains the treatment of choice in trigeminal neuralgia. It causes both a reduction in pain intensity, pain

paroxysms, and triggering stimuli. Oxcarbazepine is a newer chemically-related drug with a more favourable side effect profile.
- ◆ Drug dose range:
  - Gabapentin: day 1, 300 mg once a day; day 2, 300 mg twice a day; day 3, 300 mg three times a day. Increasing up to 800 mg three times a day.
  - Pregabalin: 75 mg twice a day, increasing to 150 mg twice a day then 300 mg twice a day if ineffective.
  - Carbamazepine: 100–400 mg twice a day.
  - Sodium valproate: 200 mg twice a day, increasing to 1 g twice a day.
  - Phenytoin: 150 mg, increasing to 500 mg once a day.
  - Mexiletine: 400–1200 mg daily in divided doses.
- **Local anaesthetics and antiarrhythmics**: suppress such hyperexcitability by means of non-specific sodium channel blockade. Additionally, low-dose lignocaine may block glutamate-evoked activity in the dorsal horn of the spinal cord.
- **Surgery**: decompression.
- **Psychological**: behavioural measures, pain management programmes.
- **Rehabilitation**.

Further reading

Jenson, T.S., Gottrup, H., Sindrup, S.H., et al. The clinical picture of neuropathic pain. *European Journal of Pharmacology* 2001; **429**:1–11.

Merksey, H. and Bogduk, N. *Classification of Chronic Pain: Descriptions of Chronic Pain Syndromes and Definitions of Pain Terms*, 2nd edn. Seattle, WA: IASP Press, 1994.

Ryder, S.-A. and Stannard, C.F. Treatment of chronic pain: antidepressant, antiepileptic and antiarrhythmic drugs. *Continuing Education in Anaesthesia Critical Care & Pain* 2005; **5**:18–21.

Clinical science

QUESTIONS

Anatomy: Intercostal nerves

1. Describe the anatomy of intercostal nerves.
2. What is the anatomical relationship between intercostal nerves and other structures in the intercostal space? Draw a typical intercostal nerve with its branches.
3. How are the intercostal muscles arranged?
4. What are the indications for an intercostal nerve block (ICNB)?
5. How is an ICNB performed?
6. What are the complications of an ICNB?
7. After you have performed a block bilaterally the patient feel unwell. What will you do?
8. How do you prevent local anaesthesia toxicity?

Physiology: Aldosterone

1. What do you know about aldosterone?
2. What are the functions of aldosterone?
3. How is the hormone release controlled from the adrenal cortex?
4. What is hyperaldosteronism?
5. What are aldosterone antagonists?

Pharmacology: Serotonin

1. What is serotonin?
2. How and where is it synthesized and metabolised?
3. What are the physiological effects of serotonin?
4. What kind of receptors are 5-HT?
5. What is the clinical relevance of serotonin?
6. What is carcinoid syndrome? What are the implications?

Physics and clinical measurements: Laminar and turbulent flow

1. Define flow. What are the units? Explain laminar and turbulent flow.
2. What is the relationship between pressure and flow (draw graphs for laminar and turbulent flow)? Explain the Hagen–Poiseuille equation.
3. What is Reynolds number? How it is calculated and what is its significance?
4. Give examples of devices used for measuring gas flow. How does a rotameter work? What are the causes of error in rotameter readings?
5. How does a pneumotachograph work?

Chapter 7

ANSWERS

Anatomy: Intercostal nerves

1. Describe the anatomy of intercostal nerves.

There are 12 pairs of thoracic anterior primary rami, the upper 11 comprises the intercostal nerves and the 12th is the subcostal nerve. They are responsible for the innervation of the muscles of the intercostal spaces and anterior abdominal wall and for the cutaneous supply of the skin of the medial aspect of the upper limb. Each nerve is connected with the adjoining ganglion of the sympathetic trunk by a grey and a white ramus communicans.

At the back of the chest they lie between the pleura and the posterior intercostal membranes, but soon pierce the latter and run between the two planes of intercostal muscles as far as the middle of the rib. They then enter the substance of the intercostales interni, and, running amidst their fibres as far as the costal cartilages, they reach the inner surfaces of the muscles and lie between them and the pleura. Near the sternum, they pierce the intercostales interni, and terminate as the anterior cutaneous branches of the thorax.

2. What is the anatomical relationship between intercostal nerves and other structures in the intercostal space? Draw a typical intercostal nerve with its branches.

Intercostal nerves lie below the blood vessels in the intercostal space (the artery is located superiorly, the vein is inferior to the artery but superior to the nerve). Each nerve (except 1st) gives off a lateral cutaneous branch anterior to the rib angles, and ends as the anterior cutaneous branch.

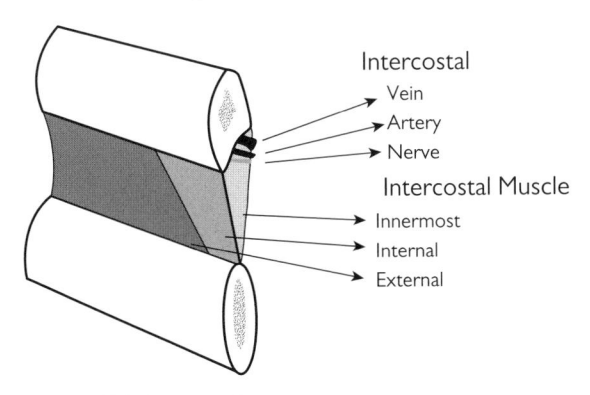

Figure 7.4 Intercostal nerve anatomy.

3. How are the intercostal muscles arranged?

Muscle layers between the ribs:
- External intercostal muscles, passing down and forward.
- Internal intercostal muscles, passing down and backward.
- Innermost intercostals, attached to the ribs' inner surface.

4. What are the indications for an intercostal nerve block (ICNB)?

ICNB provides excellent analgesia for:
- Chest trauma with multiple rib fractures (respiratory parameters typically show impressive improvements upon removal of pain).

151

- Also used as multimodal pain therapy after chest and upper abdominal surgery as:
  - Thoracotomy, thoracostomy.
  - Mastectomy.
  - Gastrostomy, and
  - Cholecystectomy.
- Neurolytic ICNB may be used to manage chronic pain conditions such as post-mastectomy pain (T2) and post-thoracotomy pain.

5. How is an ICNB performed?

Anatomy: the intercostal nerve can be blocked anywhere proximal to the mid-axillary line, where the lateral cutaneous branch originates. In adults, the most popular site for ICNB is at the angle of the rib (6–8 cm from the spinous processes). Blockade of two dermatomes above and two below the level of surgical incision is required.

Technique
- Position:
  - ICNB can be performed with the patient in the prone, sitting, or lateral position (block side up).
- Landmark:
  - At the angle of the rib, the rib is relatively superficial and easy to palpate and the subcostal groove is the widest, reducing the pleural puncture.
  - Feel for the angle of the rib at the posterior axillary line; place the index and middle fingers either side of the rib.
- Needle: a 4–5-cm 22 G to 24 G short-bevel needle.
- Site of skin is infiltrated with 1–2 ml of 1–2% lignocaine.
- The site of entry is at a 20° cephalad angle and with the bevel facing cephalad.
- The needle is advanced until it contacts the rib at a depth of <1 cm for most non-obese patients to the skin, to touch the lower border of the rib.
- Pass the needle beneath the rib, insert 3–4 mm.
- A click or loss of resistance or paraesthesia may be felt—inject 3–5 ml.
- For catheter insertion use a 16 G Tuohy needle with an oblique angulation parallel to the rib until there is loss of resistance to air/saline.

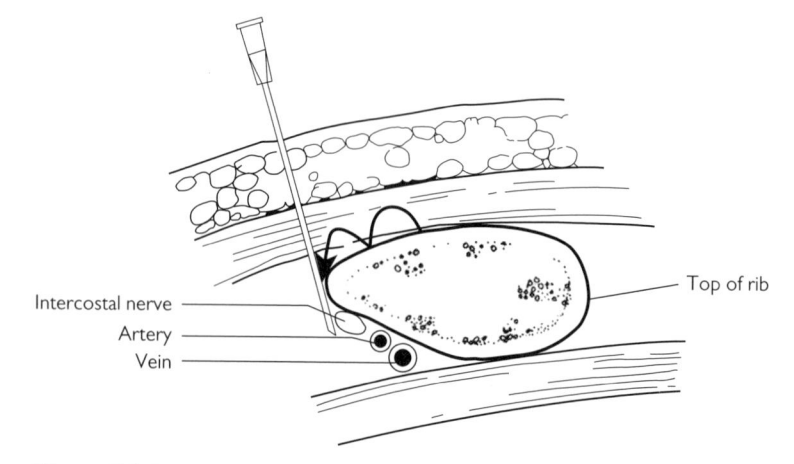

Figure 7.5 Intercostal nerve block.

6. What are the complications of an ICNB?

The complications which can occur are:
- Intravascular injection
- Bleeding
- Pneumothorax
- Local anaesthetic drug toxicity

7. After you have performed a block bilaterally the patient feel unwell. What will you do?

This is a situation which could be due to drug toxicity:
- Drug overdose.
- Direct intravascular injection.
- Rapid absorption/injection into a highly vascular area.
- Cumulative effect of multiple injections or continuous infusion.

Treatment of toxicity
- Stop injection of the patient.
- Assess patient's 'airway, breathing, circulation' and provide 100% O_2 by mask.
- If this is a drug toxicity with:
  - Mild symptoms:
    - Treat with O_2.
    - Midazolam (1–4mg) to increase the convulsant threshold.
    - Assess the patient's ventilation and continue monitoring.
  - Moderate to severe toxicity: alteration in mental status, severe agitation or loss of consciousness, with or without tonic–clonic convulsions. Convulsions followed by cardiovascular collapse.
    - Stop the local anaesthetic and call for help.
    - ABC resuscitation.
    - Prevent/treat convulsions and maintain oxygenation:
      - Use thiopental, propofol or midazolam.
      - Paralyse and intubate if convulsions recur and ventilate with 100% O_2.
- If cardiovascular collapse ensues, begin CPR.
- If cardiac arrest occurs:
  - Continue CPR throughout treatment with lipid emulsion.
  - Recovery from local anaesthetic-induced cardiac arrest may take >1 hour.
  - Propofol is not a suitable substitute for lipid emulsion.
  - Lignocaine should not be used as an anti-arrhythmic therapy.
- Give an initial intravenous bolus injection of 20% lipid emulsion 1.5 ml/kg over 1 min followed by 15 ml/kg/hour. The maximum dose should not exceed 12 mls/kg/hour.
- Early intervention leads to better outcome.

8. How do you prevent local anaesthesia toxicity?

The toxicity of local anaesthetic technique could be prevented by:
- Following the monitoring guidelines of AAGBI.
- Identifying the site to be blocked.
- Using the correct dose of local anaesthetic. The maximum dose varies depending on site to be anaesthetized, vascularity of the tissues, individual tolerance, and anaesthetic technique.

- Aspiration during regional techniques should be gentle, as the side wall of a small blood vessel is easily sucked on to the needle/catheter.
- Using adrenaline to decrease vascular re-absorption

Further reading

Association of Anaesthetists of Great Britain and Ireland. *Management of Severe Local Anaesthetic Toxicity* (Safety Guidance). London: AAGBI, 2010.

Karmakar, MK. and Ho, A.M.H. Acute pain management of patients with multiple fractured ribs. *Journal of Trauma* 2003; **54**:612–15.

Karmakar, M.K., Critchley, L.A.H., Ho, A.M.H., et al. Continuous thoracic paravertebral infusion of bupivacaine for pain management in patients with multiple fractured ribs. *Chest* 2003; **123**:424–31.

Strømskag, K.E. and Kleiven, S. Continuous intercostals and interpleural nerve blockades. *Techniques in Regional Anesthesia and Pain Management* 1998; **2**:79–89.

The New York School of Regional Anesthesia website: http://www.nysora.com

Physiology: Aldosterone

1. What do you know about aldosterone?

Aldosterone is a steroid hormone (mineralocorticoid family) produced by the outer-section (zona glomerulosa) of the adrenal cortex in the adrenal gland, and acts on the distal tubules and collecting ducts of the nephron, the functioning unit of the kidney to cause the conservation of sodium, secretion of potassium, increased water retention, and increased BP. The overall effect of aldosterone is to increase reabsorption of ions and water in the kidney.

2. What are the functions of aldosterone?

Aldosterone is the primary of several endogenous members of the class of mineralocorticoids in human. Deoxycorticosterone is another important member of this class. Aldosterone tends to promote Na^+ and water retention, and lower plasma K^+ concentration by the following mechanisms:

- Acting on the nuclear mineralocorticoid receptors (MR) within the principal cells of the distal tubule and the collecting duct of the kidney nephron, it upregulates and activates the basolateral Na^+/K^+ pumps, stimulating ATP hydrolysis leading to phosphorylation of the pump and a conformational change in the pump exposes the Na^+ ions to the outside. The phosphorylated form of the pump has a low affinity for Na^+ ions, hence reabsorbing sodium (Na^+) ions and water into the blood, and secreting potassium (K^+) ions into the urine.
- Aldosterone upregulates epithelial sodium channel increasing apical membrane permeability for Na^+.
- Cl^- is reabsorbed in conjunction with sodium cations to maintain the system's electrochemical balance.
- Aldosterone stimulates uptake of K^+ into cells.
- Aldosterone stimulates Na^+ and water reabsorption from the gut salivary and sweat glands in exchange for K^+.
- Aldosterone stimulates H^+ secretion by intercalated cells in the collecting duct, regulating plasma bicarbonate (HCO_3^-) levels and its acid/base balance.
- Aldosterone may act on the CNS via the posterior pituitary gland to release vasopressin (ADH), which serves to conserve water by direct actions on renal tubular reabsorption.

3. How is the hormone release controlled from the adrenal cortex?
- Involves the renin–angiotensin system.
- The plasma concentration of potassium.
- ACTH, a pituitary peptide, also has some stimulating effect on aldosterone probably by stimulating the formation of deoxycorticosterone, a precursor of aldosterone. Aldosterone is increased by blood loss, pregnancy, and possibly by other circumstances such as physical exertion, endotoxin shock, and burns.
- The role of sympathetic nerves via carotid artery pressure, pain, posture, and probably emotion (anxiety, fear, and hostility) (including surgical stress). Anxiety increases aldosterone, which must have evolved because of the time delay involved in migration of aldosterone into the cell nucleus.
- The role of baroreceptors:
  - Pressure in the carotid artery decreases aldosterone.
  - The role of the juxtaglomerular apparatus.

4. What is hyperaldosteronism?
This is a condition when there is excessive aldosterone secreted by the adrenal gland. This is featured with low potassium levels in blood. Clinical features are hypertension, hypokalaemia and alkalosis.

5. What are aldosterone antagonists?
Aldosterone antagonists refers to diuretic drugs which antagonize the action of aldosterone at mineralocorticoid receptors. This group of drugs is often used as adjunctive therapy, in combination with other drugs, for the management of chronic heart failure. Spironolactone, the first member of the class, is also used in the management of hyperaldosteronism (including Conn's syndrome) and female hirsutism.

Further reading
Conn, J.W. Presidential address. I. Painting background. II. Primary aldosteronism, a new clinical syndrome. *Journal of Laboratory and Clinical Medicine* 1955; **45**:3–17.
Young, W.F. Primary aldosteronism: renaissance of a syndrome. *Clinical Endocrinology (Oxford)* 2007; **66**:607–18.

Pharmacology: Serotonin

1. What is serotonin?
Serotonin (5-hydroxytryptamine, 5-HT) is a monoamine neurotransmitter synthesized in serotonergic neurons in the CNS, enterochromaffin cells in the GIT, and platelets. It is an indole monoamine which is an endogenous vasoactive substance that serves as an inhibitory neurotransmitter.

2. Where is it synthesized and metabolized?
Synthesis
Serotonin is produced by hydroxylation and decarboxylation of l-tryptophan in nerve terminals, and is stored in synaptic vesicles. It is found in the GIT, in platelets and mast cells, and in the CNS—notably the hypothalamus, limbic system, cerebellum, spinal cord, and retina.

Metabolism

After release into the synaptic cleft, 5-HT is both taken up into the presynaptic membrane by an active reuptake mechanism and metabolized by monoamine oxidase (MAO). The main metabolic product is 5-hydroxyindole acetic acid (5-HIAA), which is excreted in the urine. Neuronal 5-HT: undergoes oxidative deamination by MAO and extraneuronal 5-HT is metabolized by the liver to 5-HIAA.

3. What are the physiological effects of serotonin?

- CNS:
    - Modulates pain transmission at spinal level.
    - Contributes to hypothalamic/sympathetic regulatory mechanisms.
    - Modulates chemoreceptor trigger zone/vomiting centre.
    - Influences arousal, muscle tone, mood, and memory.
- Cardiovascular:
    - Vasoconstriction (splanchnic, renal, pulmonary, and cerebral circulations).
    - Amplification of local actions of noradrenaline, angiotensin II, and histamine.
    - Increased vascular permeability and platelet aggregation.
- Respiratory bronchoconstriction.
- Gastrointestinal role in water/electrolyte secretion.
- Alters smooth muscle contractility.
- Key role in emesis.

4. What kind of receptors are 5-HT?

All 5-HT receptors involve cAMP and G proteins, except 5-HT$_3$, which functions via a ligand-gated ion channel.

Receptor	Second messenger	Channel effects
5-HT$_{1A}$	cAMP	Increases K conductance
5-HT$_{1B}$	cAMP	Increases K conductance
5-HT$_{1C}$	IP3, DAG	Decreases K conductance
5-HT$_{1D}$	cAMP	Decreases K conductance
5-HT$_2$	IP3, DAG	
5-HT$_3$	Ion channel	Na
5-HT$_4$	cAMP	

5. What is the clinical relevance of serotonin?

Antidepressants

A CNS deficiency of serotonin is the aetiology of depression. The selective 5-HT reuptake inhibitors (SSRIs) are the first-line pharmacological treatment. Anaesthesia in patients taking SSRIs can, rarely, precipitate hypotension, arrhythmias, altered thermoregulation/postoperative shivering, and postoperative confusion.

Serotonin syndrome

Serotonin syndrome is a complex of symptoms and signs attributable to drug-induced changes in sensitivities of serotonin receptors in the CNS. The syndrome is characterized by changes in autonomic, neurological, and cognitive behavioural functions and appears to result from over-stimulation of 5-HT$_{1a}$ and 5-HT$_2$ receptors in the central grey nuclei and medulla.

Chapter 7

Migraine
Migraine is a chronic neurovascular disorder, characterized by attacks of severe headache, visual disturbance, and nausea/vomiting. Transient focal neurological signs are common. Various theories have been suggested regarding the pathophysiology of migraine. Sumatriptan is the most extensively studied agent.

Gastrointestinal tract
5-HT is thought to be a key mediator of functional gut disorder.

Postoperative nausea and vomiting
5-HT$_3$ receptor antagonists have become the treatment of choice for PONV. They are effective, safe, and well tolerated.

Carcinoid syndrome
Carcinoid syndrome is caused by tumours originating in the endocrine argentaffin cells of the small bowel mucosa. These tumours secrete, variably, peptides, kinins, prostaglandins and serotonin, resulting in flushing, hypotension, diarrhoea, and occasionally bronchospasm.

Surgical management may involve resection or debulking of primary or metastatic carcinoid tumours. The key anaesthetic consideration is prevention of mediator release.

Octreotide, a synthetic analogue of somatostatin, is used before operations to counteract serotonin and kinin activity.

Pre-eclampsia/eclampsia
Pre-eclampsia is a multisystem disorder of endothelial dysfunction. One theory (of many) is that placental ischaemia might cause trophoblastic fragmentation. Platelet aggregation on these fragments releases serotonin, resulting in diffuse vasospasm and consequent endothelial cell dysfunction. Cardiovascular, CNS, renal, respiratory, hepatic, and coagulation systems can be affected.

Cardiology
5-HT$_4$ receptors have been identified in atrial cells, and when stimulated they may cause atrial arrhythmias. Piboserod, a 5-HT$_4$-receptor antagonist, is under clinical investigation as a treatment for atrial fibrillation and cardiac failure.

6. What is carcinoid syndrome? What are the implications?
Occurs in patients with argentaffin cell tumours of the mucousa (GIT 75%) with hepatic metastases or a primary tumour with non-portal venous drainage. Occurs only in 5% cases of carcinoid tumour.

Symptoms
- Mechanical: obstructive symptoms due to the primary tumour.
- Humoural:
  - Flushing: 90%—head, neck, and torso.
  - Diarrhoea: 78%.
  - Bronchospasm: 20%.
  - Endocardial fibrosis.
  - Pulmonary and systemic effects depends on the balance between the vasoconstrictor and dilator effects of the mediators released.

Problems anticipated
- CVS: haemodynamic disturbances.
- Respiration: pulmonary hypertension and bronchospasm.
- Electrolyte imbalance due to diarrhoea.
- Delayed awakening due to serotonergic effects postoperatively.

Further reading

Chinniah, S., French, J.L.H., and Levy, D.M. Serotonin and anaesthesia. *Continuing Education in Anaesthesia Critical Care & Pain* 2008; **8**:43–5.
Linde, M. Migraine: a review and future directions for treatment. *Acta Neurologica Scandinavica* 2006; **114**:71–83.
Sanders-Bush, E. and Mayer, S.E. 5-Hydroxytryptamine (serotonin) receptor agonists and antagonists. In Hardman, J.G., Limbird, L.E., and Gilman, A.G. (eds.) *Goodman & Gillman's The Pharmacological Basis of Therapeutics* 10th edn., pp. 269–90. New York: McGraw-Hill, 2001.

Physics and clinical measurements: Laminar and turbulent flow

1. Define flow. What are the units? Explain laminar and turbulent flow.

- Flow is the mass of a substance (in this case a fluid), that passes a certain point in one second.
- The units are litres per second.

In **laminar flow**, the fluid moves in layers called laminas. Laminar flow need not be in a straight line. For laminar flow, the flow follows the curved surface of the airfoil smoothly, in layers. The closer the fluid layers are to the airfoil surface, the slower they move. Moreover, the fluid layers slide over one another without fluid being exchanged between the layers.

In **turbulent flow**, secondary random motions are superimposed on the principal flow and there is an exchange of fluid from one adjacent sector to another. Turbulence is flow dominated by recirculation, eddies, and apparent randomness. More importantly, there is an exchange of momentum such that slow-moving fluid particles speed up and fast-moving particles give up their momentum to the slower-moving particles and slow down themselves.

2. What is the relationship between pressure and flow (draw graphs for laminar and turbulent flow)? Explain the Hagen–Poiseuille equation.

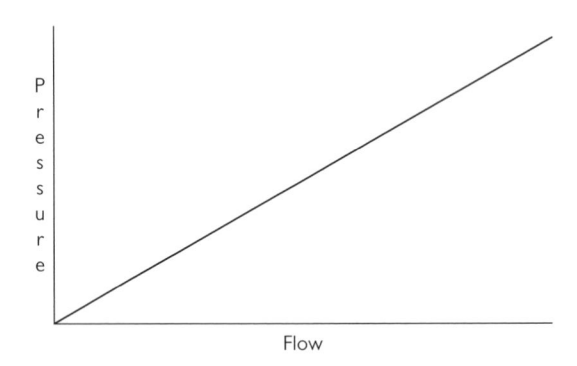

Figure 7.6 Laminar flow; relationships between flow and pressure.

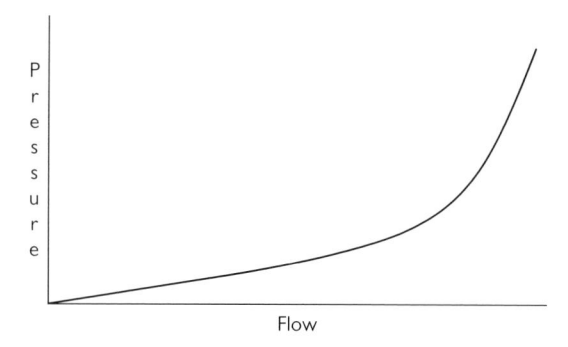

Figure 7.7 Turbulent flow, a non-linear relationship exists between flow and pressure.

For laminar flow, flow is directly proportional to pressure drop but for turbulent flow, flow is directly proportional to the square root of pressure drop.

Hagen–Poiseuille equation applies to laminar flow:

$$Q = \pi P r^4 / 8\eta l$$

where: Q = flow in litres/second; η = viscosity in Pa.s; P = Pressure in Pascals; r = radius of the tube in meters; l = length of the tube in question in metres.

3. What is Reynolds number? How is it calculated and what is its significance?

Reynolds number attempts to describe the point at which flow changes from laminar to turbulent, and the spectrum in between. The equation for Reynolds number (Re) is:

$$Re = \rho v d / \eta$$

where Re = Reynolds number; ρ = density of the liquid; v = flow velocity of the liquid; d = orifice diameter; η = viscosity.

For numbers less than 2000, the flow through a tube tends to be laminar. When the flow is between 2000 to 4000, the flow pattern is a mix of the two, and above 4000 the flow is mainly turbulent.

4. Give examples of devices used for measuring gas flow. How does a rotameter work? What are the causes of error in rotameter readings?

Pressure drop across a resistance can be used to calculate flow by: keeping the resistance constant and measuring the pressure change as the flow varies, as in a pneumotachograph or having a constant pressure drop and varying the resistance in a measurable way (e.g. bobbin rotameter).

Inaccuracies in rotameters
- The bobbin can stick in the tube due to dirt or static electricity.
- Back pressure caused by downstream resistance also leads to inaccurately low readings.
- High altitude/low atmospheric pressure.

5. How does a pneumotachograph work?

In a pneumotachograph, a resistance is put in the gas pathway and the resulting pressure drop across it measured rapidly and accurately using a differential pressure transducer, from which flow rate and volume are calculated. For improved accuracy, the resistance is usually designed to produce laminar flow, so that the flow rate is directly proportional to the measured pressure drop. This is achieved using a series of small-bore tubes arranged in parallel, through which the gas flow must pass.

A heating element is sometimes incorporated to prevent the build-up of condensation that could compromise accuracy. The total resistance added by the pneumotachograph should be small so that it can be used in a spontaneously breathing patient.

Further reading

Davis, P.D. and Kennny, G.N.C. *Basic Physics and Measurement in Anaesthesia*, 5th edn, Chapter 2: Fluid flow, pp. 14–28. Oxford: Butterworth Heinemann, 2003.

Koh, K.F. Gas, tubes and flows. *Anaesthesia and Intensive Care Medicine* 2002; **3**:214–15.

Chapter 8

Clinical anaesthesia

Long case: A young boy with Guillain–Barré syndrome   *163*
Short cases   *168*
   Questions   *168*
   Answers   *169*
      Short case 1: Pre-eclampsia   *169*
      Short case 2: A patient in recovery following TURP   *172*
      Short case 3: Autonomic neuropathy   *173*

Clinical science

Questions   *176*
Answers   *177*
   Anatomy: Femoral triangle   *177*
   Physiology: Intraocular pressure   *179*
   Pharmacology: Local anaesthetic   *181*
   Physics and clinical measurements: Tourniquets   *183*

Clinical anaesthesia

Long case: A young boy with Guillain–Barré syndrome

A 13-year-old boy is admitted with complaints of 2 days' history of malaise, lethargy, intermittent headache, and weak legs. He also complains of features suggestive of bulbar weakness. His parents are Jehovah's Witnesses. On examination, he was apyrexial.

Clinical examination	**Temperature: 36.4°C; weight: 49 kg; height 160 cm**					
	Pulse: 110/min, irregular; BP: 150/75 mmHg; respiratory rate: 26/min; SaO$_2$; 92% with 6 L/min O$_2$					
	Chest: bilateral air entry present, harsh vesicular breath sounds, crepitations over right lower lung base					
	Cardiovascular system: normal heart sound with no murmurs					
	Central nervous system: blurred vision, dysphasia, and dysarthria. Power of 3/5 in all 4 limbs areflexia in all 4 limbs					
Laboratory investigations	Hb	13.0 g/dL		Na		142 mEq/L
	MCV	89 fL		K		3.7 mEq/L
	WBC	5.1 × 10^9/L		Urea		6.6 mmol/L
	Platelets	350 × 10^9/L		Creatinine		107 μmol/L
	CRP	110		Glucose		6.4 mmol/L
	pH: 7.22	PaO$_2$: 10 kPa	PaCO$_2$: 6.5 kPa	HCO$_3^-$: 31	BE: 5	Lactate: 0.9 mmol/L
CSF	Protein >400 mg/L, no elevation in cell counts					

QUESTIONS

1. Summarize the case.
2. Do you want to know any other details from history and examination?
3. Comment on the chest X-ray and ECG.
4. What are the differential diagnoses?
5. Why is it not botulism?
6. Why is it not polio?
7. Can this be aseptic meningitis?
8. What is your probable diagnosis?
9. What are the clinical features of Guillain–Barré syndrome (GBS)?
10. What are the indications for admitting a GBS patient to ICU?
11. What are the treatment options available?
12. Which is better—plasmapheresis or immunoglobulins? Why?
13. Which treatment options are you going to use in this patient and why?
14. Can this boy decide for himself about treatment?
15. What are the supportive treatments you can provide?

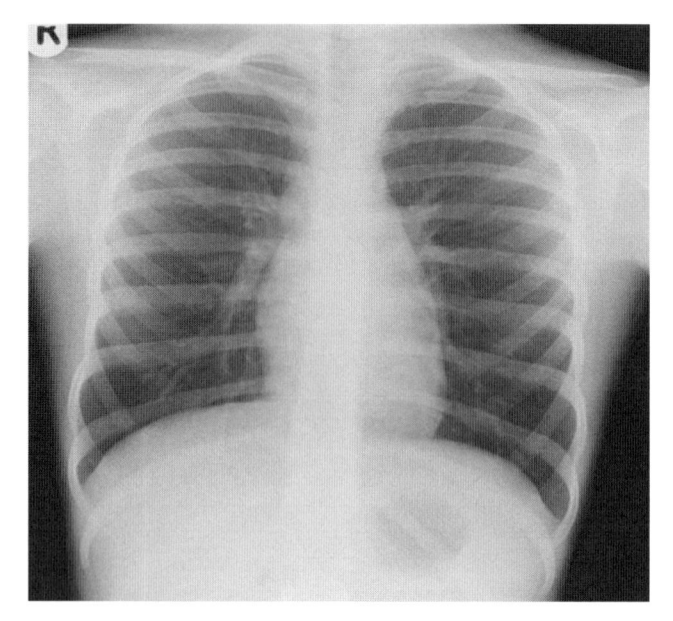

Structured Oral Examination Practice for the Final FRCA

Figure 8.1 Chest X-ray.

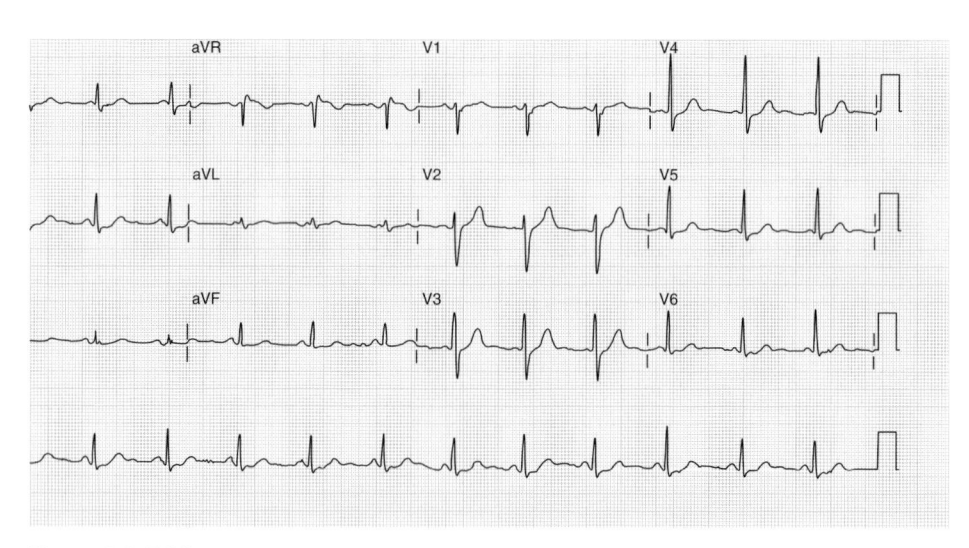

Figure 8.2 ECG.

Chapter 8

ANSWERS

1. Summarize the case

A 13-year-old boy presents with a history of lethargy, intermittent headache, weak legs and bulbar weakness. On examination all his limbs are weak 3/5 and areflexic. He is apyrexial, hypertensive, tachycardic, and blood gases show a compensated respiratory acidosis. CSF shows evidence of increased protein. Blood count and CSF show no evidence of infection.

2. Do you want to know any other details from history and examination?

History

- Any preceding illness—gastrointestinal infection/respiratory infection?
- Recent vaccines, travel, trauma, toxic ingestion.
- Any sensory symptoms, visual disturbance, problems with balance/ataxia?
- Does he have pain?
- Any difficulty voiding urine/excessive sweating?
- Degree of difficulty with coughing, swallowing, speaking.
- Previous history of similar events. Past medical history, medications, allergies, family history.

Examination

- Sensory abnormalities.
- Cranial nerve examination—facial weakness, bulbar palsy, ophthalmoplegia, reactivity of pupils.
- Ataxia.
- Ability to cough, clear secretions, vital capacity.

3. Comment on the chest X-ray and ECG.

Chest X-ray: posterio-anterior chest X-ray. Normal cardiomediastinal contour. Lungs and pleural spaces clear. Normal bones.

ECG: sinus rhythm, HR: 75 bpm, normal P waves, normal PR interval (duration of 0.12–0.2 sec), QRS complex (duration of 0.06–0.1 sec), normal axis (between 0–90°). My Impression is of a normal ECG.

4. What are the differential diagnoses?

The differential diagnosis can be subdivided into:

- **Spinal cord lesions:** trauma, transverse myelitis, epidural abscess, tumours, vascular malformations, cord infarctions, cord compression, lumbosacral disc syndromes, poliomyelitis, enteroviral infections of the anterior horn cells, Hopkins syndrome.
- **Peripheral neuropathies:** toxic neuropathy (glue sniffing, heavy metals, organophosphate pesticides, vincristine), HIV, diphtheria, Lyme disease, inborn errors of metabolism (porphyria, Leigh disease, Tangier disease), critical illness polyneuropathy.
- **Neuromuscular junction disorders:** tick paralysis, myasthenia gravis, botulism, hypercalcaemia, Lambert–Eaton syndrome.
- **Myopathies:** periodic paralysis, hypokalaemia, dermatomyositis, critical illness myopathy, benign acute childhood myositis.

5. Why is it not botulism?

- Botulism is an acute bilateral symmetrical descending paralysis, it affects neck and arms before legs unlike this patient who complains of leg weakness.
- Tendon reflexes are normally present except in severe cases of botulism.
- History of nausea, vomiting, or abdominal pain is common with botulism (not wound botulism).

6. Why is it not polio?

This is not poliomyelitis because:
- Poliomyelitis is a disease caused by one of three small RNA enteroviruses transmitted by the respiratory of faecal–oral routes.
- Polio gives a picture of meningeal symptoms and asymmetrical paralysis following an acute febrile illness. Although the patient has a headache there is no other evidence of meningeal symptoms such as confusion, decreases consciousness level, irritability.
- He also has a symmetrical paralysis which affects his arms and legs unlike polio which is mostly lower limbs and cranial nerves only.
- CSF examination in polio also differs, showing an increased number of lymphocytes and only minimal increase in protein.

7. Can this be aseptic meningitis?

No, as patients with aseptic meningitis often have flu-like symptoms and headache; they do not have focal neurological signs and are not critically unwell. This is not the case for this patient who has bulbar and limb weakness.

8. What is your probable diagnosis?

My probable diagnosis is Guillain–Barré syndrome.

9. What are the clinical features of Guillain–Barré syndrome (GBS)?

The clinical features of GBS are:
- Progressive motor weakness, usually ascending from the legs (proximal more than distal).
- Areflexia.
- Facial palsy and bulbar weakness.
- Ophthalmoplegia.
- Sensory symptoms.
- Severe pain, often affecting the girdle area.
- Weakness of the respiratory musculature leading to respiratory failure.
- Autonomic dysfunction—under/over activity of sympathetic and parasympathetic systems leading to arrhythmias, wide fluctuations in BP and pulse, urinary retention, ileus, and excessive sweating.

10. What are the indications for admitting a GBS patient to ICU?

The management of patients with GBS can be challenging because of its unpredictable course. These patients can rapidly deteriorate leading to respiratory failure. It is suggested that any patient without sound evidence of stable neuromuscular status on initial evaluation or presentation will require admission to ICU. One in three patients with GBS will need prolonged ICU monitoring and possible intubation. 25–30% need mechanical ventilation.
- A vital capacity <20 ml/kg, a maximum inspiratory pressure (PImax) <30 cmH$_2$O, and a maximum expiratory pressure (PEmax) <40 cmH$_2$O suggest the need for mechanical ventilation. (20/30/40 rule). Some also state a >30% reduction in VC from baseline.
- Presence of dysautonomia.
- Disease status and progression—Hughes Disability Score greater of equal to 3 or <3 but progressing.
- Protection of airway—the presence of bulbar dysfunction necessitates ICU admission and if evidence of aspiration, intubation.

11. What are the treatment options available?

GBS treatment includes supportive care as well as specific treatment modalities for those patients who are non-ambulatory and present within 4 weeks of onset of symptoms.

Chapter 8

The main modalities of treatment are plasma exchange and immunoglobulin therapy, CSF filtration has also been mentioned in case reports.

12. Which is better—plasmapheresis or immunoglobulins? Why?

- A 2001 Cochrane analysis of three trials indicated that IV immunoglobulin treatment was equivalent to plasma exchange.
- In 2009 the meta-analysis of five trials showed IV immunoglobulin to be as effective as plasma exchange.
- Since these trials, IV immunoglobulin has become the standard treatment for the syndrome because it can be given rapidly with fewer side effects than plasma exchange. The standard regimen of 0.4 g/kg body weight each day for 5 consecutive days is well tolerated, but side effects include dermatitis and much more rarely renal impairment and hyperviscosity effects, including strokes.

13. Which treatment options are you going to use in this patient and why?

This patient requires ITU admission for evaluation, monitoring, and supportive care. Neurologists also need to be involved in the treatment of this patient's GBS. In view of the Cochrane review and patient's religious beliefs I would start immunoglobulin therapy rather than plasma exchange.

14. Can this boy decide for himself about treatment?

Jehovah's Witnesses are individual patients whose religious beliefs prohibit accepting blood or blood products. However, use of extracorporeal circulation and plasmapheresis is acceptable to most Jehovah's Witnesses. If possible, the patient and his family should be consulted and a formal consent obtained. This boy is 13. One would have to establish whether he has so called 'Gillick' competence. Is he able to retain the information and consider the consequences and alternatives of the treatment?

Under English law a child who is deemed competent is able to agree to a treatment but cannot refuse. Communication with the child and his parents is key here. Involving Trust management early if needed.

15. What are the supportive treatments you can provide?

The supportive treatments are:

- Physiotherapy
- Occupational therapy
- Counselling
- Nutrition
- Analgesia
- Thromboembolic prophylaxis
- Respiratory support

Further reading

Hughes, R.A., Raphael, J.C., Swan, A.V., et al. Intravenous immunoglobulin for Guillain–Barré syndrome. *Cochrane Database Systematic Reviews* 2001; **2**:CD002063.

Hughes, R.A., Wijdicks, E.F., Benson, E., et al. Intravenous immunoglobulin for Guillain–Barré syndrome. *Cochrane Database Systematic Reviews* 2009; **1**:CD002063.

Richards, K and Cohen, A.T Guillain–Barré syndrome. Continuing Education in Anaesthesia Critical Care & Pain 2003; **3**:46–9.

Wenham, T. and Cohen, A. Botulism. *Continuing Education in Anaesthesia Critical Care & Pain* 2008; **8**:21–5.

Winner, J.B. Guillain–Barré syndrome. British Medical Journal 2008; **337**:a671.

Short Cases

QUESTIONS

Short case 1: Pre-eclampsia

A 39-year-old female patient, gravida 1 Para 0000 at 29 weeks' gestation was admitted to your maternity unit because of BP 182/111 mmHg. She also complains of headache. The midwife has checked for protein in the urine which is 2++.

1. What do you think the issues are in this patient?
2. When do you consider a parturient patient is hypertensive? When do you call it pre-eclampsia?
3. When would you consider it to be severe pre-eclampsia?
4. What are the risk factors for developing pre-eclampsia?
5. What is the pathogenesis of eclampsia?
6. What are the pathophysiological changes to various systems?
7. The obstetrician is not happy with the fetal heart rate and wishes to go ahead with Caesarean section. What would be your management plan?

Short case 2: A patient in recovery following TURP

A 79-year-old man had transurethral resection of prostate under general anaesthesia and is now in recovery. He has a past medical history of myocardial infraction, complicated by congestive hear failure on diuretics, beta-blockers, and calcium channel blocker. He is very restless, confused, and his BP is 180/100 mmHg. The recovery nurse has organized a blood gas and asked you to review this patient.

1. What are the differential diagnoses in your mind?
2. The blood gas shows all values normal but the Na level is 120. What does that mean to you?
3. When do you consider hyponatraemia?
4. How do you recognize TURP syndrome?
5. How would manage this patient in recovery?

Short case 3: Autonomic neuropathy

A 54-year-old lady has a known history of diabetes for 30 years. Her diabetes is not very well controlled. She has retinopathy, hypertension, and renal dysfunction. She has come for vitrectomy. She has been informed by her GP that she has autonomic neuropathy.

1. What is autonomic neuropathy?
2. What do you understand by the autonomic nervous system (ANS)?
3. What are the causes of autonomic neuropathy?
4. What are the signs and symptoms of autonomic neuropathy?
5. How would you test and diagnose autonomic neuropathy?
6. What are the implications of autonomic neuropathy in this patient?

Chapter 8

ANSWERS

Short case 1: Pre-eclampsia

1. What do you think the issues are in this patient?
We have a pre-eclamptic patient. The important issues are maternal and fetal.

2. When do consider a parturient patient is hypertensive? When do you call it pre-eclampsia?
Hypertension in pregnancy is defined as manual BP recording of ≥140 systolic and/or ≥90 diastolic on two consecutive occasions >4 hours apart or one BP reading of ≥110 diastolic. It must be noted that most automated BP monitors (Dinamap) underestimate diastolic BP and hence a manual method is preferable.

Pre-eclamptia is a multiorgan disorder characterized by development of hypertension with proteinuria after the 20th week of gestation. It is a disorder of unknown aetiology affecting approximately 8% of all pregnancies, with most cases occurring in first pregnancy.

3. When would you consider it to be severe pre-eclampsia?
Pre-eclampsia complicates 3–5% of first pregnancies with 5–10% of cases being severe. It accounts for 16% of maternal deaths in the UK.

Severe pre-eclampsia exists if one or more of the following is present:
- Arterial pressure >160 mmHg systolic or >110 mmHg diastolic on two occasions at least 6 hours apart.
- Proteinuria >5 g in 24 hours or <3 + on dipstick.
- Oliguria <400 ml/day.
- Cerebral signs: headache, blurred vision, or altered consciousness.
- Pulmonary oedema or cyanosis.
- Epigastric or right upper quadrant pain.
- Impaired liver function.
- Hepatic rupture.
- Thrombocytopenia.
- HELLP syndrome.

4. What are the risk factors for developing pre-eclampsia?
Pre-eclampsia is a disease of varied origin linked to maternal, paternal, placental, and fetal factors. The risk factors are important to identify the mothers at-risk. The risk factors are:

- First pregnancy—primigravida—or >10 years since previous pregnancy.
- Previous pregnancy requiring early delivery.
- Family history of pre-eclamptic toxaemia (PET).
- Age >40 years.
- Booking BMI >35.
- Chronic hypertension (booking BP >140 systolic).
- Multiple pregnancy.
- Hydropic fetus.
- Associated medical conditions: diabetes mellitus, renal disease and anti-phospholipid syndrome.

5. What is the pathogenesis of eclampsia?
This is a disease of heterogeneous cause of both maternal and placental origin.

- Exact aetiology is not known but there are association to immunological, genetic, endothelial, platelet, and coagulation factors.
- There is endothelial damage or altered sensitivity which leads to decreased production of vasodilatory substances, increased sensitivity to vasoconstrictors, and increased glomerular permeability. These changes leads to:
  - Increased systemic vascular resistance.
  - Increased sodium and water retention.
  - In severe conditions there is platelet aggregation, haemolysis, and hepatic dysfunction (HELLP syndrome).

6. What are the pathophysiological changes to various systems?

Pre-eclamptic toxaemia (PET) is a multisystem disorder of unknown origin but widespread endothelial dysfunction.

- **Cardiovascular system:**
  - Generalized vasoconstriction leading to increased SVR and diastolic hypertension.
  - Increased capillary permeability—peripheral oedema, intravascular depletion, and decreased colloid oncotic pressure.
  - Poor correlation between CVP and pulmonary capillary wedge pressure measurements and are prone for pulmonary and cerebral oedema.
  - Hypercoagulability, platelet activation, and activation of fibrinolytic systems are seen.
- **Respiratory system:**
  - Upper airway oedema—face, tongue, neck, and larynx may lead to difficult laryngoscopy and intubation.
  - Fluid management requires special care as the patient is prone to pulmonary oedema, especially postpartum stage.
- **Renal system:**
  - There is decreased GFR and increased permeability leading to proteinuria and hypoalbuminaemia.
  - Decreased uric acid excretion leads to increased plasma levels and acts as a marker for severity of the disease.
  - There is tubular dysfunction leading to acute renal failure.
- **Hepatic changes:**
  - Serum transaminase levels frequently increase, in extreme cases HELLP syndrome.
  - Epigastric or subcostal pain is a serious sign—indicating hepatic oedema, subcapsular haematoma, or impending hepatic rupture.
- **CNS changes:**
  - Neurological signs/symptoms like headache, visual disturbances, vomiting, confusion, hyper-reflexia indicate altered cerebral perfusion.
  - Cerebral ischaemia due to oedema and vasoconstriction may lead to seizures— eclampsia.
  - Cerebral haemorrhage due to severe hypertension is also seen and can be fatal.
- **Haematological changes:**
  - Altered coagulation, thrombocytopenia, and rarely DIC is seen.
  - Microvascular haemolysis and anaemia is seen in HELLP.
- **Feto-placental** unit: many of the changes seen are due to decreased placental perfusion. Intrauterine growth restriction (IUGR) is a serious risk and so is placental abruption.

Chapter 8

7. The obstetrician is not happy with the fetal heart rate and wishes to go ahead with Caesarean section. What would be your management plan?

My plan depends on the urgency of the delivery. This appears to be Grade I Caesarean section and I would go ahead with general anaesthesia and as this is a high-risk case I would have a senior help. I would consider the following issues:

- Potentially difficult intubation, laryngeal oedema may not become apparent until laryngoscopy.
- Exaggerated hypertensive response to intubation may increase the risk of cerebrovascular accident, increase myocardial oxygen requirement, induce cardiac arrhythmias, induce pulmonary oedema, and reduce uterine blood flow.
- $MgSO_4$ has been used to control both catecholamine release and the pressor response. It was found that pre-treatment with 40 mg/kg is superior to either lignocaine or alfentanil. Short-acting opioids have been used at induction of anaesthesia, e.g. fentanyl 2.5 mcg/kg and alfentanil 10 mcg/kg. Esmolol proved to be useful not only for intubation but also for extubation due to its rapid onset and short duration of action.
- Impaired intervillous blood supply.
- Difficulties related to neuromuscular blockers in the mother receiving magnesium sulphate. Fasciculations may not occur after suxamethonium, with potentiation if from the action of non-depolarizing agents.
- Potential aspiration of gastric content.

My technique would be:

- Aspiration prophylaxis: sodium citrate.
- Pre-oxygenation for 5 min.
- Induction of anaesthesia with cricoid pressure (rapid sequence).
- Use a smaller ETT (7 or 7.5).
- Place an arterial line to monitor the BP and take special precautions for pressor response to intubation. Use a high-dose of a fast-onset opioid like fentanyl or remifentanil
- Continue IV magnesium sulphate infusion and labetalol.

Further reading

Allman, K.G. and Wilson, I.H. *Oxford Handbook of Anaesthesia*, 2nd edn. Chapter 32: Obstetric anaesthesia and analgesia, pp.695–754. Oxford: Oxford University Press, 2006.

Dommisse, J. Magnesium sulphate in the management of eclampsia and severe pre-eclampsia. *International Journal of Obstetric Anesthesia* 1992; **1**:177–8.

NICE. *Hypertension in pregnancy: The management of hypertensive disorders during pregnancy* (Clinical Guideline 107). London: NICE, 2010. Available at: http: http://www.nice.org.uk/guidance/CG107

Sibai, B.M. Hypertension. In: Gabbe, S.G., Niebyl, J.R., Simpson, J.L (eds.) *Obstetrics – Normal and Problem Pregnancies* 5th edn, pp. 322–43. Philadelphia, PA: Elsevier Churchill Livingstone, 2007.

Visintin, C., Mugglestone, M.A., Almerie, M.Q., et al. Management of hypertensive disorders during pregnancy: summary of NICE guidance. *British Medical Journal* 2010; **341**:C2207.

Short case 2: A patient in recovery following TURP

1. What are the differential diagnoses in your mind?
- TURP syndrome
- Postoperative confusion
- Acute myocardial infarction
- Bladder perforation
- Adrenal insufficiency and adrenal crisis
- Congestive heart failure and pulmonary oedema
- Gastroenteritis
- Hypothyroidism and myxoedema
- Coma
- Renal failure—acute, chronic, and dialysis complications
- Syndrome of inappropriate antidiuretic hormone secretion
- Cirrhosis
- Nephrotic syndrome
- Psychogenic polydipsia
- Pseudohyponatraemia (falsely low sodium reading due to presence of excessive high -weight molecules in the serum, such as lipids or protein)

2. The blood gas shows all values normal but the Na level is 118. What does that mean to you?
This is a condition which is called transurethral resection of prostate (TURP) syndrome and there is hyponatraemia. The TURP syndrome is due to rapid absorption of a large volume of irrigation solution leading to hyponatraemia and fluid overload. It is characterized by intravascular shift and plasma-solute effect. Glycine, which is an inhibitory neurotransmitter, may contribute to the syndrome.

3. When do you consider hyponatraemia?
Serum sodium concentration is maintained by a homeostatic mechanism that involves thirst, antidiuretic hormone (ADH) secretion, and the renal handling of sodium. This is defined as a serum sodium <135 mmol/L. A level <120 mmol/L is considered severe.

4. How do you recognize TURP syndrome?
The TURP syndrome could be identified by:

Symptoms
- Mild: anorexia, headache, nausea, vomiting, lethargy.
- Moderate: personality change, muscle cramps and weakness, confusion, ataxia.
- Severe: drowsiness.

Signs
These are highly variable and depend on the level and rate of fall of the serum sodium. They may include:
- Neurological signs:
    - Decreased level of consciousness.
    - Cognitive impairment (e.g. short-term memory loss, disorientation, confusion depression).
    - Focal or generalized seizures.
    - Brainstem herniation: seen in severe acute hyponatraemia; signs include coma; fixed, unilateral, dilated pupil, decorticate or decerebrate posturing, respiratory arrest.

Chapter 8

- Signs of hypovolaemia: dry mucous membranes, tachycardia, diminished skin turgor.
- Signs of hypervolaemia: pulmonary rales, S3 gallop (3rd heart sound), jugular venous distention, peripheral oedema, ascites.

The common symptoms are headache, restlessness, nausea and vomiting, convulsions, coma, tachypnoea, hypertension, dyspnoea secondary to pulmonary oedema. Haematological: hyperglycinaemia, hyperammonaemia, hyponatraemia, hypo-osmolality haemolysis, acute renal failure.

5. How would you manage this patient in recovery?

This is a medical emergency where Na is <120 mmol/L. and requires resuscitation.

My aim is to immediately follow the ABC and transfer the patient to CCU with intensivist involved for further management.

- Supporting respiration (if necessary, with intubation and ventilation).
- Support the circulation.
- Treat bradycardia and hypotension with atropine and adrenergic drugs.
- Monitoring:
  - ECG.
  - Arterial line.
  - Central line.
  - Bloods to investigate sodium, osmolality, and haemoglobin.
- Correction of hyponatraemia slowly at around 0.5–1 mmol/L/hour. The rate of infusion of 3% NaCl (ml/hour) = body weight (kg) × desired rate of correction (mmol/L/hour).
- Too rapid correction of serum sodium can cause central pontine myelinolysis (also known as osmotic demyelination syndrome). It is always associated with rapid correction to normal levels (therefore stop at 120 mmol/L and allow more gradual correction subsequently).

Further reading

Hahn, R.G. Fluid absorption in endoscopic surgery. *British Journal of Anaesthesia* 2006; **96**:8–20.
O'Donnel, A.M. and Foo, I.T.H. Anaesthesia for transurethral resection of the prostate. Continuing Education in Anaesthesia Critical Care & Pain 9:92–6.
Upadhyay, A., Jaber, B.L., and Madias, N.E. Incidence and prevalence of hyponatremia. *American Journal of Medicine* 2006; **119**(7 suppl 1):S30–5.

Short case 3: Autonomic neuropathy

1. What is autonomic neuropathy?

Autonomic neuropathy is a nerve disorder that affects involuntary body functions, including heart rate, BP, perspiration, and digestion. This damage disrupts signals between the brain and portions of the autonomic nervous system, such as the heart, blood vessels, and sweat glands, resulting in decreased or abnormal performance of one or more involuntary body functions. Autonomic neuropathy can be a complication of a number of diseases and conditions.

2. What do you understand by the autonomic nervous system (ANS)?

The ANS conveys all output from the CNS and thus controls homeostasis of the body. There are three components:

- The sympathetic system.
- The parasympathetic system.
- The enteric nervous system: the enteric system is able to function independently of the CNS, but the other two cannot function without it.

3. What are the causes of autonomic neuropathy?

Autonomic neuropathy can be caused by a large number of diseases and conditions or as a side effect of treatment for diseases unrelated to the nervous system. Some common causes of autonomic neuropathy include:

- **Alcoholism:** a chronic, progressive disease that can lead to nerve damage.
- **Abnormal protein build-up** in organs (amyloidosis), which affects the organs and the nervous system.
- **Autoimmune diseases:** in which your immune system attacks and damages parts of your body, including your nerves. Examples include Sjögren's syndrome, systemic lupus erythematosus, and rheumatoid arthritis. Autonomic neuropathy may also be caused by an abnormal attack by the immune system that occurs as a result of some cancers (paraneoplastic syndrome).
- **Diabetes:** which is the most common cause of autonomic neuropathy; can gradually cause nerve damage throughout the body.
- **Multiple system atrophy:** a degenerative disorder that leads to loss and malfunction of some portions of the CNS.
- **Injury to nerves:** caused by surgery or trauma.
- **Treatment with certain medications:** including some drugs used in cancer chemotherapy and anticholinergic drugs, sometimes used to treat irritable bowel syndrome and overactive bladder.
- **Other chronic illnesses:** such as Parkinson's disease and HIV/AIDS.

4. What are the signs and symptoms of autonomic neuropathy?

Signs and symptoms of autonomic neuropathy vary, depending on which parts of autonomic nervous system are affected. They may include:

- Dizziness and fainting upon standing (orthostatic, or postural, hypotension), caused by a drop in BP
- Urinary problems, including difficulty starting urination, overflow incontinence and inability to empty bladder completely, which can lead to urinary tract infections
- Sexual difficulties, including erectile dysfunction in men, and vaginal dryness.
- Difficulty digesting food, due to abnormal digestive function and slow emptying of the stomach (gastroparesis), there is a feeling of fullness leading to loss of appetite, diarrhoea, constipation, abdominal bloating, nausea, vomiting and heartburn
- Sweating abnormalities, such as excessive or decreased sweating, which affects the ability to regulate body temperature
- Sluggish pupil reaction, making it difficult to adjust from light to dark and causing problems with driving at night.
- Exercise intolerance, which may occur if your heart rate remains unchanged instead of appropriately increasing and decreasing in response to your activity level

5. How would you test and diagnose autonomic neuropathy?

The diagnosis is mainly clinical by the GP. But following test can be used to confirm the diagnosis

- **Breathing tests**: these tests measure how your heart rate and BP respond to breathing exercises such as the Valsalva test.

- **Tilt-table test**: this test monitors the BP and heart rate respond to changes in posture and position. Postural hypotension: drop of > 30 mmHg indicates autonomic dysfunction.
- **Gastrointestinal tests**: gastric-emptying tests are the most common tests to check for slowed movement of food through system, delayed emptying of the stomach and other abnormalities.
- **Thermoregulatory sweat test.**
- **Urinalysis and bladder function (urodynamic) tests**: if the bladder or urinary symptoms, a series of urine tests can evaluate bladder function.
- **Ultrasound**: of the bladder.

What are the implications of autonomic neuropathy in this patient?

Autonomic neuropathy occurs in approximately 1 in 10 diabetic patients. The implication of autonomic neuropathy is increased morbidity and mortality. Orthostatic hypotension in the perioperative period is common and may be severe in immediately postoperatively.

Myocardial ischaemia is often painless with risk of arrest.

These patients are at risk of:

- Severe hypotension during anaesthesia (particularly with SAB/epidural anaesthesia or IPPV).
- Reduced response to hypoglycaemia.
- Increased risk of aspiration of gastric contents.
- Hypothermia.
- Perioperative cardiac or respiratory arrest (especially diabetic patients).

Further reading

Allman, K.G. and Wilson, I.H. *Oxford Handbook of Anaesthesia*, 2nd edn. Chapter 8: Endocrine and metabolic disease, pp. 150–5. Oxford: Oxford University Press, 2006.

Craig, R.G. and Hunter; J.M. Recent developments in the perioperative management of adult patients with chronic kidney disease. *British Journal of Anaesthesia* 2008; **101**:296–310.

Jermendy, G. Clinical consequences of cardiovascular autonomic neuropathy in diabetic patients. *Acta Diabetology* 2003; **40**(Suppl 2):S370–4.

Marks, J.B. Perioperative management of diabetes. *American Family Physician* 2003; **67**:93–100.

Weimer, L.H. Autonomic testing: common techniques and clinical applications. *Neurologist* 2010; **16**(4):215–22.

Clinical science

QUESTIONS

Anatomy: Femoral triangle

1. Describe the anatomy of the femoral triangle.
2. Describe the course of the femoral nerve from its origin to the terminal branches.
3. How do you perform a femoral nerve block?
4. What is fascia iliaca compartment block?
5. What type of operations can it be used for?
6. If there is local anaesthetic toxicity how would you know?
7. How would you manage local anaesthetic toxicity?

Physiology: Intraocular pressure

1. How and where is aqueous humour secreted?
2. What are the functions of aqueous humour?
3. What is the normal intraocular pressure (IOP)?
4. What are the factors influencing IOP?
5. Describe the drainage of the aqueous humour.
6. What are the effects of anaesthetic drugs on IOP?
7. How can you reduce the IOP?

Pharmacology: Local anaesthetic

1. What are local anaesthetics?
2. Classify local anaesthetic agents.
3. How are pH and local anaesthetics related?
4. What determine the different characteristics of local anaesthetics?
5. What are the types of toxicity with bupivacaine?
6. What factors affect toxicity?

Physics and clinical measurements: Tourniquets

1. What are the principles of tourniquets?
2. What are the local effects of tourniquets?
3. What are the systemic effects of tourniquets?
4. Enumerate the complications secondary to use of a tourniquet.
5. How is a tourniquet applied?

Chapter 8

ANSWERS

Anatomy: Femoral triangle

1. Describe the anatomy of the femoral triangle.

The femoral triangle is situated in the upper medial aspect of the thigh. It is bounded superiorly by inguinal ligament, laterally to medially by medial border of the sartorius, iliopsoas, pectineus, and adductor longus. The floor is formed by the adductor longus, pectineus, psoas, and the iliacus.

Content: it contains femoral nerve and branches, femoral sheath containing femoral artery and its branches, femoral vein and its tributaries, and deep inguinal lymph nodes.

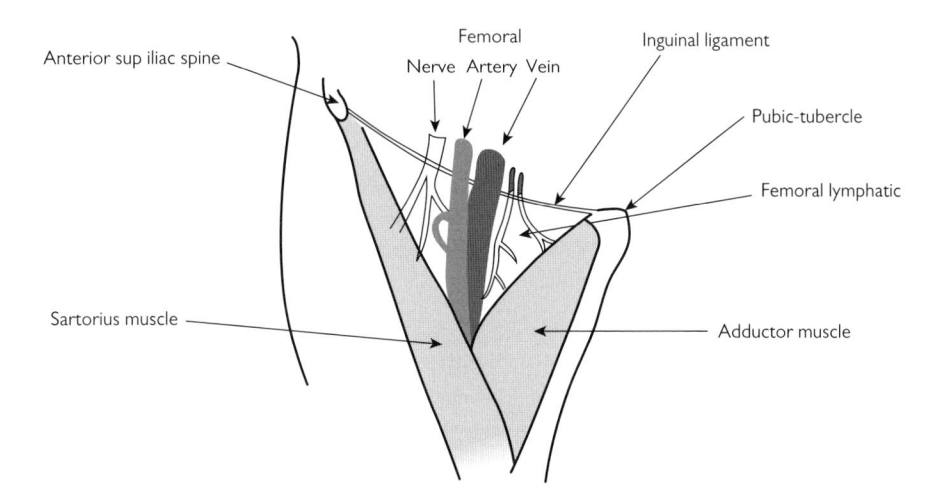

Figure 8.3 The femoral triangle.

2. Describe the course of the femoral nerve from its origin to the terminal branches.

The femoral nerve is the largest branch of the lumbar plexus. It arises from L2, L3, and L4 nerve roots. It descends through the fibres of the psoas muscle, emerging from the psoas at the lower part of its border, and passes down between the psoas and the iliacus. The nerve passes underneath the inguinal ligament into the thigh. As it passes underneath the inguinal ligament, it is lateral and slightly deeper than the femoral artery, separated from it by a portion of the psoas major. At the femoral crease, the nerve is covered by the fascia iliaca and separated from the femoral artery and vein by a portion of the psoas muscle and the ligamentum ileopectineum.

Branches of the femoral nerve
- Anterior division:
  - Middle cutaneous branches.
  - Medial cutaneous supplying the anteromedial thigh.
  - Muscular: pectineus, sartorius, quadriceps femoris.
- Posterior division:
  - Muscular (individual heads of the quadriceps muscle).
  - Articular branches (hip and knee).

- Saphenous nerve accompanies the great saphenous vein and gives off an infrapatellar branch. The saphenous nerve is distributed to the medial side of the leg and foot.

3. How do you perform a femoral nerve block?

- **Consent:** from the patient with full information.
  - In theatre with full resuscitation facilities, monitoring, and trained staff.
  - Aseptic technique, peripheral nerve stimulator, Stimuplex—insulated needle size 50 mm.
  - Ultrasound machine with appropriate size probe.
- **Positioning:**
  - Patient supine with both legs extended.
  - For obese patients, if a pillow placed underneath patient's hips this may facilitate palpation of the femoral artery and block performance.
- **Anatomical landmarks:**
  - Inguinal ligament and femoral artery.
  - Landmarks for the femoral nerve block are easily recognizable in all patients and include: femoral crease and femoral artery pulse
- **Technique:**
  - The short bevelled needle is introduced parallel and immediately lateral to the border of the artery and advanced in the sagittal and slightly cephalad plane.
  - A visible or palpable twitch of the quadriceps muscle (patella twitch) at 0.2–0.5 mA current is the optimal response.

4. What is fascia iliaca compartment block?

Fascia iliaca compartment block is performed by injection of local anaesthetic solution behind the fascia iliaca into a compartment between the iliacus and the psoas muscle.

Surface landmarks technique: feel the needle as it passes the fascia lata and the iliacus fascia. There will be two pops which indicates correct position of the needle.

Ultrasound technique: ultrasound will locate the superficial fascial layer of the iliopsoas muscle at the anterior edge of the ilium. Introduce a needle just beneath that fascia. Local anaesthetic solution is then injected, creating a local anaesthetic-filled space below the fascia. As this local-filled space increases in size during injection, the fluid travels cephalad beneath the fascia and contacts the nerves of the lumbar plexus which are located there. These nerves are the lateral femoral cutaneous nerve, the femoral nerve, and the obturator nerves.

5. What type of operations can it be used for?

- Surgery on the anterior thigh, knee, and quadriceps tendon repair.
- For analgesia for femoral shaft fracture.
- Postoperative pain management after femur and knee surgery.
- When combined with a block of the sciatic nerve, anaesthesia of almost the entire lower extremity from the mid-thigh level can be achieved.

Chapter 8

6. If there is local anaesthetic toxicity how would you know?

Toxicity due to excessive local anaesthetic blood levels is always a possibility and it presents as:

CNS signs	CVS respiratory signs
Light headedness, dizziness, drowsiness	Bradycardia
Tingling around lips, fingers, or generalized	Hypotension
Metallic taste, tinnitus, blurred vision	Cardiovascular collapse
Confusion, restlessness, incoherent speech	ECG changes (prolongation of QRS and PR interval, AV block and/or changes in T-wave amplitude)
Tremors or twitching leading to convulsions with loss of consciousness and coma	
	Respiratory arrest

7. How would you manage local anaesthetic toxicity?

My immediate management would be to:

- Discontinue injection of local anaesthetic.
- Call for help with AAGBI guideline available to hand.
- ABC approach with 100% O_2 to ensure adequate ventilation.
- Intravenous assessment in view of resuscitation.
- Control seizures: give a benzodiazepine, thiopental, or propofol in small incremental doses.
- If patient continues to shows signs of severe toxicity:
    - Intubate and ventilate if required to prevent hypoxic cardiovascular collapse.
    - Hyperventilation may help by increasing pH in the presence of metabolic acidosis.
    - CPR, if pulseless start ALS protocol.
- Consider treatment with lipid emulsion. Continue CPR throughout treatment.
- Recovery from local anaesthetic-induced cardiac arrest may take >1 hour.
- Further follow the AAGBI guideline.

Further reading

Association of Anaesthetists of Great Britain and Ireland. *Management of Severe Local Anaesthetic Toxicity* (Safety Guidance). London: AAGBI, 2010.
Capdevila, X., Biboulet, P., Bouregba, M., et al. Comparison of the three-in-one and fascia iliaca compartment blocks in adults: clinical and radiographic analysis. *Anesthesia & Analgesia* 1998; **86**(5):1039–44.
Lopez S. Fascia iliaca compartment block for femoral bone fractures in prehospital care. *Regional Anesthesia and Pain Medicine* 2003; **28**(3):203–7.
The New York School of Regional Anesthesia website: http://www.nysora.com
Tran, D., Clemente, A., and Finlayson, R.J. A review of approaches and techniques for lower extremity nerve blocks. *Canadian Journal of Anaesthesia* 2007; **54**:922–34.

Physiology: Intraocular pressure

1. How and where is aqueous humour secreted?

Aqueous humour is secreted from plasma into the posterior chamber by the ciliary body, specifically the non-pigmented epithelium of the ciliary body (pars plicata). There are three mechanisms of production: active transport, diffusion, and ultrafiltration.

2. What are the functions of aqueous humour?
- Maintains the intraocular pressure and inflates the globe of the eye.
- Provides nutrition (e.g. amino acids and glucose) for the avascular ocular tissues; posterior cornea, trabecular meshwork, lens, and anterior vitreous.
- May serve to transport ascorbate in the anterior segment to act as an antioxidant agent.
- Presence of immunoglobulins indicates a role in immune response to defend against pathogens.

3. What is the normal intraocular pressure (IOP)?
The tissue pressure of the intraocular contents is called the IOP. The normal range for IOP is 10–20 mmHg and it is maintained at this level throughout life and between the sexes, though there is some diurnal and seasonal variation, 10–22 mmHg.

4. What are the factors influencing IOP?

Intra-global	Extra-global
Aqueous humour volume	Anaesthetic regional blocks
Blood volume	Extraocular compression devices
Foreign bodies	Honan balloon
Sulphur hexafluoride or carbon octafluoride bubble	Extraocular muscle tone
Tumours	Scleral strapping (for retinal detachment)
Haemorrhage	Retrobulbar or peribulbar
Vitreous humour volume	Haematoma
Scleral rigidity	Abscess
	Tumour
	Face mask
	Prone positioning

5. Describe the drainage of the aqueous humour.
Aqueous humour flows through the narrow cleft between the front of the lens and the back of the iris, to escape through the pupil into the anterior chamber, and then to drain out of the eye via the trabecular meshwork. From here, it drains into Schlemm's canal by one of two ways: directly, via aqueous vein to the episcleral vein, or indirectly, via collector channels to the episcleral vein by intrascleral plexus and eventually into the veins of the orbit. The mydriatics cause papillary dilation, this impedes outflow and the miotics cause the pupillary constriction, improving trabecular outflow.

6. What are the effects of anaesthetic drugs on IOP?
- Induction agents (apart from ketamine) and all inhalational anaesthetic agents reduce IOP. This fall in IOP is independent of their effect on BP, CVP, and extraocular muscle tone and is more likely to be a direct action on central control mechanisms.
- Opioids have no direct effect on IOP, but attenuate the elevation in pressure due to intubation.
- Non-depolarizing muscle relaxants have a minimal effect on IOP.
- Succinylcholine leads to an increase in IOP of up to 10 mmHg for 10 min but, as has been debated frequently, it is also the drug of choice to provide rapid, short acting and ideal intubation conditions in an emergency situation where there is a risk of aspiration. Suxamethonium: increased in IOP secondary to tonic contracture of EOMs, choroidal vessel dilatation, relaxation of orbital smooth muscles. Lasts ~7 min, up to 8 mmHg increase in IOP. Non-depolarizer pre-treatment only partly effective. Acetazolamide, propranolol have been tried to reduce IOP.

7. How can you reduce the IOP?

Therapeutic intraocular pressure reduction can be achieved by:
- Intravenous:
  - Acetazolamide: carbonic anhydrase inhibition leads to a reduction in aqueous humour production.
  - Mannitol: osmotic diuretic dehydrates the vitreous chamber.
- Topical:
  - Parasympathomimetics: cholinergic and anticholinesterase medication contract the ciliary body and increase aqueous humour drainage through the trabecular network.
  - Sympathomimetics: epinephrine reduces aqueous humour production and increases drainage, possibly through ciliary body vasoconstriction and adenylate cyclase inhibition beta-adrenoceptor antagonists timolol reduces aqueous humour production through adenylate cyclase inhibition.
- Prostaglandin analogues: increase aqueous humour drainage via uveoscleral route.

Further reading

Murgatroyd, H. and Bembridge, J. Intraocular pressure. *Continuing Education in Anaesthesia, Critical Care & Pain* 2008; **8**:100–3.

Pharmacology: Local anaesthetic

1. What are local anaesthetics?

A local anaesthetic can be defined as a drug which reversibly prevents transmission of the nerve impulse in the region to which it is applied, without affecting consciousness.

Local anaesthetic mechanism of action has two steps:
- Firstly, the drug enters the neuron by simple diffusion. The rate of entry is governed by Fick's law.
- Secondly, it becomes protonated (ionized) and interacts with the sodium channel. Local anaesthetics may also affect the lipid membrane directly. This prevents propagation of nerve action potentials and stops neuronal transmission of nociceptive (and other) impulses.

2. Classify local anaesthetic agents.

The local anaesthetics generally have a lipid-soluble hydrophobic aromatic group and a charged, hydrophilic amide group. The bond between these two groups determines the class of the drug, and may be amide or ester. Examples:
- Amide group: lignocaine, bupivacaine, and prilocaine.
- Esters group: cocaine and amethocaine.

3. How are pH and local anaesthetics related?

The local anaesthetic and pH can be explained by the Henderson–Hasselbach equation:

$$pKa = pH + \log [BH^+]/[B]$$

The permeability of the membrane depends on the ionization. The drug molecule exists as weak acids or bases. The drug could be in ionized or unionized form. The ratio of the two forms depends on the pH of the environment.

- **Weak base:** $BH^+ = B + H^+$
- **Acid environment:** the equation will shift towards left and the ionized form will be more.
- **Alkaline environment:** the equation would be on the right sided and unionized form will be more.

A base in an alkaline solution will be non-ionized and have a greater ability to cross lipid membranes. However, in an acid environment, it will be trapped, as it is ionized. The result is that an alkaline drug will be concentrated in a compartment with a low pH.

Local anaesthetics as an example of the situation above
- Local anaesthetics block action potential generated by blocking Na^+ channels.
- Most local anaesthetics are weak bases, with a pKa between 8 and 9, so that they are mainly but not completely ionized at physiological pH. The un-charged species (B) penetrates the nerve sheath and axonal membrane and is then converted to the BH^+ active form, which then blocks the Na^+ channels. Increasing the acidity of the external solution would favour ionization and render local anaesthetics ineffective.

4. What determine the different characteristics of local anaesthetics?
- Molecular weight: increased chain size and lipid solubility.
- Lipid solubility: greater penetration of nerve membrane, greater potency.
- pKa: increased pKa increases ionized proportion, so more drug exists intracellularly in the active state.
- pH: acidosis increases ionization. Less drug crossing the cell membrane.
- Protein binding: greater binding increases duration of action.

5. What are the types of toxicity with bupivacaine?
- CNS: causes stimulation, restlessness, tremor and toxicity manifesting in convulsions even and CNS depression (including respiratory depression)
- CVS: myocardial depression (inhibition of Na^+ current in cardiac muscle, thereby reducing intracellular Ca^{2+} stores) and vasodilatation (direct effect on smooth muscle and inhibition of sympathetic nervous system). Cardiac toxicity manifesting in cardiac depression and arrhythmias.
- Toxicity associated with blockade of neuronal and cardiac voltage-gated sodium channels. Also disrupt metabotropic and ionotropic signal transduction.
- They can also inhibit each of the four components of oxidative phosphorylation—i.e. substrate transport, electron transport, proton motive force maintenance, and ATP synthesis.

6. What factors affect toxicity?
- Mass of drug administered: the dose given.
- Site of injection: in increasing order of magnitude for absorption: subcutaneous <peripheral<plexus <epidural <intercostals.
- Vascularity of site.
- Protein binding and metabolism.

Further reading
Calvey, N. and Williams, N. *Principles and Practice of Pharmacology for Anaesthetists* 5th edn. Oxford: Wiley-Blackwell, 2008.

Physics and clinical measurements: Tourniquets

1. What are the principles of tourniquets?

Arterial tourniquets apply mechanical compression, and reduce arterial circulation to, and venous drainage from, a limb. They are widely used in orthopaedic, plastic, and reconstructive surgery where they are invaluable in providing excellent operating conditions and reducing blood loss. The equipment includes padding and tape, a special pneumatic tourniquet, a supply of compressed gas, and a pressure regulator and display.

2. What are the local effects of tourniquets?

Local effects are the result of tissue ischaemia distal to the inflated tourniquet and a combination of ischaemia and compression of the tissues beneath it.

- **Muscle:**
    - There is a progressive decrease in PO_2 and an increase in PCO_2 within muscle cells.
    - Energy stores steadily decline with time and intracellular stores of ATP and creatine phosphate are exhausted after 2 and 3 hours, respectively.
    - Lactate concentration increases with the switch to anaerobic metabolism and, with the increasing PCO_2, contributes to the development of an intracellular acidosis.
    - Microvascular injury occurs in muscle after ischaemia of greater than >2 hours' duration.
- **Nerve:**
    - A physiological conduction block develops between 15–45 min after inflation of a cuff around the arm to a suprasystolic pressure. The conduction block affects both motor and sensory modalities and is reversible after deflation of the cuff.
    - Higher cuff pressures can cause morphological changes within the larger myelinated nerves.

3. What are the systemic effects of tourniquets?

- **Cardiovascular:**
    - Increase in preload and systemic vascular resistance, this leads to an increase in circulating blood volume, resulting in a transient increase in CVP and BP.
    - Increase HR and BP after 30–60 min (tourniquet pain); may not respond to analgesics or increasing depth of anaesthesia.
    - Decrease systemic vascular resistance and venous return on deflation, during reperfusion.
    - Application may dislodge intravascular material leading to venous or arterial emboli.
- **Haematological:**
    - Systemic hypercoagulability: This is attributable to increased platelet aggregation caused by catecholamines released in response to pain from surgery and the tourniquet itself.
    - May precipitate sickling in susceptible individuals
- **Metabolism:**
    - >30 min, anaerobic metabolism may lead to metabolic acidosis, hypoxia, hypercarbia, and tachycardia.
    - Deflation of the tourniquet after 1–2 hours of ischaemia is associated with small increases in plasma concentrations of potassium and lactate. Peak increases of 0.3 and 2 mmol/L, respectively, occur 3 min after deflation.
- **Respiratory:**
    - Deflation of the tourniquet is followed almost immediately by an increase in end-tidal carbon dioxide concentration which usually peaks within 1 min. The peak increase in end-tidal CO_2 concentration is greater with deflation of lower limb tourniquets (0.7–2.4 kPa) than with upper limb tourniquets (0.1–1.6 kPa).

- **CNS:**
  - Pain (awake patients may not tolerate prolonged usage).
  - Increase in cerebral blood flow.

4. Enumerate the complications secondary to use of a tourniquet.

- **Neurological injuries:**
  - Lower limb tourniquets >upper limb tourniquets to produce neurological complications.
  - The nerves most commonly affected are the sciatic nerve in the lower limb and the radial nerve in the upper limb.
  - Large size nerve more susceptible.
- **Muscle injury:**
  - The post-tourniquet syndrome results in a swollen, stiff, weak limb. Very rarely post-ischaemic swelling and oedema, in combination with reperfusion hyperaemia.
  - Rhabdomyolysis is rare.
- **Skin injury:**
  - Chemical burns are the most common when alcohol-based solutions used.
  - Vascular injury is rare.
- **Tourniquet pain:**
  - Inflation of a tourniquet is followed by the development of a dull, aching pain. It is thought that tourniquet pain is predominantly mediated by unmyelinated, slowly conducting C-fibres.

5. How is a tourniquet applied?

- Apply an appropriately sized cuff above the surgical site, using soft padding underneath.
- Aim for even pressure, and ensure that the skin is not pinched. Use adhesive tape as a barrier to surgical skin preparation solutions (which can cause chemical burns if they soak through the padding).
- Exsanguination of limb may be passive (by elevation) or active (Esmarch bandage or Rhys Davies exsanguinator). Once the limb is exsanguinated just prior to surgery, inflate the cuff.
- The inflation pressures are:
  - Lower limb: ≥100 mmHg above systolic BP (usually around 300 mmHg).
  - Upper limb: ≥50 mmHg above systolic BP (usually around 250 mmHg).

Limit inflation time to ≤2 hour. In practice, safe inflation time will be determined by the patient's age, physical health, and integrity of the vascular supply to the limb. Most recommendations in the literature suggest a period of 1.5–2 hours in a healthy adult, which corresponds to the point at which muscle ATP stores are depleted.

If surgery is prolonged, consider deflation for 10 min every 2 hours to allow reperfusion. Longer ischaemic times increase the risk of nerve and soft tissue damage.

The Anaesthetic Record should have record inflation and deflation times on the anaesthetic chart.

Further reading

Deloughry, J.L. and Griffiths, R. Arterial tourniquets. *Continuing Education in Anaesthesia, Critical Care & Pain* 2009; **9**:56–60.

Chapter 9

Clinical anaesthesia

Long case: A patient for elective open AAA repair   *187*
Short cases   *192*
    Questions   *192*
    Answers   *193*
        Short case 1: Emergency burn   *193*
        Short case 2: Carotid endarterectomy   *193*
        Short case 3: Day-care laryngospasm   *196*

Clinical science

Questions   *200*
Answers   *201*
    Anatomy: Circle of Willis   *201*
    Physiology: Cerebral perfusion pressure   *203*
    Pharmacology: Magnesium   *206*
    Physics and clinical measurements: Laser   *208*

Clinical anaesthesia

Long case: A patient for elective open AAA repair

You have a 67-year-old male patient for elective open abdominal aortic aneurysm repair. He has COPD, with controlled hypertension on ACE inhibitors, a history of ischaemic heart disease, and renal dysfunction.
Drug history: furosemide, ACE inhibitors, aspirin, and occasionally requires GTN spray.

Clinical examination	Temperature: 38.2°C; weight: 85 kg; height: 160 cm		
	Pulse: 78/min; regular; BP: 160/95 mmHg; respiratory rate: 12/min		
	Chest: clear, no crepitations/rhonchi		
	Cardiovascular system: normal heart sound with no murmurs		
	Central nervous system: no neurological deficit		
Laboratory investigations	Hb	13.6 g/dl	Na	149 mEq/L
	MCV	89 fL	K	3.9 mEq/L
	WBC	12.1×10^9/L	Urea	14 mmol/L
	Platelets	236×10^9/L	Creatinine	180 µmol/L
	pH: 7.51	pO_2: 9.1	pCO_2: 6.4	HCO_3^-: 29

QUESTIONS

1. Summarize the information you have.
2. Comment on the ECG and chest X-ray findings.
3. Will you use beta-blockers in this patient? Elaborate.
4. Can you go through the blood gas results?
5. What are the implications of metabolic alkalosis in this patient?
6. How will you evaluate the COPD status of this patient?
7. Will you operate on this patient? If not, why? How will you go about it?
8. Do you need any further investigation in this patient?
9. This patient comes back after 8 weeks with controlled hypertension. How will you manage him for elective open AAA repair?
10. What are the important stages in the procedure?
11. During aortic cross-clamping, what are the changes?
12. When do you give heparin?
13. What are the main postoperative issues?
14. When would you extubate?
15. What is the transfusion trigger for you in this gentleman?

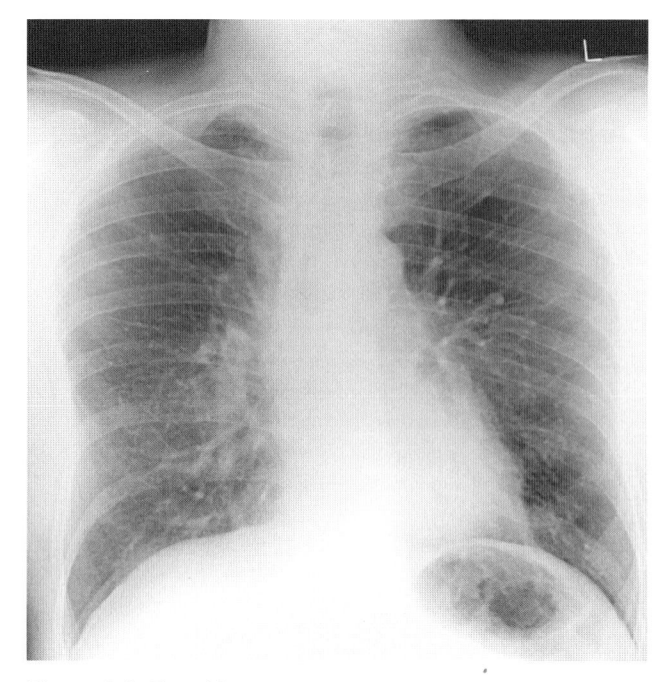

Figure 9.1 Chest X-ray.

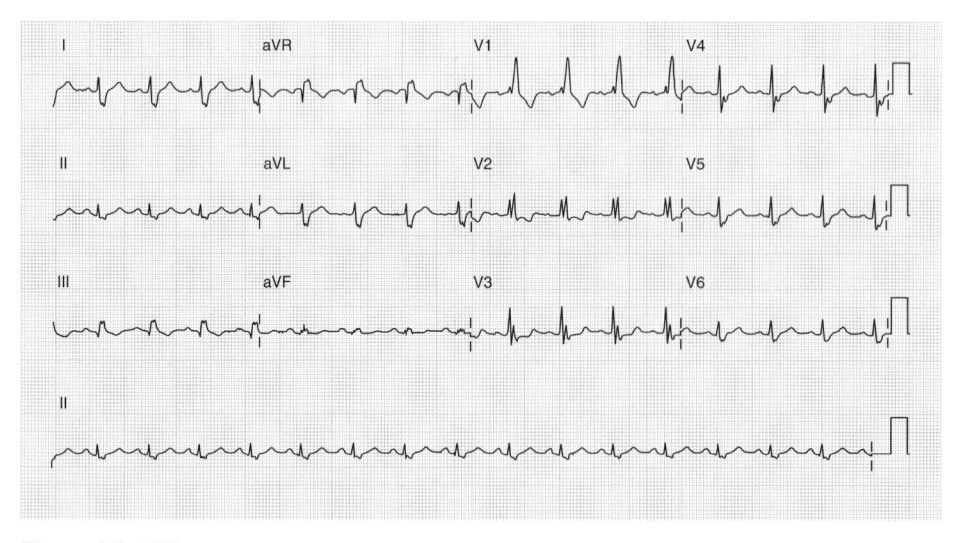

Figure 9.2 ECG.

Chapter 9

ANSWERS

1. Summarize the information you have.
We have a middle-aged gentleman with a complex medical history for elective major vascular surgery. He has poorly controlled hypertension, long-standing respiratory disease, and ischaemic heart disease.

2. Comment on the chest X-ray and ECG findings.
Chest X-ray: posterior–anterior CXR. The lungs are hyperexpanded with flattening of the hemidiaphragms. There are disorganized vascular markings and paucity of lung markings and small bullae in the right upper lobe. No focal collapse or consolidation. The appearances are in keeping with COPD. Normal cardiomediastinal contour with heart size is normal. The chest X-ray shows emphysema.

ECG: this shows sinus rhythm, QRS >0.12 sec, slurred S wave in lead I, no q waves in I and V6, RSR pattern in lead V1. This ECG shows left bundle branch block, left axis deviation.

3. Will you use beta-blockers in this patient? Elaborate.
Yes I will use perioperative beta-blockade based on recent guidelines from both the European Society of Cardiologists and American Heart Association. Regarding perioperative beta-blockade:

- The aim is to titration HR (60–80 bpm) and BP.
- It is important to balance the risks against the benefits for individual patients
- High-risk cardiac patients undergoing major surgery are likely to benefit.
- Beta-blockade should be continued in patients who are already on treatment.
- If indicated perioperatively, it should be started about 30 to 7 days preoperatively.

4. Can you go through the blood gas results?
The blood gas results show a picture of metabolic alkalosis. This may be due to chronic diuretic administration.

5. What are the implications of metabolic alkalosis in this patient?
Metabolic alkalosis can cause hypokalaemia, decreased concentration of ionized calcium, compensatory CO_2 retention, and shift to the left of oxygen–Hb dissociation curve.

6. How will you evaluate the COPD status of this patient?
Assessment of the respiratory system by:

History

- Cough with or without sputum production.
- Determination of exercise tolerance.
- Smoking.
- Frequency of exacerbations, hospital admissions, and previous requirements for invasive and non-invasive ventilation.
- Need for nebulizations at home or episodes of ventilatory support.
- Medication patient is on.

Clinical examination

- Examination of chest for added sound presence of prolonged expiration, rales, wheeze, or rhonchi.
- Signs of chest infection.
- Poor nutritional status.

Investigation
- Spirometry.
- Lung function tests, PFT before and after bronchodilator.
- ECG for right heart status.
- Blood gas and chest X-ray.

7. Will you operate on this patient? If not, why? How will you go about it?

No, I will not go ahead with this patient as the BP needs to optimized. For this I would refer him to his GP. He probably requires addition of other antihypertensives like a calcium channel blocker. This will require BP monitoring in primary care for about 4–6 weeks. When the BP is reasonably controlled then the patient should be considered for surgery. This should be communicated to the medical team, surgical team, and the GP.

8. Do you need any further investigation in this patient?

I would require a coagulation profile, echocardiogram resting, and a stress echocardiogram. Given the history of IHD we should also have a MIBI (myocardial perfusion) scan to look at reversible ischaemic areas in the heart and if they can be reversed before a major vascular procedure.

9. This patient comes back after 8 weeks with controlled hypertension. How will you manage him for elective open AAA repair?

I would have an informed discussion with the patient about the different plans for anaesthetic, including explaining the use of invasive lines such as an arterial line and CV catheter, and informing about admission to critical care or HDU depending on the operation and other factors. Furthermore, I would explain the risks and benefits of epidural analgesia for postoperative use. My plan for this patient would be:

- Premedication: beta-blockers, anxiolytic, normal antianginals, hypertensive.
- Consider a general anaesthetic technique supplemented with thoracic epidural.
- Monitoring: 5-lead ECG, ST analysis, IBP, CVP, consider PA catheter, urine output, temperature, consider TOE.
- Management of cross-clamp application and release:
  - Protection of organs—heart, kidneys, spinal cord.
  - Intravascular volume and perfusion pressure most important for renal function: furosemide, mannitol, dopamine—no evidence of benefit.
  - Cross-clamp—may need GTN, inotrope depending on response.
- Preparation for major blood loss: use cell saver, level 1 transfuser.
- Extubate if:
  - Stable haemodynamic parameters.
  - Normal temperature.
  - Blood gas: PaO_2, base excess.
  - Clotting—postoperative HDU care.

10. What are the important stages in the procedure?

- Induction/intubation
- Aortic cross-clamping and unclamping
- Extubation

11. What are the changes due to aortic cross-clamping?

Aortic cross-clamping causes proximal hypertension due to increase in SVR which increases myocardial workload and O_2 consumption. The rise in BP can be controlled by an infusion of labetalol, GTN, or a top-up of epidural. A point of note here is that it is the higher BP which is driving blood flow through collaterals to the areas which are distal to the cross-clamp.

12. When do you give heparin?

Heparin is given about 5–10 min before the cross-clamp is applied. This helps to prevent clotting distal to the cross-clamp due to sluggish circulation.

13. What are the main postoperative issues?

- Postoperative invasive monitoring CVP and arterial:
  - Fluid balance.
  - Distal pedal pulse monitoring (Doppler).
  - 12-lead ECG on day 1 and day 3 as they are prone to perioperative myocardial infarction.
- Analgesia:
  - A good working epidural is an ideal analgesic.
  - PCA morphine.
  - Oxycodone supplemented with regular paracetamol.

14. When would you extubate?

Once the patient is reasonably fit and with good exercise tolerance as assessed preoperatively, haemodynamically stable, warm, with adequate analgesia on board (good working epidural), and good gas exchange, then we can extubate the patient.

15. What is the transfusion trigger for you in this gentleman?

In this patient who has had a recent major vascular operation and history of IHD, my trigger point would be haemoglobin of 9–10 g/dL. Blood transfusion should be carefully planned in view of the patient's cardiac status. I'd assess the patient for symptoms of anaemia (shortness of breath, dizziness, new or worsening of angina.) and try to quantify the blood loss (such as 15% or 20% of circulating volume lost).

Further reading

Allman, K.G. and Wilson, I.H. *Oxford Handbook of Anaesthesia*, 2nd edn. Oxford: Oxford University Press, 2006.

Edrich, T. and Sadovnikoff, N. Anesthesia for patients with severe chronic obstructive pulmonary disease. *Current Opinion in Anaesthesiology* 2010; **23**:18–24.

Howell, S.J., Sear, J.W., and Foëx, P. Hypertension, hypertensive heart disease and perioperative cardiac risk; *British Journal of Anaesthesia* 2004; **92**:570–83.

NICE. *Hypertension: management of hypertension in adults in primary care* (Clinical Guideline 34). London: NICE, 2006. Available at: http:// http://www.nice.org.uk/CG034

Structured Oral Examination Practice for the Final FRCA

Short cases

QUESTIONS

Short case 1: Emergency burn

A 5-year-old is admitted to the A&E department of your hospital. He has fallen against the cooker and has been scalded by a saucepan of hot water.

1. What is your immediate management and primary concerns?
2. How would you assess a burn patient?
3. How would you estimate the total body surface area (TBSA) of a burn patient?
4. What are the fluid requirements in the first 24 hours?

Short case 2: Carotid endarterectomy

A 75-year-old lady is scheduled for a right carotid endarterectomy for asymptomatic right carotid stenosis. She has 90% occlusion of the right carotid artery. She has a past medical history of hypertension, insulin-dependent diabetes mellitus, and coronary artery disease with angioplasty 2 years ago.

1. What are the presenting symptoms of carotid stenosis?
2. What are the other comorbidities you expect?
3. What are the indications for surgery and risk factors for carotid endarterectomy?
4. What are the anaesthetic options?
5. How would you monitor the patient?
6. How would you know that the patient's cerebral perfusion is adequate during surgery?
7. What are the concerns in the postoperative period?
8. What is hyperperfusion syndrome?

Short case 3: Day-care laryngospasm

You are in day care and have just anaesthetized a patient for knee arthroscopy using a laryngeal mask. As soon as the surgeon puts the scope into the knee you notice there is no carbon dioxide on the monitoring screen. The patient cannot be ventilated and saturation is falling.

1. What are the possible causes of no end-tidal carbon-dioxide?
2. What is the probable cause?
3. What is laryngospasm?
4. What are you going to do know?
5. You have tried but could not intubate and saturation is 70%. What are you going to do?
6. How will you perform cricothyroidotomy?

Chapter 9

ANSWERS

Short case 1: Emergency burn

1. What is your immediate management and primary concerns?

The primary concern is the primary survey ABCDE, it is unlikely in this case that there will be other associated injuries; however, with other burns victims there may be other injuries that can be life threatening. IV access to start fluid replacement, cover the wounds with cling film as evaporative losses are approximately 2 ml/kg/hour.

The child is 5 years old, hence their estimated weight would be ([2 × age] + 9) = 19 kg and oral ETT size (internal diameter in mm) is (4 + [age/4]).

2. How would you assess a burn patient?

Grading of burns is based on:

- Type (electrical, chemical, thermal).
- Depth (degree):
  - 1st degree: superficial thickness; heals in 3–4 days.
  - 2nd degree: partial thickness; heals in 2–3 weeks.
  - 3rd degree: full thickness; dermis is destroyed, dry, leathery, brown/white
- Size (rule of 9s—modified for paediatric patients).
- Location of burns (airways, facial, perineal).

3. How would you estimate the total body surface area (TBSA) of a burn patient?

The rule of 9s is used. Each upper limb is 9%; each lower limb is 18%; trunk front is 18%; trunk back is 18%. Head is 9% and neck is 1%.

Paediatric age group head is 18%. Changes with paediatric age group would be available in A&E.

4. What are the fluid requirements in the first 24 hours?

The fluid requirement for first 24 hours can be calculated as:

- Modified Parklands formula: 4ml/kg per %TBSA/24 hours
- Hypertonic saline 0.3ml/kg per %TBSA in first 24 hours, then adjust to urine output.
- Mount Vernon formula: 0.5 × weight in kg × %TBSA (ml) of 4.5 % human albumin in each six periods over 36 hours.

Further reading

Fenlon, S. and Nene, S. Burns in children. *Continuing Education in Anaesthesia Critical Care & Pain* 2007; **7**: 76–80.

Short case 2: Carotid endarterectomy

1. What are the presenting symptoms of carotid stenosis?

Carotid stenosis is commonly asymptomatic but can present as transient ischaemic attacks (TIAs) with or without severe permanent strokes, particularly within the first 2 days. TIAs by definition last less than 24 hours (and usually last a few minutes), and usually take the form of a weakness or loss of sensation of a limb or the trunk on one side of the body, or loss of sight (amaurosis fugax) in one eye. Less common symptoms are artery sounds (bruits), or ringing in the ear (tinnitus).

Carotid endarterectomy is preventative surgery aimed at reducing the rate of stroke in patients at high risk of such an event.

2. What are the other comorbidities you expect?

These are elderly patients with geriatric changes along with significant disease which are:

- TIAs with or without stroke
- Diabetic autoneuropathy and neuropathy
- IHD and hypertension
- Respiratory changes
- Endocrine diabetes
- Multiples medications and anticoagulants

3. What are the indications for surgery and risk factors for carotid endarterectomy?

Indications

- TIAs with without stroke
- Reversible ischaemic neurological deficit with >70% stenosis
- Unstable neurological status

Risk factors

- Age >75 years
- Female sex
- Systolic hypertension
- Peripheral vascular disease—marker for coronary artery disease
- Experience of the surgeon
- Ipsilateral cerebral symptoms

4. What are the anaesthetic options?

The anaesthetic options are:

- Local anaesthesia: cervical plexus block ± sedation + arterial line.
- General anaesthesia: IPPV, ETT with arterial line.

The GALA trial did not show any benefit for general vs. local anaesthetic. The local anaesthetic technique has the advantage of being able to tell that patients are affected by the clamping of the carotid. Anaesthesia is standard and the emphasis is on careful control of BP.

Principles of anaesthetic management

- Ensure optimization of BP—preferable to avoid ACE inhibitors.
- Maintain BP within 20% of the baseline readings from that of the ward.
- Higher systolic pressures preferable during cross-clamp application.
- Induction during general anaesthesia, cross-clamp period, and extubation are the periods of high vigilance for cardiovascular instability.
- Keep communication channels open (awake patient)—monitor speech, contralateral hand grip and mentation throughout the surgical period.
- Patient will need a longer stay in recovery for cardiovascular monitoring.

Chapter 9

Advantages	Disadvantages
Local anaesthesia: cervical plexus block ± sedation + arterial line	
Awake patients—gold standard/best CNS monitoring	Technical difficulties—competence with performing block
Maintenance of CPP and cerebral autoregulation	Patients discomfort—supine for prolonged period
Selective shunting (avoids adverse effects of shunts)	Sedation or analgesic supplementation required usually
Avoids minor complications of general anaesthesia	Lack of airway protection
	Difficult access to patient—if neurological or cardiovascular complications
General anaesthesia: IPPV, ETT with arterial line	
Patient comfort	Will need cerebral blood flow monitoring
Airway protection	Minor complications of general anaesthesia will have to be accepted—nausea, vomiting, sore throat, delirium, adverse drug reaction/interactions
Reduced cerebral metabolic requirement of O_2 ($CMRO_2$)	
Autoregulation maintained by low-dose inhalational agents or TIVA	
Therapeutic manipulation of $PaCO_2$ possible	

5. How would you monitor the patient?

Patients who are about to undergo carotid endarterectomy are monitored with routine measurements of cardiovascular, pulmonary, and metabolic functions which include ECG, non-invasive /invasive BP monitoring, pulse-oximetry, end-tidal capnometry, and temperature.

6. How would you know that the patient's cerebral perfusion is adequate during surgery?

In awake patients undergoing carotid endarterectomy under local anaesthesia, repeated neurological examination can be performed to assess the adequacy of cerebral perfusion.

In patients under general anaesthesia, the cerebral perfusion or function should be monitored. There is no gold standard but a number of monitors are used, such as EEG, somatosensory evoked potential, internal carotid pressure, jugular venous oxygen saturation, cerebral oximetry.

Cerebral oximetry: near-infrared spectroscopy (NIRS) is a non-invasive method of estimating regional cerebral oxygenation. It shows the differences with cerebral oxygenation during surgery. Used in carotid endarterectomy for estimates of cerebral oxygenation—a desaturation of >50% is an indication for shunt insertion. It may have some use but 'Monitoring SO_2 with INVOS-3100 to detect cerebral ischaemia during carotid endarterectomy has a high negative predictive value, but the positive predictive value is low'.

Transcranial Doppler is a non-invasive monitor that calculates red cell flow velocity (RCFV) from the shift in frequency spectra of the Doppler signal—an indirect estimate of cerebral blood flow (CBF). Changes in flow velocity correlate with changes in CBF when the direction of ultrasound beam, diameter of the vessel, and minimal changes with $PaCO_2$ and BP remains reasonably constant.

7. What are the concerns in the postoperative period?

In the postoperative period the objective is a smooth and prompt emergence with optimal systemic and cerebral haemodynamics. Concerns in the immediate postoperative period include:

- Hypertension: may occur as a result of damage or local anaesthesia to the carotid sinus or its nerves. Patients with hypertension are at greater risk of developing a neurologic deficit than those patients who remain normotensive.

- Hyperperfusion: is most likely to occur in patients with high-grade carotid artery stenosis who develop >100% increase in CBF after carotid endarterectomy. Normo-tension should be maintained in patients at risk for hyperperfusion.
- Hypotension: after the removal of atheromatous plaques, increased stimulation to baroreceptors may result in bradycardia and hypotension. Regional anaesthesia may be associated with a higher incidence of postoperative hypotension while general anaesthesia is more often associated with postoperative hypertension.
- Myocardial infarction: the most frequent cause of morbidity and mortality.
- Stroke: most often is embolic in origin.
- Bleeding and haematoma can lead to airway obstruction. Soft tissue swelling with oedematous supraglottic mucosal folds can compromise the airway.
- Cranial nerve injury: occurs in approximately 10% of patients.
- Carotid body damage: results in reduced ventilatory response to hypoxemia and hypercapnia.
- Neurological dysfunction are associated with carotid endarterectomy, per se, and postoperative

8. What is hyperperfusion syndrome?

This may occur due to cerebral haemorrhage or cerebral oedema and can occur in up to one-third of the patients but is symptomatic in very few. Impaired autoregulation may be the mechanism. Ipsilateral headache, cognitive impairment, seizures, and cerebral haemorrhage, peaking at 6–12 hours postoperatively, but may last longer. Transcranial Doppler ultrasound is useful. Careful perioperative control of BP is required with any change in neurological deficit needs urgent review.

Further reading

Allman, K.G. and Wilson, I.H. *Oxford Handbook of Anaesthesia*, 2nd edn. Oxford: Oxford University Press, 2006.
GALA trial: www.dcn.ed.ac.uk/gala/
Murkin, J.M. and Arango, M. Near-infrared spectroscopy as an index of brain and tissue oxygenation. *British Journal of Anaesthesia* 2009; **103**(Suppl 1):i3–13.
Oxford Stroke Prevention Research Unit. Model for predicting the risk of ipsilateral ischaemic stroke in patients with recently symptomatic carotid bifurcation stenosis. Available at: http://www.stroke.ox.ac.uk/model/form1.html

Short case 3: Day-care laryngospasm

1. What are the possible causes of no end-tidal carbon dioxide?

Equipment fault	Reduced respiratory compliance
Incorrect ventilator settings	Breathing against the inspiratory phase of the ventilator
Ventilator disconnection, leak, or failure	Coughing and breath-holding
Incorrect switch placement between controlled and spontaneous modes	Inadequate anaesthesia
Failure of pressure regulators or valves	Chest: pulmonary oedema, infection, fibrosing alveolitis, ARDS, or a pneumothorax
ETT displacement, kinking, or blockage	Chest wall rigidity (opioids)
Obstruction in the breathing circuit (foreign bodies, kinked tubing)	Pneumoperitoneum, distension
Oxygen flush jammed in the 'on' position	Position: steep head-down
Closed PEEP valve	Direct pressure from the surgical team

Increased airway resistance	Obstruction
Bronchospasm, excessive secretions, and pulmonary aspiration	Airway: blood, secretions, foreign body
Atelectasis	ETT: kinking, displacement, endobronchial intubation, cuff herniation, patient biting
Aspiration	Laryngospasm (with supraglottic airway)
Pulmonary oedema	
Pneumothorax or haemothorax	
Laryngospasm	

2. What is the probable cause?

This could be laryngospasm as it presents with a sound readily recognized by:
- Stridor or 'crowing' indicate partial obstruction and
- Heard during inspiration.

During severe laryngospasm the airway is completely obstructed and is silent. There can be signs of respiratory distress:
- Tracheal tug.
- Suprasternal and/or intercostal recession.
- Abdominal muscles contraction.
- Ventilation is difficult or impossible with a flat capnograph and rapidly progressive hypoxaemia.

3. What is laryngospasm?

This is defined as glottic closure resulting from the reflex constriction of the laryngeal muscles. It is common in the paediatric age group. It occurs during anaesthesia for two reasons:
- Lack of inhibition of glottic reflexes.
- Increased number of stimuli such as manipulation of airway, secretion, blood irritating the cords, visceral stimuli.

4. What are you going to do?

This is an acute emergency and I will immediately look, listen, and feel for respiratory movement and check the circuit along with machine.

Immediate management
- Stop surgery or other stimulation. Suction secretions.
- Open and clear the airway as much as possible and remove airway devices that may be stimulating the larynx.
- Increase oxygen flow to give 100% oxygen. Apply CPAP with 100% oxygen via bag and mask.
- A firm jaw thrust may 'break' the spasm.
- Visualize and clear pharynx and airway. Exclude supraglottic obstruction (e.g. base of tongue, foreign body, clot, or tumour).
- If desaturation continues:
  - Call for help for immediate assistance.
  - Deepen anaesthesia with IV anaesthetic agent (20% of induction dose of propofol).
  - Continue CPAP.
- If CPAP fails, saturation continues to decrease:
  - Give suxamethonium (0.5 mg/kg IV; 2–4 mg/kg may be given IM).

- Give atropine (10 mcg/kg). About 1 in 20 cases overall—and 1 in 4 infants—will develop bradycardia.
  - Once airway patency is established, consider whether to continue bag-mask ventilation or use another airway device.
- Occasionally, hypoxia due to laryngospasm may become life threatening, perhaps where intubation has not been possible.
- If the patient continues to deteriorate:
  - Intubation will secure and protect the airway; however, an ETT may precipitate further spasm when it is removed.
- If severe laryngospasm:
  - Be prepared to move to a needle cricothyroidotomy or
  - Surgical airway—it may be life-saving.
- Subsequently management according to the progress:
  - Monitoring until patient's condition is stable.
  - Chest X-ray to rule out negative pressure pulmonary oedema.

5. You have tried but could not intubate and saturation is 70%. What are you going to do?

This is a situation called 'can't intubate, can't ventilate'. It is an acute emergency and I will call for help with a difficult airway trolley with a plan of performing a cricothyroidotomy to oxygenate the patient.

6. How will you perform cricothyroidotomy?

When the trachea cannot be intubated, a surgical airway must be made. Cricothyroid membrane puncture is a safe and simple method for establishing an airway when this occurs.

- Place the patient in a supine position and feel for the cricothyroid membrane. The membrane stretches between the thyroid cartilage and the cricoid cartilage.
- The cricothyroid membrane is felt as an indentation between the two cartilages.
- Assemble the 12- or 14-G IV cannula to the 10-ml syringe with saline.
- Puncture the skin midline and directly over the cricothyroid membrane with the needle directed 45° caudally; aspirate as you advance the needle. Entry into the trachea is indicated by aspiration of air.
- Withdraw the needle from the IV cannula and advance the soft catheter further into the trachea.
- Attach the hub of the cannula to the 3-mm paediatric ETT adapter (or the 3-ml syringe body).
- Connect to oxygen tubing with a Y connector and turn on the oxygen source at 15 L/min (50 psi).

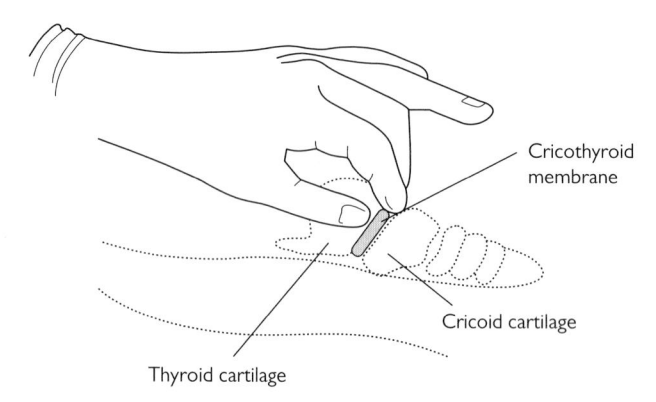

Figure 9.3 Landmarks: between the thyroid and cricoid cartilage, at the cricothyroid membrane.

- Positive pressure ventilation is delivered through the IV catheter by placing the thumb over the open end of the Y connector, 1 sec on and 4 sec off.
- Observe chest expansion and auscultate for adequate ventilation.

Further reading

Benumof, J.L. and Scheller, M.S. The importance of transtracheal jet ventilation in the management of the difficult airway. *Anesthesiology* 1989; **71**: 769–78.

Greig, H.J., Schnider, T., and Heidegger, T. Prophylactic percutaneous transtracheal catheterisation in the management of patients with anticipated difficult airways: a case series. *Anaesthesia* 2005; **60**:801–5.

Henderson, J.J., Popat, T.M., Latto, I.P., *et al*. Difficult airway society guidelines for the management of the unanticipated difficult intubation. *Anaesthesia* 2004; **59**:675–94.

Larson, C.P. Laryngospasm – the best treatment. *Anesthesiology* 1998; **89**:1293–4.

Clinical science

QUESTIONS

Anatomy: Circle of Willis

1. What is the blood supply to the brain? What are the areas supplied by the different arteries?
2. What is the physiological significance of the circle of Willis?
3. What are the common locations of intracranial vascular aneurysms?
4. What is the clinical presentation of subarachnoid haemorrhage (SAH)?
5. What is the mortality from SAH? What factors influence morbidity and mortality?

Physiology: Cerebral perfusion pressure

1. What is cerebral perfusion pressure (CPP)? Why is it important?
2. What is normal cerebral blood flow?
3. How is cerebral blood flow maintained?
4. What is the effect of head trauma on autoregulation?
5. Draw the relationship between intracranial pressure and volume. Why is it that shape? What are the implications of this shape?
6. How can you decrease raised ICP?

Pharmacology: Magnesium

1. What can you tell me about magnesium and its importance?
2. What are the uses of magnesium?
3. What are normal plasma and therapeutic magnesium levels?
4. How is magnesium sulphate administered?
5. What are the manifestations of magnesium toxicity?

Physics and clinical measurements: Laser

A 21-year-old patient with a history of recurrent respiratory papillomatosis is scheduled for direct laryngoscopy and possible excision.

1. What is a laser and how does it work?
2. What are the physical characteristics of a laser?
3. Enumerate different types of laser beams and give examples of the types of surgery they are used for.
4. What are the risks associated with the use of a laser?
5. What precautions should be taken while using a laser in the operating theatre?

Chapter 9

ANSWERS

Anatomy: Circle of Willis

1. What is the blood supply to the brain? What are the areas supplied by the different arteries?

The arterial blood supply of brain includes:
- **Internal carotid arteries** and
- **Vertebral arteries**.
- These two systems are joined by the **anterior** and **posterior communicating arteries**.
- This anastomosis is called the **circle of Willis**.

The **anterior cerebral artery** supplies the frontal lobes and medial aspects of the parietal and occipital lobes.

The **middle cerebral artery**, also called the artery of stroke, supplies the lateral side of the hemisphere (frontoparietal somatosensory cortex). Infarcts in its territory result in contralateral hemiparesis.

The **posterior cerebral artery** supplies the occipital lobe and medial side of temporal lobe.

The medulla is supplied by the **vertebral arteries**. The anterior spinal artery arises at the bifurcation of the vertebrals and descends to supply the spinal cord.

The vertebral arteries fuse at the pontomedullary junction to form the **basilar artery**. The posterior **inferior cerebellar artery** arises from the caudal aspect of the basilar artery. Penetrators from the basilar artery supply the pons.

The **superior cerebellar artery** arises superiorly from the basilar artery. The basilar artery then bifurcates into the posterior cerebral arteries.

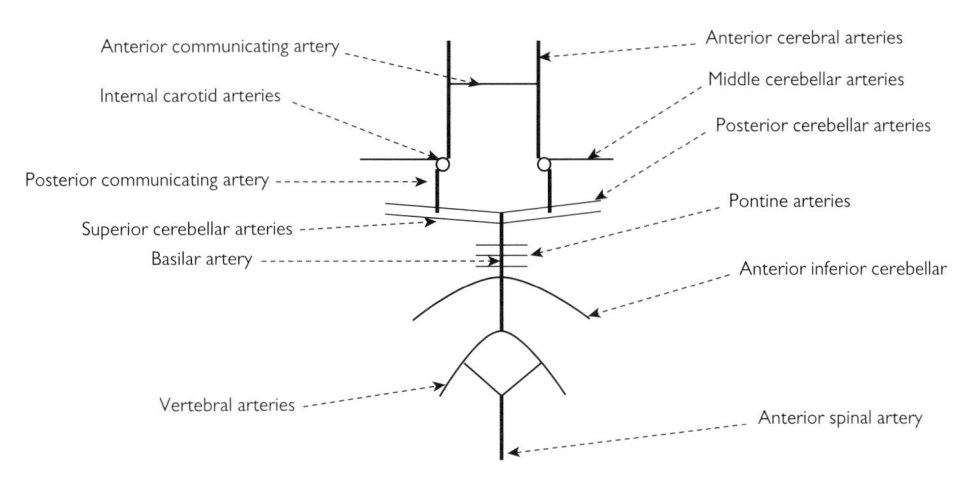

Figure 9.4 Diagram of blood supply to the brain.

2. What is the physiological significance of the circle of Willis?

If any one of the arteries in the circle become blocked or narrowed (stenosed) or one of the arteries supplying the circle is blocked or narrowed, blood flow from the other blood vessels is usually insufficient to maintain cerebral perfusion.

3. What are the common locations of intracranial vascular aneurysms?

Most aneurysms are located in the anterior circulation with the junction of anterior communicating and anterior cerebral arteries. Approximately 85% of cerebral aneurysms develop in the anterior part of the circle of willis, and involve the internal carotid arteries and their major branches that supply the anterior and middle sections of the brain.

The most common sites include:

- The anterior communicating artery (39%).
- The bifurcation of the internal carotid and posterior communicating artery (30%).
- The bifurcation of the middle cerebral artery (22%).
- The bifurcation of the basilar artery, and the posterior circulation: posterior cerebral, basilar, and vertebral arteries (8%).

4. What is the clinical presentation of subarachnoid haemorrhage (SAH)?

- Headache occurs in 85–95% of patients
- Nausea and vomiting
- Stiff neck or neck pain
- Blurred vision or double vision
- Pain above and behind the eye
- Dilated pupils
- Sensitivity to light
- Loss of sensation
- Loss of consciousness
- Transient neurological deficits: depend upon site & size of aneurysm—extent of intracerebral haematoma

5. What is the mortality from subarachnoid haemorrhage (SAH)? What factors influence morbidity and mortality?

Mortality is 40–50% overall.

In a multivariable analysis, unfavourable outcome was associated with increasing age, worsening neurological grade, ruptured posterior circulation aneurysm, larger aneurysm size, more SAH on admission CT, intracerebral haematoma or intraventricular haemorrhage, elevated systolic BP on admission, and previous diagnosis of hypertension, myocardial infarction, liver disease, or SAH.

Further reading

Allman, K.G. and Wilson, I.H. *Oxford Handbook of Anaesthesia*, 2nd edn. Chapter 16: Neurosurgery, see pp. 408–9. Oxford: Oxford University Press, 2006.

Kasell, N.F., Torner, J.C., Haley, C., et al. The international cooperative study on the timing of aneurysm surgery. Part I, overall management results. Journal of Neurosurgery 1990; **73**:18–32.

Rosengart, A.J., Schultheiss, K.E., Tolentino, J., et al. Prognostic factors for outcome in patients with aneurysmal subarachnoid hemorrhage. *Stroke* 2007; **38**:2315–21.

Physiology: Cerebral perfusion pressure

1. What is cerebral perfusion pressure (CPP)? Why is it important?

CPP is defined as the difference between the mean arterial pressure (MAP) and the intracranial pressure (ICP) or central venous pressure (CVP) (whichever is greater), so:

$$CPP = MAP - CVP \text{ or } ICP \text{ (whichever is the greater)}$$

It represents the pressure gradient driving cerebral blood flow (CBF) and hence oxygen and metabolite delivery.

CPP is the pressure gradient across the cerebral circulation: when the ICP is greater than the CVP, the cerebral circulation can be considered to behave as a Starling resistor.

2. What is normal cerebral blood flow?

Normal CBF is 50 ml/min/100 g (i.e. 750 ml/min), approximately 15% of the cardiac output. Flow rates vary little, allowing maintenance of normal brain function under variable systemic conditions.

3. How is cerebral blood flow maintained?

Autoregulation provides a constant flow regardless of CPP by altering the resistance of cerebral blood vessels. CBF varies in an analogous manner to Ohm's law ($V = I \times R$) and is determined by CPP and cerebral vascular resistance (CVR):

$$CBF = CPP/CVR$$

Proposed mechanisms: metabolic, myogenic (Laplace law), neurogenic.

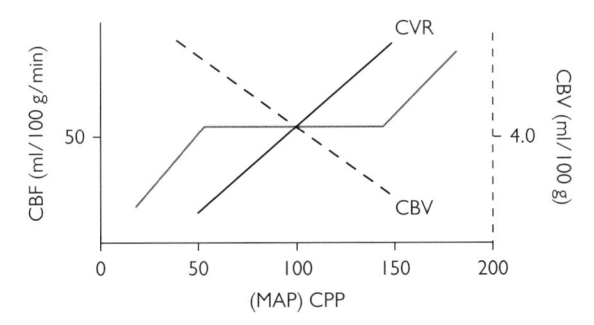

Figure 9.5 Maintenance of CBF.

The autoregulation is maintained by:

- **Metabolic autoregulation**: this is an extremely important control mechanism for the cerebral circulation. When an area of brain is active, locally released vasodilator metabolites cause an increase in vessel calibre and therefore CBF.
- **Pressure autoregulation**: this enables CBF to remain constant at MAP values of 50–150 mmHg. Increased intravascular pressure tends to stretch vessels; they respond by contraction of smooth muscle. This reduces vessel diameter, increases CVR, and reduces CBF.
- **Response to carbon dioxide**: there is a linear relationship between CBF and PCO_2 over a wide range (pCO_2 7–12 kPa). Hyperventilation (reduction in PCO_2) increases CVR and reduces the blood volume, and therefore the pressure, inside the skull. However, the vasoconstriction response lasts <6 hours; bicarbonate crosses the blood–brain barrier, returning interstitial pH to normal. Subsequent elevation (normalization) of PCO_2 then causes vasodilatation and worsening

of ICP. This may explain why routine hyperventilation for head-injured patients results in worse outcomes.
- **Response to oxygen:** reduction in cerebral oxygen delivery results in vasodilatation. The shape of the oxygen dissociation curve influences the shape of this graph: when saturations fall below 90%, oxygen content falls away sharply.
- **Nervous system control:** the sympathetic system alters CVR by only a very small amount. However, it has a major influence on CBF by virtue of its effect on the performance of the systemic circulation, and therefore CPP.

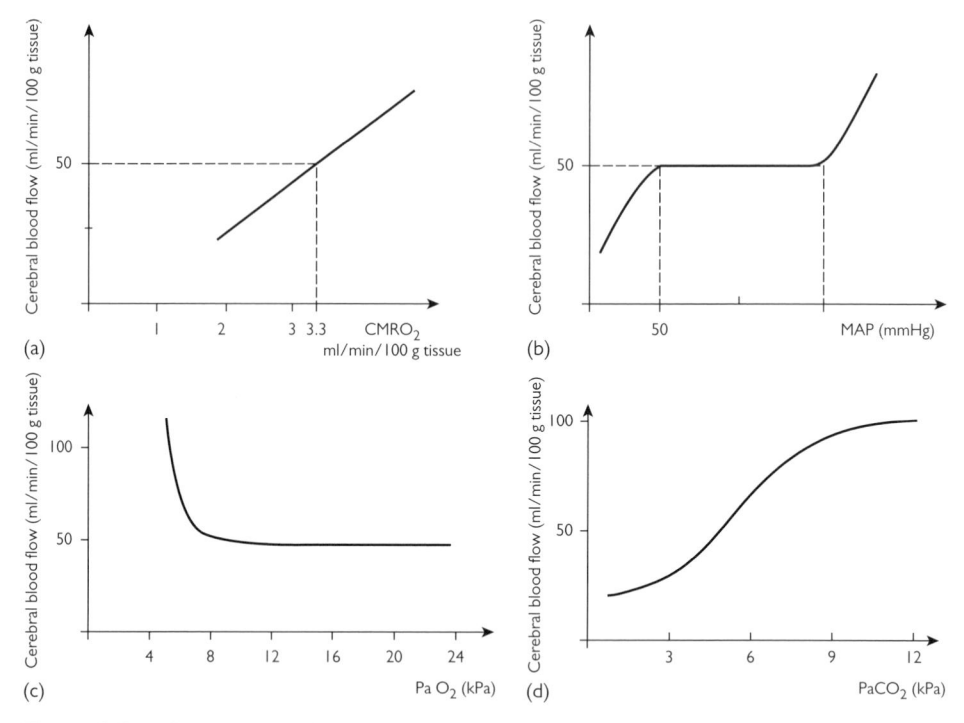

Figure 9.6 a) Cerebral blood flow vs. cerebral metabolic rate. b) Cerebral blood flow vs. mean arterial pressure. c) Cerebral blood flow vs. PaO_2. d) Cerebral blood flow vs. $PaCO_2$.

4. What is the effect of head trauma on autoregulation?

Autoregulation is lost after head trauma (CVR is usually increased)—the brain becomes susceptible to changes in BP. Those areas of the brain that are ischaemic, or at risk of ischaemia are critically dependent on adequate CBF and therefore CPP.

Chapter 9

5. Draw the relationship between intracranial pressure and volume. Why is it that shape? What are the implications of this shape?

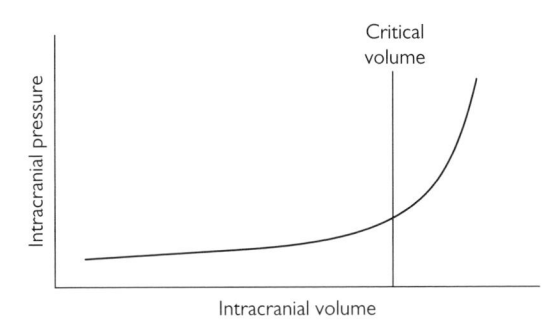

Figure 9.7 The relationship between intracranial pressure and volume.

As the cranial vault is essentially a closed, fixed bony box, its volume is constant.

Monro–Kellie doctrine: v.intracranial (constant) = v.brain + v.CSF + v.blood (+ v.mass lesion)

As all these components are fluids, and non-compressible, once the cranial vault is filled, ICP rises and this can the lead to interruption of CBF by reducing the CPP.

As an intracranial mass lesion or oedematous brain expands, some compensation is possible as cerebrospinal fluid (CSF) and blood move into the spinal canal and extracranial vasculature respectively. Beyond this point, further compensation is impossible and ICP rises dramatically.

Patients who are on the cusp of the graph have exaggerated ICP responses to events such as tracheal intubation, coughing, or fighting a ventilator.

6. How can you decrease raised ICP?

Aim is to reduce increased ICP which is assumed when there is neurological deterioration or if ICP monitoring is available and the ICP goes above 25 cm of H_2O.

Intracranial vascular blood volume

- CBF:
  - Avoid hypoxia.
  - Avoid hypercapnia/hypocapnia.
  - Avoid venous increase in volume; positioning/ETT tie.
  - Avoid rise in $CMRO_2$; sedate/paralyse/anticonvulsants hypothermia/normoglycaemia (adenosine/EAA).
- CPP:
  - Treat mean arterial pressure (MAP) (fluids/inotropes – CPP >70mmHg).

Brain volume

- Surgical: operative removal of haematomas/tumours/decompression.
- Hyperosmolar therapy: mannitol/hypertonic saline.

CSF volume

Drainage.

General measures
- Ensure adequate ABC (keep CPP above 70 mmHg).
- Decrease cerebral metabolic requirements by using sedatives and analgesics.
- Prevent coughing/patient-ventilator asynchrony by using muscle relaxants.
- Induced cerebral vasoconstriction—hyperventilation, hypothermia.
- Diuretics and osmotherapy—mannitol, glycerol, urea.
- Anaesthetic agents—barbiturates.
- Surgical decompression.

Further reading
Allman, K.G. and Wilson, I.H. *Oxford Handbook of Anaesthesia*, 2nd edn. Chapter 16: Neurosurgery, pp. 385–94. Oxford: Oxford University Press, 2006.
Werner, C. and Engelhard, K. Pathophysiology of traumatic brain injury. *British Journal of Anaesthesia* 2007; **99**(1):4–9.

Pharmacology: Magnesium

1. What can you tell me about magnesium and its importance?

Magnesium is a cofactor in numerous enzymatic reactions in the human body. Magnesium is the fourth most abundant cation in the body and second most important intracellular cation.

- Mg regulates Na-K-ATPase activity.
- K channels activity.
- It is a natural calcium channel blocking agent. These properties explain its important place in electrophysiology of myocardial cells and the effects on the tension of smooth muscles, resulting in a vasodilation and a bronchodilation respectively.
- The antagonistic effect of magnesium on calcium decreases the presynaptic release of acetylcholine at the neuromuscular junction and the release of epinephrine at the peripheral sympathetic nerves and the adrenals.
- Magnesium potentiates the effect of non-depolarizing muscle relaxants.
- Biosynthesis of DNA and RNA.

2. What are the uses of magnesium?

- **Pre-eclampsia and eclampsia:** magnesium stabilizes the membranes, vasodilates cerebral vessels, and reduces CNS excitability. Magnesium has strong advantages over diazepam and phenytoin in reducing the incidence of primary eclampsia by 60% as well as preventing recurrence of seizures.
- **Antiarrhythmic:** magnesium treatment may reduce the incidence of ventricular fibrillation, ventricular tachycardia, severe arrhythmia needing treatment, especially digoxin-mediated dysrhythmias and torsades de pointes.
- Systematic use of magnesium seems to decrease mortality of acute myocardial infarction and is justified during cardiac surgery, often associated with hypomagnesaemia, because of vasodilation of coronary arteries and in order to prevent occurrence of arrhythmias.
- **Tetanus:** magnesium infusion is used to treat muscle spasm and autonomic instability.
- **Status epilepticus.**
- **Status asthmaticus.**

Chapter 9

- **Perioperative management of phaeochromocytoma:** magnesium, because of its calcium channel blocking properties and as it lowers the release of epinephrine, is indicated for surgery of phaeochromocytoma.

3. What are normal plasma and therapeutic magnesium levels?
- Normal: 0.7–1.0 mmol/L.
- Therapeutic: 2.0–3.5 mmol/L.

4. How is magnesium sulphate administered?
Bolus followed by infusion, about 0.5–1.0 mmol/kg/day. Therapeutic level 2 mmol/L.

5. What are the manifestations of magnesium toxicity?
- Decreased reflexes: knee reflex monitoring is used as an indicator of magnesium toxicity.
- Respiratory paralysis at around 15 mmol/L.
- Cardiac dysrhythmias at levels between 15–25 mmol/L.
- Magnesium crosses placenta rapidly—therefore it can exert similar effects in the neonate, who may exhibit hypotonia and apnoea.

Toxicity

Blood level	Signs
4.0–6.5 mmol/L	Somnolence
	Nausea and vomiting
	Double vision
	Slurred speech
	Loss of patellar reflex
6.5–7.5 mmol/L	Muscle paralysis
	Respiratory arrest
>10 mmol/L	Cardiac arrest

Monitoring

When $MgSO_4$ is used, monitoring should include:

- Regular measurement of plasma concentration of magnesium and assessment of tendon reflexes for hypotonia.
- Vital signs, oxygen saturation, deep tendon reflexes, and level of consciousness.
- Assess patient for signs of toxicity (e.g. visual changes, somnolence, flushing, muscle paralysis, loss of patellar reflexes) or pulmonary oedema.
- Assessment intervals of 15 min for the first hour following a bolus and should be in one-to-one care.

Further reading
Altman, D., Carroli, G., Duley, L., et al. Do women with pre-eclampsia, and their babies, benefit from magnesium sulfate? The Magpie Trial: a randomised, placebo-controlled trial. *Lancet* 2002; **359**:1877–90.
Belfort, M.A., Anthony, J., Saade, G.R., et al. A comparison of magnesium sulfate and nimodipine for the prevention of eclampsia. *New England Journal of Medicine* 2003; **348**:304–11.
Lazarus, S.C. Emergency treatment of asthma. *New England Journal of Medicine* 2010; **3b63**:755–64.
Lucas, M.J., Leveno, K.J., and Cunningham, F.G. A comparison of magnesium sulfate with phenytoin for the prevention of eclampsia. *New England Journal of Medicine* 1995; **333**:201–6.
Shechter, M., Hod, H., Marks, N., et al. Beneficial effect of magnesium sulfate in acute myocardial infarction. *American Journal of Cardiology* 1990; **66**:271–4.

Physics and clinical measurements: Laser

1. What is a laser and how does it work?

Electromagnetic radiation consistent of photons; photons have properties consistent with both particles and waves. LASER is an acronym for 'light amplification by stimulated emission of radiation'. What makes laser distinctive is the high-energy density that it provides, and the ability to transfer large quantities of energy rapidly to remote locations. It involves stimulation of atoms, ions, or molecules in a tube using a high voltage. Photons of energy are absorbed by atoms, which drives the atoms to a higher energy level. As the excited atoms fall back to their original stable state, they emit photons of energy. These photons are reflected back by mirrors to encounter other excited atoms—more photons are emitted, which are parallel and in phase i.e. laser radiation.

2. What are the physical characteristics of a laser?

The high-energy density of a laser is the result of the following characteristics:

- There is a high degree of mono-chromaticity.
- The electromagnetic field of all photons in the laser beam oscillate synchronously in the same phase.
- Laser light remains in a narrow collimated beam.

These characteristics of monochromatic light (all waves of same wavelength), parallel, coherent, and in phase allow for a very concentrated energy delivery, often producing heat.

3. Enumerate different types of laser beams and give examples of the types of surgery they are used for.

The effect of laser on tissues depend on wavelength:

- **Argon**: wavelength 488–515 nm; colour blue green, used for photocoagulation in ophthalmology (diabetic retinopathy) and dermatology.
- **Nd:YAG (neodymium-doped yttrium aluminium garnet)**: wavelength 1064 nm; used for debulking of tumours and photocoagulation—penetrates 1 cm into tissues, airway neoplasms, vascular malformation.
- **CO_2**: wavelength 10,600 nm; far-infrared, used for precise cutting and coagulation, e.g. facial surgery, ENT surgery, neurosurgery.

4. What are the risks associated with the use of a laser?

- Danger to eye, skin: CO_2 laser damage cornea, Nd:YAG laser damage retina.
- Ignition: upper airway fires, explosion as NO_2 support combustion.

5. What precautions should be taken while using a laser in the operating theatre?

- A laser safety officer should be present at all times.
- Laser light can be reflected so special equipment should be used with a matt finish.
- An illuminated sign placed outside theatre: 'Laser surgery in progress'.
- Protection for eyes: appropriate wavelength goggles.
- Skin: patient's skin covered, non-combustible skin preparation.
- Airway: laser tubes (special flexible, metal tracheal tubes without cuffs or metallic tubes). Avoidance of intubation: Sander injector with jet ventilation along with TIVA.
- Saline-soaked swabs on face covering eye.
- Intermittent use of laser beams.

- Use of tracer beam.
- Lowest possible concentration of O_2 and avoid N_2O to reduce chance of fire.

Further reading

Allman, K.G. and Wilson, I.H. *Oxford Handbook of Anaesthesia*, 2nd edn. Chapter 29: Laser surgery, pp. 673–7. Oxford: Oxford University Press, 2006.

Ramphil, I.J. Anaesthesia for laser surgery. In Miller, R.D. (ed.) *Millers's Anaesthesia* 6th edn, pp. 2573–88. Philadelphia, PA: Elsevier Churchill Livingstone, 2005.

Chapter 10

Clinical anaesthesia

Long case: A patient in Accident and Emergency   *213*
Short cases   *219*
   Questions   *219*
   Answers   *220*
      Short case 1: Post-tonsillectomy bleeding   *220*
      Short case 2: Direct laryngoscopy   *221*
      Short case 3: Penetrating eye injury   *223*

Clinical science

Questions   *225*
Answers   *226*
   Anatomy: Heart circulation   *226*
   Physiology: Prone position   *228*
   Pharmacology: Deep vein thrombosis   *229*
   Physics and clinical measurements: Defibrillators   *231*

Clinical anaesthesia

Long case: A patient in Accident and Emergency

A 21-year male has been brought to A&E with a suspected drug overdose. He is drowsy and the paramedics think that he may have consumed a mixture of drugs. In A&E his Glasgow Coma Scale (GCS) is E4V3M4. He has a past medical history of depression, heavy alcohol intake, and drug abuse. He responds to IV naloxone but becomes agitated

Clinical examination	Temperature: 38.2°C; weight: 85 kg; height: 160 cm			
	Pulse: 56/min, regular; BP: 80/40 mmHg; respiratory rate: 8/min; SaO_2 86% (on room air)			
	Chest: clear, no crepitations/rhonchi			
	Cardiovascular system: normal heart sound with no murmurs			
	Central nervous system: agitated, GCS is E4V3M4. No neurological deficit			
Laboratory investigations	Hb	13.6 g/dL	Na	131 mEq/L
	MCV	89 fL	K	7.8 mEq/L
	WBC	12.1×10^9/L	Urea	10.3 mmol/L
	Platelets	236×10^9/L	Creatinine	270 μmol/L
			Creatinine kinase	49,000 IU
ABGs	pH: 7.2	pO_2: 8.2	pCO_2: 5.9	HCO_3^-: 23. BE: 6

QUESTIONS

1. Summarize the case.
2. What are the issues in this case and how would you proceed?
3. Comment on the biochemistry.
4. Comment on the chest X-ray.
5. What further investigations would be helpful?
6. What does the ECG show?
7. So potassium is 7.8 and there are ECG changes. What would you do now?
8. What are the options to treat hyperkalaemia?
9. What is rhabdomyolysis and how it is caused?
10. How is rhabdomyolysis diagnosed?
11. What is the mechanism of renal injury in rhabdomyolysis?
12. How can renal injury be attenuated or prevented in patients with rhabdomyolysis?
13. What are the indications for renal replacement therapy in this patient?

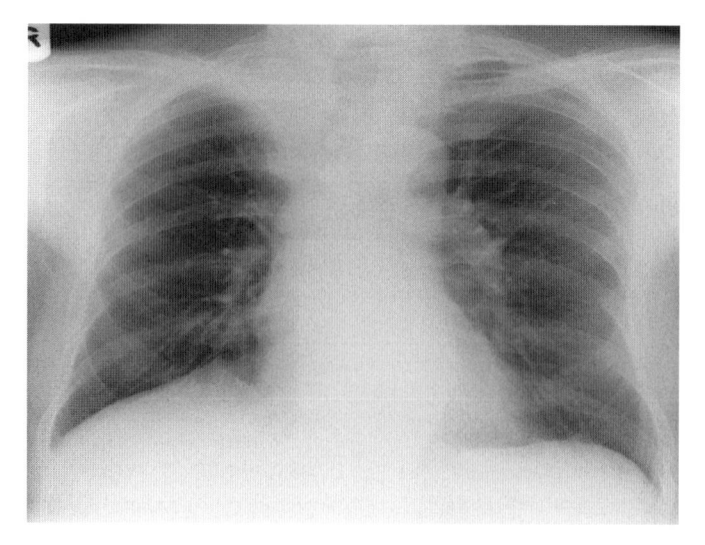

Structured Oral Examination Practice for the Final FRCA

Figure 10.1 Chest X-ray.

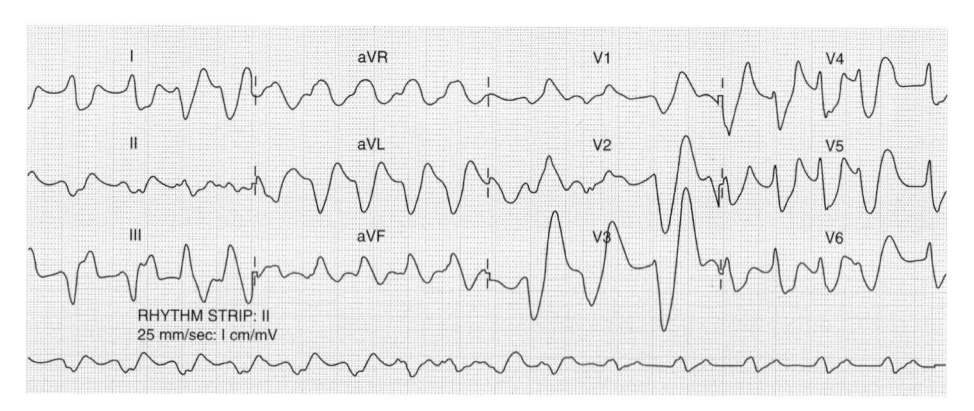

Figure 10.2 ECG.

ANSWERS

1. Summarize the case.

A young adult patient with drug overdose has presented with a depressed GCS. He is hypoxic and acidotic with abnormal renal function. He is also hyperkalaemic and hyponatraemic with associated ECG changes. Increased creatinine kinase suggests rhabdomyolysis to be the main cause of the acid–base and electrolyte imbalance.

2. What are the issues here and how would you proceed?

This is an acute emergency and the issues are:

- Drug overdose
- Hyperkalaemia

My aim here would be:
- ABC approach.
- Intubation and ventilation.
- Correction of high potassium.
- This patient requires a multidisciplinary approach with management in a critical care unit.

3. Comment on the biochemistry.

The biochemistry of the patient gives a picture of raised urea and creatinine which means the patient is in acute renal failure. The serum potassium is very high which requires immediate correction as this could lead to cardiac arrest.
- Electrolytes:
  - Serum potassium is very high
  - Serum sodium is low
- Serum creatinine kinase is high which signifies skeletal muscle damage.
- The blood gases show a metabolic acidosis with poor respiratory compensation. This could be due to the suppressed conscious state due to opioid overdose. The patient is also hypoxaemic which could be due to chest sepsis or ARDS.

4. Comment on the chest X-ray.

Posterior–anterior chest X-ray. There is loss of volume of the right hemithorax with tenting of the right hemidiaphragm. The right horizontal fissure is pulled superiorly and bowed with opacification of the right apex in keeping with right upper lobe collapse. The right hilum is pulled superiorly due to the loss of volume although the mediastinal contour is otherwise normal although a small hilar lesion can not be excluded on this chest X-ray.

5. What further investigations would be helpful?

Along with resuscitation I would like to
- Perform a toxic screen.
- Check alcohol levels.
- Liver function tests.
- Haematology screen along with coagulation.
- Echocardiography once the patient is stable.

6. What does the ECG show?

The ECG shows prolonged QRS, tall T waves, no P waves, showing signs of hyperkalaemia.

7. So potassium is 7.8 and there are ECG changes. What would you do now?

Hyperkalaemia with ECG changes is a medical emergency which can cause life-threatening arrhythmias. My aim is to reduce serum potassium by 1–2 mmols/l over 30 minutes, hence I would treat with the following:
- Step I: calcium gluconate 10%, 10–20 ml IV over 5–10 min.
- Step II: soluble insulin 10–20 units in 50 ml of 50% glucose IV over 15 min.
- Step III: salbutamol 5–10 mg nebulized every 30 min and calcium resonium 15 mg three times a day oral or PR.

I would continue monitoring the patient's potassium level.

8. What are the options to treat hyperkalaemia?

The options for management are as follows.
- **Physiologically antagonize K^+:** IV calcium antagonizes the effects of hyperkalaemia:

- Decreases membrane excitability within minutes but the effect is relatively short-lived (20–30 min). Dose is 10 ml 10% calcium gluconate given IV over 3 min repeated after 5–10 min if ECG changes persist. If there are signs of circulatory compromise, calcium chloride may be preferred. Calcium chloride is hypertonic (2000 mosmol/L) and ideally should be given through a central vein.
- **Shift K^+ into cells by using**:
- Glucose–insulin bolus: a bolus of 50 ml of 50% glucose containing soluble insulin (5–10 units) over 5–10 min. This can be repeated if necessary.
- Beta-2 adrenergic agonist: 10–20 mg of nebulized salbutamol decreases the plasma K^+ levels in 30 min.
- **Shift K^+ into cells by using $NaHCO_3$**: sodium bicarbonate ($NaHCO_3$) cause the shift of K^+ to intracellular fluid. HCO_3 delivered to the cortical collecting duct promotes K^+ excretion in the presence of aldosterone. Typically, 50 mmol is given over 5–10 min, repeated 30 min later if necessary. Used as emergency treatment.
- **Increase K^+ loss from the ECF** by either increased urinary or GIT losses.
  - **Urinary K^+ loss:** a loop diuretic can promote potassium loss.
  - **GIT K^+ loss** can be promoted by using K^+ binding exchange resins such as polystyrene sulfonate. Rectally administered resins work more rapidly as the rate of secretion of K^+ in the colon exceeds that in the proximal GIT.
- **Insufficient renal function for K^+** excretion is an indication for renal replacement therapy. Haemodialysis or haemofiltration is more efficient at removing K^+ than peritoneal dialysis.

Therapy	Dose	Onset of effect	Duration of effect	Mechanism of action
Calcium chloride	5–10 ml IV of 10% solution (500–1000 mg)	1–3 min	30–60 min	Physiological antagonism
Sodium bicarbonate	1 mEq/kg IV bolus	5–10 min	1–2 hours	Stimulate exchange of cellular H^+ for Na^+, thus leading to stimulation of the Na-K ATPase
Insulin plus glucose (use 1 unit of insulin/2.5 g glucose)	Regular insulin 10 U IV plus 50 ml D_{50} (25 g glucose) IV bolus	30 min	4–6 hours	Promotes intracellular K transfer
Nebulized salbutamol	10–20 mg nebulized over 15 min	15 min	15–90 min	Promotes intracellular K transfer
Hyperventilation	Aim for $PaCO_2$ ~4 kPa	Immediate	Duration of hyperventilation	Promotes intracellular K transfer
Furosemide	40–80 mg IV bolus	With onset of diuresis	Until diuretic effect ends	K excretion
Kayexalate	15–50 g PO or PR, plus sorbitol	1–2 hours	4–6 hours	Reduced K absorption
Peritoneal dialysis or haemodialysis		Immediate	Until dialysis completed	K removal

9. What is rhabdomyolysis and how it is caused?

Rhabdomyolysis is the breakdown of muscle fibres resulting in the release of myoglobin leading to acute tubular necrosis and kidney failure.

- Trauma: direct injury to muscle resulting in disruption of the sarcolemma and leakage of cell content.
- Infection:
  - *Legionella* is the bacterium most commonly reported to cause rhabdomyolysis. The pathogenesis of it is believed to be due to direct invasion and toxic degeneration of muscle fibres.
  - Group A beta haemolytic streptococcal infection is another known bacterial cause.
  - Viral influenza A and B.
- Metabolic and genetic factors:
  - Genetic defects of muscle where there is either inability to use ATP or inadequate ATP.
  - Hypophosphataemia.
  - Hypokalaemia creates a negative potassium balance, which causes rhabdomyolysis.
- Drugs and certain toxins:
  - Ethanol causes metabolic derangement by direct toxic effect and disruption of the blood supply due to immobilization. Ethanol abuse may cause hypophosphataemia and hypokalaemia, which are additive causes of rhabdomyolysis.
  - Patients who overdose on narcotics and sedative hypnotics and remain immobilized for extended periods may have pressure necrosis that results in rhabdomyolysis.

10. How is rhabdomyolysis diagnosed?

The diagnosis of rhabdomyolysis can be confirmed by means of certain laboratory variables. The most reliable indicator is creatine kinase (CK).

- Assessing CK is most useful because of its ease of detection from serum and its presence in serum immediately after muscle injury.
- The CK peaks in 24–36 hours and decreases at a rate of 36–40% per day. The serum half-life of CK is approximately 36 hours.
- Failure of CK to decrease suggests ongoing muscle injury.
- CK levels 5 times higher than normal suggests rhabdomyolysis and are frequently 100 times above normal or even higher.

Myoglobin

- Measuring plasma myoglobin is not reliable because its half-life is 1–3 hours and it is cleared from plasma within 6 hours.
- The result may be false negative if myoglobin is not measured at the right time. A positive test result may help to confirm the diagnosis.
- Urine myoglobin is presumed if the urine is positive for blood but negative for red blood cells.

11. What is the mechanism of renal injury in rhabdomyolysis?

Perhaps the most significant complication of rhabdomyolysis is acute renal failure (ARF), seen in about 30% of patients. It may be caused by:

- Direct nephrotoxic effects of myoglobin, by its precipitation in renal tubules, or by its conversion to ferrihaemate at a pH <5.6, which is toxic to renal tubules and also precipitates.
- Recently a potential role for oxygen-free radicals has been suggested in renal injury in myoglobinuria, as well as haemoglobinuria. The laboratory values, as described above, are typical of ARF of any aetiology, except that hyperkalaemia and hyperphosphataemia tend to occur early,

and serum creatinine concentration tends to be higher than expected for a given level of azotaemia, because of the release of previously formed creatinine from damaged muscle. Dialysis may be required in 50–70 % of patients.

12. What can you do to prevent renal injury in the patients with rhabdomyolysis?

The renal injury could be prevented with rapid hydration and high urine output.
- Early and aggressive fluids (hydration) may prevent kidney damage by rapidly flushing myoglobin out of the kidneys.
- Following the correction of hypovolaemia, administration of mannitol to induce diuresis.
- Some patients may need kidney dialysis.
- Alkalinization of urine prevents the dissociation of myoglobulin into globin and ferrihaemate, which are toxic to the renal tubules. The possibility of aggravation of hypocalcaemia by large doses of bicarbonate should be borne in mind, although this is rather uncommon, especially if hypovolaemia is corrected.
- It is essential to maintain a urine output of 200 ml/hour or more.

13. What are the indications for renal replacement therapy in this patient?

- I would consider renal replacement therapy when the conservative management has failed.
- Potassium >6 mmol/L or H^+ >80 nmol/L or creatinine > 200 µmol/L.

Further reading

Bagley, W.H., Yang, H., Shah, K.H., et al. Rhabdomyolysis. *Internal and Emergency Medicine* 2007; **2**:210–18.

de Meijer, A.R., Fikkers, B.G., de Keijzer, M.H., et al. Serum creatine kinase as predictor of clinical course in rhabdomyolysis: a 5-year intensive care survey. *Intensive Care Medicine* 2003; **29**:1121–5.

Hall, A.P. and Henry, J.A. Acute toxic effects of 'Ecstasy' (MDMA) and related compounds: overview of pathophysiology and clinical management. *British Journal of Anaesthesia* 2006; **96**:678–85.

Chapter 10

Short cases

QUESTIONS

Short case 1: Post-tonsillectomy bleeding

The ENT registrar call you for a 4-year-old child who had tonsillectomy as a day-care procedure and who is now bleeding. He wishes you to assess the patient and would like to re-explore in theatre.

1. What are the main concerns in this case?
2. How would you manage this patient?
3. How would you assess blood loss?
4. How would you proceed if the surgeon wished to re-explore?

Short case 2: Direct laryngoscopy

A 76-year-old male patient requires direct laryngoscopy along with pharyngoscopy with biopsy under anaesthesia.

1. What are the key issues in your anaesthetic assessment?
2. The ENT surgeon has requested you to use a microlaryngeal tube (MLT). How would you anaesthetize this patient?
3. What can you tell me about MLTs?
4. The surgeon is unable to take a biopsy and would like to take the tube out. How would you proceed?
5. What is jet ventilation and how will you conduct jet ventilation?
6. How would you maintain anaesthesia during the biopsy?
7. What are the complications of this technique?

Short case 3: Penetrating eye injury

A 35-year-old man presented to A&E with a fishhook embedded in his eyes. He had a full meal before the accident.

1. What are your concerns in this case?
2. What are the determinants of intraocular pressure?
3. Is this a surgical emergency?
4. The patient has a full stomach. Outline management of anaesthesia for a penetrating eye injury.

ANSWERS

Short case 1: Post-tonsillectomy bleeding

1. What are the main concerns in this case?

This is a case of a postoperative bleeding tonsil. This is a medical emergency. My main concerns in this case of a bleeding tonsil are:

- Full stomach with swallowing of blood; risk of aspiration.
- Blood loss with low haemoglobin and hypovolaemia.
- Potential for difficult airway due to:
  - Bleeding.
  - Oedema of oropharynx.
  - Poor visualization of larynx.
- Residual anaesthetic effects.
- Stressed and anxious patient and parents.
- Poor venous access.

2. How would you manage this patient?

We have a 4-year-old patient who had tonsillectomy who is now readmitted with bleeding. This is a medical emergency my aim would be to:

- Immediately call for senior help (consultant on call).
- Assess the patient with a view to resuscitation.
- If child can tolerate, provide oxygen by mask.
- Send bloods for haemoglobin, coagulation, and cross-match.
- Reassure the patient and the parents.
- Review the patient's anaesthetic chart for the size of ETT and grade of airway.
- Alert the theatre team and get the theatre ready with experienced staff.

3. How would you assess blood loss?

Post-tonsillectomy bleeds are difficult to estimate for blood loss. The patients tend to swallow the blood and can vomit some blood as well. Hence the blood loss is underestimated. In situations like this my aim is to assess the blood loss based on the following clinical signs of hypovolaemia:

- Initial hypovolaemia:
  - Tachycardia
  - Tachypnoea
  - Low pulse volume
  - Delayed capillary refill time
  - Decreased urine output
- Advanced hypovolaemia:
  - Pallor
  - Hypotension (late sign)
  - Deteriorating level of consciousness or altered sensorium

4. How would you proceed if the surgeon wished to re-explore?

I would proceed with the following plan:

Preoperatively in theatre

- Resuscitation with quick anaesthetic assessment along with review of previous anaesthetic chart.

- Resuscitation is essential with adequate IV access or insertion of an interosseous needle.
- Preoperatively, cross-matched packed red blood cells available and transfused as necessary.
- Consultant anaesthetist in theatre.
- Paediatric airway trolley available with ETT (internal diameter) one size smaller at 4.5 mm (ETT size = 4 + age/4).
- Before induction, a selection of laryngoscope blades, and two suction catheters should be immediately available.

Anaesthetic
- Anaesthesia is induced once the child is haemodynamically stable.
- Preoxygenation and rapid sequence induction with slight head-down positioning of the patient ensures rapid control of the airway and protection from pulmonary aspiration.
- Consideration should be given to adopting the left lateral position if bleeding is excessive.
- Controlled ventilation provides good conditions for haemostasis.

Intraoperatively
- Fluid resuscitation and transfusion of blood and blood products should continue intraoperatively as necessary.
- Once haemostasis is achieved, a large-bore stomach tube is passed under direct vision and the stomach emptied.
- Neuromuscular block is antagonized and the trachea is extubated, with the child fully awake in the recovery position.
- A combination of ondansetron 0.1–0.2 mg/kg and dexamethasone 0.1–0.5 mg/kg (maximum 8 mg) intraoperatively have been shown to greatly reduce the incidence of PONV.

Postoperatively
- Extended stay in recovery for close monitoring.
- Pain-relief.
- Rescue cyclizine 0.5–1 mg/kg.
- Check postoperative haemoglobin.
- Update the parents.

Further reading

Allman, K.G. and Wilson, I.H. *Oxford Handbook of Anaesthesia*, 2nd edn. Chapter 25: Ear, nose, and throat surgery, see pp. 612–14. Oxford: Oxford University Press, 2006.

Ravi, R. and Howell, T. Anaesthesia for paediatric ear, nose, and throat surgery. *Continuing Education in Anaesthesia Critical Care & Pain* 2007; **7**:33–7.

Short case 2: Direct laryngoscopy

1. What are the key issues in your anaesthetic assessment?

- Assessment of airway:
    - History: stridor, hoarseness, dyspnoea.
    - Examination: Mallampati score, large mandible, tongue, and epiglottis, MP grading.
    - Investigations: CT and indirect laryngoscopy by surgeon may be useful.
    - Evaluation of location, size, extent, and mobility of any lesion.

- Previous anaesthetic and surgical findings.
- Geriatric age and pathophysiology.
- Evaluation of coexisting cardiovascular and respiratory morbidity.
- Shared airway.
- Very still operating environment with paralysis but rapid return of consciousness and airway reflexes to reduce postoperative problems.

2. The ENT surgeon has requested you to use a microlaryngeal tube (MLT). How would you anaesthesia this patient?

I will use an IV anaesthetic technique with full muscular paralysis and full monitoring using a MLT to provide an optimal position for the surgeon to perform the procedure with extension of the neck.

3. What can you tell me about MLTs?

A MLT is a long, narrow, cuffed tracheal tube (e.g. 31 cm long, 4–6 mm internal diameter).

Advantages: the MLT gives the surgeon better operating conditions and still permits conventional IPPV without excessive increases in ventilation pressure; further permitting use of conventional anaesthetic equipment.

Disadvantages: tube obscures the posterior 1/3rd of the glottis, operative field is relatively mobile.

4. The surgeon is unable to take a biopsy and would like to take the tube out. How would you proceed?

This is a common situation when the ETT obstructs the view of the surgeon or the surgeon would like to biopsy below the glottis. This is possible using:

- **Jet ventilation technique:**
  - Advantages: good view, decreased stimulation.
  - Disadvantages: no airway protection, possibility of barotraumas, may not be able to humidify and warm inspired gases, risk of gastric insufflation.
- **Intermittent apnoea without intubation:**
  - Advantages: unobstructed surgical view.
  - Disadvantages: poor airway protection, poor control of anaesthetic depth.

5. What is jet ventilation and how will you conduct jet ventilation?

Jet ventilation is a technique of airway ventilation for upper airway surgery introduced by Sanders. Driving pressure can be adjusted between zero and 4 bar and is connected to a stiff narrow cannula positioned at the inlet of the laryngoscope. A Sanders injector with pressure gauge and adjustable driving pressure controls the pressure required for the oxygen boluses delivered. Due to the Venturi effect of a high-velocity stream of oxygen the ambient air is entrained through the laryngoscope entrance. The jet injector provides a simple approach to deliver physiological tidal volume.

6. How would you maintain anaesthesia during the biopsy?

I will use total intravenous venous anaesthesia (TIVA) using propofol, remifentanil and atracurium with neuromuscular monitoring.
Monitoring: pulse oximetry, NIBP, ECG, end-tidal carbon-dioxide.

7. What are the complications of this technique?

- Problems with a rigid scope:
  - Maximal extension of atlanto-axial joint.
  - Damage to teeth.

Chapter 10

- ◆ Bleeding.
- ◆ Airway oedema.
- Anaesthetic issues:
  - ◆ No airway protection.
  - ◆ Possibility of barotraumas; pneumomediastinum and pneumothorax.
  - ◆ Dehydration of mucosa as unable to humidify and warm inspired gases.
  - ◆ Risk of gastric distension insufflation and regurgitation.
  - ◆ Laryngospasm and laryngeal incompetence postoperatively.

Further reading

Hunsaker, D.H. Anesthesia for microlaryngeal surgery: the case for subglottic jet ventilation. *Laryngoscope* 1994; **104**(8 Pt 2 Suppl 65):1–30.

Nagler, J. and Bachur, R.G. Advanced airway management. *Current Opinion in Pediatrics* 2009; **21**:299–305.

Short case 3: Penetrating eye injury

1. What are your concerns in this case?

- Emergency surgery.
- Full stomach.
- Penetrating eye injury.
- Anaesthetic manoeuvre may alter the intraocular pressure (IOP) leading to extrusion of vitreous humour and loss of vision.

2. What are the determinants of intraocular pressure?

The IOP is determined by the balance between production and drainage of aqueous humour. This is possible by:

- Changes in choroidal blood flow volume.
- Vitreous volume.
- Extra-ocular tone.

Normal IOP is 12–20 mmHg.

3. Is this a surgical emergency?

The situation is not always an emergency and some time can be spent in adequately preparing the patient for anaesthesia and surgery. The surgery should be performed within 12 hours to minimize the risk of infection. Risk:benefit ratio should be appropriately balanced based on the multidisciplinary discussion with the surgeon.

4. The patient has a full stomach. Outline management of anaesthesia for a penetrating eye injury.

Anaesthetic assessment

- Full history and examination.
- Trauma:
  - ◆ Associated injuries: extensive trauma managed appropriately.

- ABCDE if required.
- Fasting status.
• Eye:
  - Nature of injury, acuity.

Preoperative

- Premedication:
  - Sodium citrate.
  - Antacid: IV—ranitidine.
  - H2 blocker.
  - Prokinetic: metoclopramide.
- Prevention of vitreous herniation:
  - Avoid pressure on the eye ball via face mask.
  - Appropriate dosage to prevent coughing or bucking.

Intraoperative

- Monitoring and access:
  - Routine: IV, ECG, SpO_2, NIBP, gas analysis, disconnect, etc.
- Induction—modified rapid sequence induction:
  - Preoxygenation.
  - Predosing with lidocaine, remifentanil, beta-blocker IV.
  - Induction with thiopentone or propofol.
  - Relaxation options:
    - Suxamethonium.
    - Predose with NDB followed by suxamethonium.
    - High-dose NDB (e.g. rocuronium).
    - Trade-off between risk of coughing and increased IOP with suxamethonium.

Maintenance

- Lower IOP:
  - Mild hyperventilation.
  - Beta-blocker.
  - Acetazolamide.
  - Mannitol.
  - Hypotension.
- Monitor muscle relaxation to prevent coughing.
- Prophylaxis: antibiotics, tetanus.

Emergence

- Prevention of coughing/vomiting and protection of airway are conflicting priorities.
- Extubate awake in lateral position.
- Give narcotic and antiemetic before emergence.

Further reading

Murgatroyd, H. and Bembridge, J. Intraocular pressure. *Continuing Education in Anaesthesia Critical Care & Pain* 2008; **8**:100–3.

Vinik, H.R. Intra ocular pressure changes during rapid sequence induction and intubation: A comparison of rocuronium, atracurium and succinylcholine. *Journal of Clinical Anaesthesia* 1999; **11**:95–100.

Clinical science

QUESTIONS

Anatomy: Heart circulation

1. Describe the arterial supply to the heart.
2. What are the regional supplies to the heart?
3. What is the normal myocardial blood supply?
4. How is coronary perfusion maintained?
5. How is coronary blood flow and autoregulation maintained?

Physiology: Prone position

1. What are the indications for the prone position?
2. What are the physiological changes associated with the prone position?
3. What could be the mechanism to improve oxygenation in the prone position?
4. What are the complications of a prolonged prone position?
5. Are there any alternatives to prone ventilation?

Pharmacology: Deep vein thrombosis

1. What are the important components which can lead to intravascular thrombosis?
2. What preoperative groups of patients are at high risk of deep vein thrombosis (DVT)?
3. What physiological mechanisms regulate clotting?
4. What interventions can be used to prevent DVT in a patient?
5. There is a patient who has a suspected pulmonary embolism (PE). How would you practically set up treatment for PE?
6. What are the recommendations for timing of dosages of anticoagulants with regards to epidural insertion/withdrawal?

Physics and clinical measurements: Defibrillator

1. Define the terms: resistance, inductance, and capacitance. What are their units?
2. What is a defibrillator and its components?
3. When would you use a defibrillator?
4. What are the differences between monophasic and biphasic defibrillators?
5. What are implantable cardioverter defibrillators (ICDs)?

ANSWERS

Anatomy: Heart circulation

1. Describe the arterial supply to the heart.

Right coronary artery (RCA) originates from the **anterior** aortic sinus, runs forward between the pulmonary artery (PA), and right atrial appendage; in the right atrioventricular groove branches include the:
- Anterior cardiac artery.
- Acute marginal branch—inferior border of the heart (right ventricle, RV).
- Posterior interventricular artery, or posterior descending artery (PDA).
- Branch to the SA node.

RCA anastomoses with,
- The circumflex artery—in the atrioventricular groove
- The left anterior descending artery (LAD) via the PDA branch—in the interventricular septum dominant in 85–90% of patients, it supplies the:
  - Posterior septum.
  - The posterior and inferior parts of the left ventricle (LV).
  - The atrioventricular node in 85% of individuals.

Left coronary artery (LCA) arises from the posterior aortic sinus and passes forward behind the pulmonary trunk. It divides in the space between the aorta and the pulmonary artery into:

- **The LAD**: this passes along the anterior interventricular groove towards the apex, turns round the lower border, and anastomoses with the posterior interventricular artery. Supplies the LV, anterior septum and some RV, also branches to form the:
  - Septal perforators.
  - Diagonal branches—variable number.
- **The circumflex branch**: this passes around the left border of the heart to reach the posterior interventricular groove branches to form the **obtuse marginal**—supplies the posterior LV wall. It supplies:
  - The SA node in 40% of individuals.
  - The lateral wall of the ventricle via the marginal arteries.

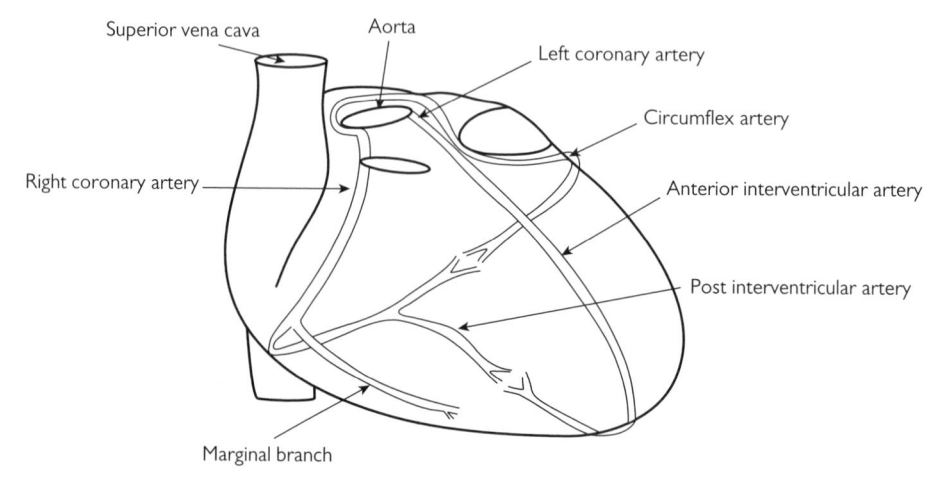

Figure 10.3 Coronary circulation.

Chapter 10

2. What are the regional arterial supplies to the heart?
- Right ventricle: branch of RCA except the upper anterior border.
- Left ventricle: branch of LCA except small diaphragmatic area.
- Interventricular septum: equally from RCA and LCA.
- Atria: variable supply from the same side.
- SA node: 65% from RCA and 35% from LCA.
- Atrioventricular node: 80% RCA and 20% LCA.

3. What is the normal myocardial blood supply?
Basal blood flow is 70–80 ml/100 g/min. Maximum flow is 300–400 ml/100 g/min. The blood supply to the myocardium flows from the left and right coronary arteries. Because of the high intramural pressure during systole, most of the flow takes place during diastole.

4. How is coronary perfusion maintained?
The coronary perfusion pressure is the difference between aortic root diastolic pressure and left ventricular end diastolic pressure (LVED). In effect, myocardial capillaries function as a Starling resistor. In systole, driving pressure and LV pressure are the same, so flow to the LV will cease. In the RV, pressures are lower so some flow will take place during systole. Systolic pressure is not transmitted equally to all parts of the ventricular wall and the epicardial arteries are slightly removed from this intraventricular pressure. This may further impact on flow. Systemic vasoactive agents (e.g. adrenaline, AVP) may influence the tone of large and small coronary vessels. Platelets (serotonin, ADP) also release substances that affect vascular tone.

5. How is coronary blood flow and autoregulation maintained?
At rest the heart extracts 70–80% of the oxygen delivered to it. Myocardial metabolism can only increase with increased coronary blood flow and supply of oxygen.

The coronary circulation shows considerable autoregulation. The calibre of the vessels and the blood flow is influenced by:
- Pressure changes in the aorta.
- By chemical factors.
- By neural factors.

Chemical factors
The products of metabolism cause coronary vasodilatation due to oxygen deficiency and increased local concentrations of CO_2, H^+, K^+, lactate, prostaglandins, adenine nucleotides, and adenosine. Asphyxia, hypoxia and intracoronary injections of cyanide all increase coronary blood flow by 200–300% in both denervated and intact hearts. This is due to the direct action of the vasomotor tone but also releases adenosine and opens ATP-sensitive potassium channels.

Neural factors
The coronary arterioles contain:
- Alpha-adrenoceptors, which mediate vasoconstriction.
- Beta-adrenoceptors, which mediate vasodilatation.

Humoral control
- The peptide hormones include antidiuretic hormone, atrial natriuretic peptide, vasoactive intestinal peptide, and calcitonin gene-related peptide. Antidiuretic hormone causes coronary constriction in stressed patients.
- The peptides cause endothelium-mediated vasodilatation.

- Angiotensin II causes coronary vasoconstriction and enhances calcium influx and releases endothelin, which is the strongest vasoconstrictor peptide.
- Angiotensin-converting enzyme (ACE) inactivates bradykinin, a vasodilator.

Special features of the coronary circulation
There are small muscle fibres with high capillary density so have a shorter diffusion distance.
- High basal oxygen extraction (>60%); this can increase to >90% during exercise.
- Well-developed autoregulation.
- Metabolic vasodilatation dominates regulation (possibly adenosine, K^+, and acidosis).
- Beta-adrenoceptors ensure that adrenaline causes vasodilatation.

Further reading
Kaplan, J.A., Reich, D.L., Konstadt, S.N. (eds.) *Cardiac Anaesthesia*, 4th edn. Philadelphia, PA: WB Saunders, 1999.
Ramanathan, T. and Skinner, H. Coronary blood flow. *Continuing Education in Anaesthesia, Critical Care & Pain* 2005; **5**:61–4.

Physiology: Prone position

1. What are the indications for the prone position?
- **Theatre:** operations requiring prone position for surgical access (posterior fossa, spine, etc.).
- **ICU:** improvement in oxygenation in severe ARDS.

2. What are the physiological changes associated with the prone position?
- **Cardiovascular:** increased intra-abdominal pressure can cause decreased venous return, hypotension.
- **Renal and splanchnic:** decreased perfusion.
- **Respiratory:** altered ventilation and perfusion distribution, effects on respiratory mechanics—decreased thoraco-abdominal compliance, changes in regional diaphragmatic motion.

3. What could be the mechanism to improve oxygenation in the prone position?
Various mechanisms have been proposed to explain the improvement of oxygenation when a patient is turned prone. These include:
- Redirecting the compressive forces of the heart weight on the lungs.
- Redistribution of secretions, atelectasis, and interstitial oedema away from the posterior areas.
- Redistribution of pulmonary perfusion to less oedematous areas.
- Increasing alveolar recruitment.
- Increasing the end-expiratory volume.
- Changes in regional diaphragmatic excursion. Improved respiratory mechanics.
- Reduction in mechanical factors associated with ventilator associated lung injury.

4. What are the complications of a prolonged prone position?
- Facial oedema, injury to eye to extent of blindness.
- Pressure sores: ulcerations frequently involving the chin, ears, anterior region of the chest, iliac crests, and knees.

Chapter 10

- Airway obstruction and accidental extubation leading to loss of airway.
- Transient decrease in oxygen saturation.
- Apical atelectasis due to incorrect positioning of the tracheal tube.
- Hypotension, arrhythmias, and difficulty in resuscitation if required.
- Loss of access to vascular catheters, drains, other catheters.
- Increased need for sedation: this can increase the occurrence of neuromuscular paresis which frequently appears in critically ill patients in ICUs.
- Difficulties with enteral feeding due to vomiting or an increase in gastric residue.

5. Are there any alternatives to prone ventilation?

Rotational (kinetic) therapy can be used—patients are turned laterally from horizontal to about 40°, often several times an hour on a rotational bed. Compared with rotational ventilation, there is less chance of accidental displacement of tubes etc., pressure sores, cardiovascular instability. Access to the patient is also better.

Further reading

Chatte, G., Sab, J.M., Dubois, J.M., et al. Prone position in mechanically ventilated patients with severe acute respiratory failure. *American Journal of Respiratory and Critical Care Medicine* 1997; **155**:473–8.

Fridrich, P., Krafft, P., Hochleuthner, H., et al. The effects of long-term prone positioning in patients with trauma-induced adult respiratory distress syndrome. *Anesthesia & Analgesia* 1996; **83**:1206–11.

Ware, L.B. and Matthay, M.A. The acute respiratory distress syndrome. *New England Journal of Medicine* 2000; **342**: 1334–9.

Pharmacology: Deep vein thrombosis

1. What are the important components which can lead to intravascular thrombosis?

Virchow's triad refers to factors predisposing to vascular thrombosis. These factors are:

- Changes in the vessel wall.
- Changes in the pattern of blood flow (flow volume).
- Changes in the constituents of blood (hypercoagulability).

2. What preoperative groups of patients are at high risk of deep vein thrombosis (DVT)?

- **Venous stasis:** recent surgery, trauma, lack of ambulation, pregnancy, stroke.
- **Abnormality of vessel wall:** varicose veins, drug-induced irritation, previous DVT.
- **Hypercoagulable state:** malignancy, inflammatory bowel disease, obesity, advanced age, deficiencies of endogenous anticoagulants.

3. What physiological mechanisms regulate clotting?

Physiologically the clotting mechanism is balanced by opposing reactions preventing coagulation, e.g. anti-thrombin III which inhibits active factors II, IX, X, XI and XII. Prostacyclin secreted by vascular endothelium inhibits platelet aggregation.

4. What interventions can be used to prevent DVT in a patient?

The interventions which are commonly employed to prevent DVT are:
- **Low-risk group:** graduated compression stockings, early ambulation.
- **Medium-risk group:** external pneumatic compression, minidose heparin.
- **High-risk group:** external pneumatic compression, heparin, warfarin, intracaval filter in patients with known DVT.

5. There is a patient who has suspected pulmonary embolism (PE). How would you practically set up treatment for PE?

- Heparin should be given to patients with intermediate or high clinical probability before imaging.
- Unfractionated heparin should be considered as a first-dose bolus, in massive PE, or where rapid reversal of effect may be needed.
- Low-molecular-weight heparin (LMWH) should be considered as preferable to unfractionated heparin, having equal efficacy and safety and being easier to use.
- Oral anticoagulation should only be commenced once venous thromboembolism (VTE) is diagnosed.
- The target INR should be 2.0–3.0; when this is achieved, heparin can be discontinued.
- The standard duration of oral anticoagulation is:
  - 4–6 weeks for temporary risk factors.
  - 3 months for first idiopathic PE, and
  - At least 6 months for other; the risk of bleeding should be balanced with that of further VTE.

BTS guidelines: DVT with or without pulmonary embolism

Enoxaparin 1 mg/kg/12 hours or enoxaparin 1.5 mg/kg/24 hours as a 'bridge' to warfarin. Treatment with the 24-hour regimen is FDA approved only for inpatients.

6. What are the recommendations for timing of dosages of anticoagulants with regards to epidural insertion and catheter withdrawal?

American Society of Regional Anaesthesia and Pain Medicine guidelines:
- **Antiplatelet medications:**
  - No contraindication with NSAIDs.
  - Stop:
    - Ticlopidine: 14 days pre-block.
    - Clopidogrel: 7 days pre-block.
- **Unfractionated heparin:**
  - Subcutaneous: no contraindication, consider delaying heparin until after block if technical difficulty anticipated.
  - Intravenous: IV heparin > 1 hour after neuraxial technique, remove catheter 4 hours after last heparin dose; no mandatory delay if traumatic.
- **Low-molecular-weight heparin:** LMWH 24 hours after surgery, regardless of technique; remove neuraxial catheter 2 hours before first LMWH dose.
- **Preoperative dose of LMWH:**
  - Needle placement 10–12 hours after LMWH.
  - First postoperative dose 6–8 hours.
  - Epidural catheters removed 10–12 hours after LMWH and 4 hours prior to next dose.
  - Postpone LMWH for 24 hours if traumatic.
- **Warfarin:** document normal INR after discontinuation (prior to neuraxial technique); remove catheter when INR <1.5 (initiation of therapy).

Chapter 10

- **Thrombolytics:**
  - No data on safety interval for performance of neuraxial technique or catheter removal.
  - Follow fibrinogen level.

Further reading

Allman, K.G. and Wilson, I.H. *Oxford Handbook of Anaesthesia*, 2nd edn. Chapter 1: General consideration, see pp.10–13; Chapter 41: Regional anaesthesia, see pp. 1058–60. Oxford: Oxford University Press, 2006.

BTS Guidelines for the Management of Suspected Acute Pulmonary Embolism, 2003. Available at: http://www.brit-thoracic.org.uk/clinical-information/pulmonary-embolism/pulmonary-embolism-guidelines.aspx

Green, L. and Machin, S.J. Managing anticoagulated patients during neuraxial anaesthesia. *British Journal of Haematology* 2010; **149**:195–208.

Gogarten, W., Vandermeulen, E., Van Aken, H., et al. Regional anaesthesia and antithrombotic agents: recommendations of the European Society of Anaesthesiology. *European Journal of Anaesthesiology* 2010; **27**:999–1015.

NICE. *Reducing the risk of venous thromboembolism (deep vein thrombosis and pulmonary embolism) in patients admitted to hospital* (Clinical Guidance 92). London: NICE, 2010. Available at: http://www.nice.org.uk/guidance/CG92

Physics and clinical measurements: Defibrillators

1. Define the terms: resistance, inductance, and capacitance. What are their units?

Resistance: resistance along a conductor to the flow of current. It is measured in ohms (Ω). It is defined as the resistance which allows a current of one ampere to flow under the influence of a potential of 1 volt (V).

Capacitance: the ability of an object to hold electrical charge. Capacitance is measured in farads. The farad is the capacitance of an object when its electric potential increases by 1 V when one coulomb of charge is added to it.

Inductance: electrical current is induced in a wire by movement of the wire relative to a magnetic field (Fleming's right hand rule). Inductance is a measure of the amount of magnetic flux produced for a given electric current. The SI unit is henry (H).

2. What is a defibrillator and its components?

Defibrillators are used to apply a short direct current across the myocardium to terminate arrhythmias. The intention of defibrillation is to stop the heart's electrical activity momentarily in the hope that normal sinus rhythm will resume. The central component of a defibrillator is a capacitor. This is used to store the required charge before discharging across the patient's heart.

Other components include a transformer (to step up the mains voltage), a rectifier (to convert mains AC current into DC current, allowing charge to accumulate on the capacitor), a switch for defibrillation itself, and an inductor which alters the waveform pattern of current delivery.

There also needs to be a connection to the patient. With external defibrillators, this is via a set of two paddles. Skin impedance must be overcome, so gel pads can be put onto the chest or hands-free paddles incorporating adhesive and gel can be used. A defibrillator system typically delivers a current of 50 A into a resistance of 50 Ω. Since $V = IR$, the voltage required is 2.5 kV.

3. When would you use a defibrillator?
- Emergency defibrillation (VF, pulseless VT): 200–360 J.
- Elective or semi-elective cardioversion (AF, VT with pulse): 50–150 J depending on response.
- Internal defibrillation during cardiothoracic surgery: 10–25 J.
- Implantable internal defibrillator: 25 J.

4. What are the difference between monophasic and biphasic defibrillators?

Monophasic: until the late 1980s, external defibrillators delivered a Lown type waveform, a heavily damped sinusoidal impulse having a mainly uniphasic characteristic.

Biphasic: the biphasic defibrillator alternates the direction of the pulses, completing one cycle in approximately 10 ms. When applied to external defibrillators, biphasic defibrillation significantly decreases the energy level necessary for successful defibrillation. This, in turn, decreases risk of burns and myocardial damage.

VF could be returned to normal sinus rhythm in 60% of cardiac arrest patients treated with a single shock from a monophasic defibrillator. Most biphasic defibrillators have a first-shock success rate of >90%.

5. What are implantable cardioverter defibrillators (ICDs)?

Also known as automatic internal cardiac defibrillator (AICDs). These devices are implants, similar to pacemakers (and many can also perform the pacemaking function). They constantly monitor the patient's heart rhythm, and automatically administer shocks for various life-threatening arrhythmias, according to the device's programming.

Many modern devices can distinguish between VF, VT, and more benign arrhythmias like SVT and AF. Some devices may attempt overdrive pacing prior to synchronized cardioversion. When the life threatening arrhythmia is ventricular fibrillation, the device is programmed to proceed immediately to an unsynchronized shock.

Defibrillator mode codes

In 1993, a NASPE/BPEG (North American Society of Pacing and Electrophysiology and British Pacing and Electrophysiology Group) defibrillator code was approved. The four position code describes defibrillator, arrhythmia diagnostic, and data storage capabilities:

- The first position of the code indicates the shock chamber—none, atrium, ventricle, or dual (*O, A, V,* or *D*).
- The second position indicates the chamber in which antitachycardia pacing is delivered—also coded *O, A, V,* or *D*.
- Position three indicates the means by which tachyarrhythmia is detected, either with the intracardiac electrogram (*E*) or by haemodynamic means (*H*). It is assumed that haemodynamic monitors include electrogram diagnostics.
- The fourth position of the code is the three- or five-letter code for the pacemaker capability of the device. For example, a ventricular defibrillator with haemodynamic or ECG tachyarrhythmia detection and with adaptive rate ventricular antibradycardia pacing would be labelled VOH-VVIR.

Further reading

Saluke, T.V., Dob, D., and Sutton, R. Pacemakers and defibrillators: Anaesthetic implications. *British Journal of Anaesthesia* 2004: **93**:95–104.

Chapter 11

Clinical anaesthesia

Long case: A patient with multiple medical issues *235*
Short cases *240*
   Questions *240*
   Answers *241*
      Short case 1: Postoperative nausea and vomiting *241*
      Short case 2: Obstructive sleep apnoea *242*
      Short case 3: Ventilator-associated pneumonia *243*

Clinical science

Questions *245*
Answers *246*
   Anatomy: Vagus nerve and recurrent laryngeal nerve *246*
   Physiology: Nutrition in a critically ill patient *247*
   Pharmacology: Adrenaline *248*
   Physics and clinical measurements: Hagen–Poiseuille equation, Heliox *250*

Clinical anaesthesia

Long case: A patient with multiple medical issues

A 64-year-old lady is booked for urgent lumbar discectomy. Past medical history includes alcohol dependency and malnutrition. She has been hospitalized for 2 weeks with severe back pain. Following a lumbar MRI on admission, she was diagnosed with L4/5 discitis. She has been receiving appropriate IV antibiotics. During this time she has suffered from recurrent episodes of diarrhoea. Four days earlier a pleural effusion was diagnosed via chest X-ray. A sample was aspirated under ultrasound guidance. Two hours ago the patient reported new sensory deficits in her left leg and inability to pass urine. An emergency lumbar MRI has been performed which supports the clinical diagnosis of cauda equina syndrome.

On examination: a thin, restless lady, with severe pain.

Clinical examination	**Temperature: 37.7°C; weight: 51 kg; height: 162cm**			
	Pulse: 105/min, regular; BP: 110/70 mmHg; respiratory rate: 24/min; SpO$_2$ 0.93 (FiO$_2$ 0.21)			
	Chest: dull to percussion at right base with reduced breath sounds throughout the right chest. Vesicular breath sounds on the left side. Apex palpable in the 5th left interspace in the mid-clavicular line			
	Cardiovascular system: heart sounds normal			
	Focal tenderness over lower lumbar spine. Numbness below left knee, posterior thigh and saddle area. Otherwise grossly normal on examination.			
	Allergies: no known drug allergies			
	Medication: regular paracetamol, thiamine, and IV antibiotics, with PRN codeine			
Laboratory investigations	Hb	9.2 g/dL	Na	138 mEq/L
	MCV	106 fL	K	2.8 mEq/L
	WBC	11.4 × 10^9/L	Urea	3.4 mmol/L
	Platelets	119 × 10^9/L	Creatinine	68 μmol/L
			Albumin	21 g/L
	PT	14.2 sec	Total bilirubin	22 μmol/L
	APTT	32.4 sec	ALP	183 IU/L
	Fibrinogen	1.7 g/L	ALT	59 IU/L
			Glucose (random)	5.7 mmol/L
Pleural fluid	Gross appearance		Straw-coloured	
	Protein		19 g/L	
	LDH		23 IU/L	
	Serum LDH		91 IU/L	
	pH		7.51	
	Microscopy/culture/Gram stain		Negative	

QUESTIONS

1. Summarize the case.
2. How urgent is this operation?
3. Comment on the chest X-ray.
4. What does the ECG show?
5. Would you take this patient to theatre immediately? Why/why not?
6. Which method should be used for chest drain insertion? What size drain would you insert?
7. Why do you think the patient is hypokalaemic?
8. Would you correct the hypokalaemia preoperatively? Why/why not?
9. What are the implications of her alcoholism on the perioperative management?
10. How would you anaesthetize this patient?
11. What are the risks and precautions for prone surgery?
12. How would you manage the chest drain during positioning of the patient?
13. How would you manage this patient postoperatively?

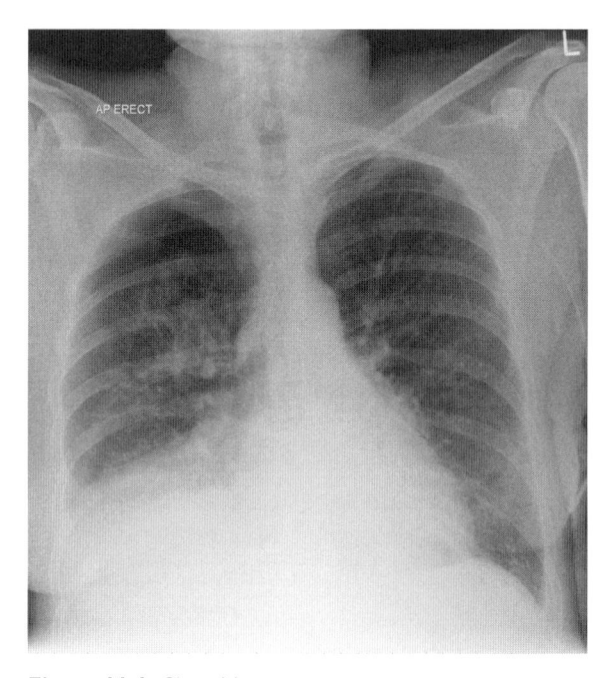

Figure 11.1 Chest-X-ray.

Chapter 11

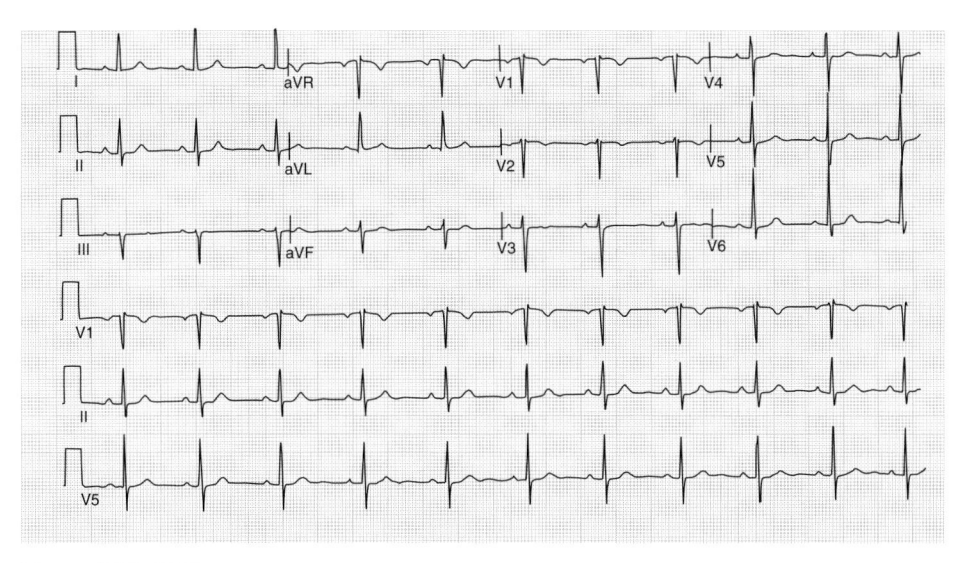

Figure 11.2 ECG.

ANSWERS

1. Summarize the case.

This is a 64-year-old lady who has acute neurological symptoms with urinary retention. Her past medical history includes alcohol dependency and malnutrition. She has been hospitalized for 2 weeks with severe back pain and was diagnosed with pleural effusion which was aspirated under ultrasound guidance.

2. How urgent is this operation?

Decompression for cauda equina syndrome is a surgical emergency; complete loss of function for more than four hours is unlikely to recover.

3. Comment on the chest X-ray.

Anterior–posterior chest X-ray. Demonstrates a right-sided hydropneumothorax, with a >2-cm iatrogenic pneumothorax resulting from pleural fluid aspiration (results consistent with transudate). The left lung is clear.

4. What does the ECG show?

The ECG is normal, with no evidence of hypokalaemia.

5. Would you take this patient to theatre immediately? Why/why not?

Despite the surgical urgency, this patient may not go to theatre immediately. An un-drained pneumothorax may expand and tension under positive pressure ventilation; a chest drain is mandatory preoperatively. This lady has evidence of impaired oxygenation (SpO$_2$ 0.93), which is likely to improve following chest drain insertion and resolution of pneumothorax and pleural effusion. Whilst proning can be used to improve oxygenation on ITU, it makes the diagnosis and treatment of hypoxia more difficult in theatre.

6. Which method should be used for chest drain insertion? What size drain would you insert?

A small drain (10–14 French) inserted via the Seldinger technique is preferred for pneumothorax, also for pleural effusion not caused by haemothorax or empyema.

7. Why do you think the patient is hypokalaemic?

The hypokalaemia is probably due to chronic diarrhoea. Other potential causes include vomiting, malnutrition, alcoholism, alkalosis (respiratory), coexistent hypomagnesaemia, and diuretic use.

8. Would you correct the hypokalaemia preoperatively? Why/why not?

As the hypokalaemia is mild, probably chronic, and not associated with ECG abnormalities, it should not delay the surgery.

9. What are the implications of her alcoholism on the perioperative management?

With alcoholism, particular attention should be given to the neurological and cardiovascular systems, and evidence of liver disease should be sought. Blood tests may reveal coagulopathy, pancytopenia, and electrolyte disturbance. An ECHO should be performed if cardiac dysfunction is suspected. Preoperative parenteral B vitamins may be necessary and coagulopathy should be corrected. Dose requirements for induction agents, volatile anaesthetics, opioids, and possibly neuromuscular blockers increase, but higher doses may exacerbate cardiovascular instability. The majority of postoperative complications are more common in alcoholism, notably delirium as a distinct but similar condition to alcohol withdrawal syndrome.

10. How would you anaesthetize this patient?

A variety of anaesthetic techniques are acceptable; stability is the goal irrespective of the technique chosen.

11. What are the risks and precautions for prone surgery?

Proning may lead to hypotension from abdominal compression and poor venous return, and airway pressures may increase following diaphragmatic compression. Most complications from proning are injuries caused by poor positioning, affecting eyes, face, head and neck, brachial plexus and peripheral nerves, breasts, and genitalia.

12. How would you manage the chest drain during positioning of the patient?

The chest drain should be briefly clamped for turning prone and later supine to avoid raising the open drain above the patient.

13. How would you manage this patient postoperatively?

This patient is at particular risk for respiratory, cardiovascular, and neurological complications postoperatively, with chest drain management required in addition to neurological observations and standard postoperative care. A high-dependency bed is appropriate.

Further reading

Chapman, R. and Plaat, F. Alcohol and anaesthesia. *Continuing Education in Anaesthesia, Critical Care & Pain* 2009; **9**:10–13.

Henry, M., Arnold, T., and Harvey, J., Iatrogenic pneumothorax. In 'BTS guidelines for the management of spontaneous pneumothorax'. *Thorax* 2003; **58**(Suppl II):ii39–ii52.

Knight, D.J.W. and Mahajan, R.P. Patient positioning in anaesthesia. *Continuing Education in Anaesthesia, Critical Care & Pain* 2004; **4**:160–3.

Laws, D., Neville, E., Duffy, J. BTS guidelines for the insertion of a chest drain. *Thorax* 2003; **58**(Suppl II): ii53–ii59.

Paramasivam, E. and Bodenham, A. Air leaks, pneumothorax, and chest drains. *Continuing Education in Anaesthesia, Critical Care & Pain* 2008; **8**:204–9.

Reddy, V.G. Potassium and anaesthesia. *Singapore Medical Journal* 1998, **39**(11):511–16.

Short cases

QUESTIONS

Short case 1: Postoperative nausea and vomiting

A 35-year-old woman is scheduled for a minor gynaecological procedure in the day surgery unit under general anaesthesia. She is anxious that she will be sick afterwards.

1. What are the risk factors for postoperative nausea and vomiting (PONV), and how could you estimate her risk?
2. What steps could you take to avoid PONV—how effective are these measures?
3. Can you assure her she will not be sick afterwards?
4. She suffers from PONV despite antiemetic prophylaxis. How would you treat established PONV?

Short case 2: Obstructive sleep apnoea

You are asked to anaesthetize a 55-year-old man for umbilical hernia repair. He has recently been diagnosed with sleep apnoea.

1. How does central sleep apnoea differ from obstructive sleep apnoea (OSA)?
2. What is the mechanism underlying OSA?
3. What are the predisposing factors to OSA?
4. Which medical conditions may result from OSA?
5. How would you anaesthetize this patient?
6. How would you manage this patient postoperatively?

Short case 3: Ventilator-associated pneumonia

A ventilated patient on the ICU has an increasing oxygen requirement over the last 12 hours.

1. What is the differential diagnosis?
2. You suspect ventilator-associated pneumonia (VAP)—how would you confirm the diagnosis?
3. What are the risk factors for VAP
4. How might VAP be prevented?
5. What methods are there to obtain microbiology specimens from the lung? Which method is best?
6. How would you treat VAP?
7. What proportion of patients with VAP die? How does VAP affect overall ITU mortality?

Chapter 11

ANSWERS

Short case 1: Postoperative nausea and vomiting

1. What are the risk factors for postoperative nausea and vomiting (PONV), and how could you estimate her risk?

The major risk factors for PONV are female sex, history of PONV or motion sickness, being a non-smoker, and the use of postoperative opioids. The type of surgery probably does not affect PONV risk. Other factors such as length of surgery are minor risk factors. The risk of PONV can be estimated (Apfel score):

Risk factors	Risk of PONV
0	10%
1	20%
2	40%
3	60%
4	80%

2. What steps could you take to avoid PONV—how effective are these measures?

The IMPACT trial showed that ondansetron, dexamethasone, or droperidol, reduce the estimated risk by 25%, with multiple interventions having a cumulative effect. Avoiding volatile anaesthesia via propofol infusion reduced the risk by 20%, and avoiding nitrous oxide decreases risk by 10%. Cyclizine has been shown to be an effective antiemetic in other studies, with metoclopramide 10 mg having no benefit over placebo and 20 mg having excessive side effects.

3. Can you assure her she will not be sick afterwards?

It is not possible to guarantee any patient that they will not experience PONV. But certainly I would like to reassure her that I would avoid emetogenic medications and give prophylaxis.

4. She suffers from PONV despite antiemetic prophylaxis. How would you treat established PONV?

Where prophylaxis fails, the treatment of established PONV is challenging. 'Surgical' causes such as airway bleeding or abdominal distension should be excluded, and the patient should receive adequate hydration and analgesia. Opioid-sparing methods of analgesia should be considered. If PONV prophylaxis was not administered intraoperatively, the commonly used antiemetics should be given. Alternative antiemetics acting via different mechanisms should then be considered, for instance, prochlorperazine. There is evidence that low doses of either propofol or midazolam are effective in refractory PONV.

Further reading

Apfel, C.C., Läärä, E., Koivuranta, M., et al. A simplified risk score for predicting postoperative nausea and vomiting: conclusions from cross-validations between two centers. Anesthesiology 1999; **91**:693–700.

Apfel, C.C., Korttila, K., Abdalla, M., et al. A factorial trial of six interventions for the prevention of postoperative nausea and vomiting. New England Journal of Medicine 2004; **350**:2441–51.

Gan, T.J., Meyer, T.A., Apfel, C.C., et al. Society for Ambulatory Anaesthesia Guidelines for the Management of postoperative nausea and vomiting. Anaesthesia & Analgesia 2007; **105**:1615–28.

Short case 2: Obstructive sleep apnoea

1. How does central sleep apnoea differ from obstructive sleep apnoea (OSA)?

Central sleep apnoea (CSA) is loss of respiratory drive, whereas obstructive sleep apnoea (OSA) features respiratory effort against an obstructed airway. Mixed pictures may exist. CSA may result from neuromuscular disorders, abnormal peripheral chemoreceptors, loss of central ventilatory control, or excessive respiratory demands.

2. What is the mechanism underlying OSA?

OSA results from a narrow floppy airway, obstructing under negative pressure when airway dilator muscles fail. Partial collapse of the pharyngeal airway causes snoring. Complete obstruction causes apnoea with subsequent arousal, deep inspiration, tachycardia, and hypertension.

3. What are the predisposing factors to OSA?

Increasing age, male gender, smoking and drinking, nasal/pharyngeal/laryngeal obstruction, and facial abnormalities predispose to OSA. Chronic renal failure is associated, along with certain endocrine, neuromuscular, and connective tissue storage disorders. OSA should be suspected in obese patients with a neck circumference >17 cm, in whom you might otherwise suspect a difficult intubation.

4. Which medical conditions may result from OSA?

OSA predisposes to respiratory failure and pulmonary hypertension, ischaemic heart disease, heart failure and hypertension, diabetes, and gastro-oesophageal reflux. These conditions should be considered at the preoperative visit.

5. How would you anaesthetize this patient?

Difficult intubation should be considered. Drugs with prolonged sedative effects should be avoided, including opioid analgesics where possible. Recovery in the lateral position may be considered. Surgery affecting the thorax, neck, and upper airway carries particular risks, as does packing the nose or having a nasogastric tube postoperatively.

6. How would you manage this patient postoperatively?

Prescribing supplementary oxygen alone is insufficient where apnoea and airway obstruction occur. Patients with established nasal CPAP should bring and self-administer this equipment into hospital. Those patients with previously undiagnosed OSA, or who require high doses of opioid analgesia may require closer monitoring in the HDU. A breathing circuit which can deliver CPAP should be immediately available.

Further reading

Loadsman, J.A. and Hillman, D.R. Anaesthesia and sleep apnoea. *British Journal of Anaesthesia* 2001; **86**:254–66.
Williams, J.M. and Hanning, C. D. Obstructive sleep apnoea. *Continuing Education in Anaesthesia, Critical Care & Pain* 2003; **3**:75–8.

Short case 3: Ventilator-associated pneumonia

1. What is the differential diagnosis?
The differential diagnosis includes pneumonia, ARDS, pulmonary oedema, pulmonary contusions, pulmonary embolism, atelectasis, aspiration, hypoventilation, endotracheal/tracheostomy tube displacement.

2. You suspect ventilator associated pneumonia (VAP)—how would you confirm the diagnosis?
The diagnosis of VAP is controversial with no test or diagnostic criteria widely accepted. Vigilance is essential, with other evidence assisting the diagnosis:

- Markers of systemic infection (pyrexia, leucocytosis/leucopenia, raised CRP).
- Markers of chest pathology (physical examination, increased sputum production, purulent sputum, deteriorating oxygenation—decreased PaO_2/FiO_2).
- Radiological evidence (infiltrates on chest X-ray or CT chest).
- Microbiological evidence (sputum culture and occasionally blood culture).

Scoring systems exist based upon similar criteria, e.g. clinical pulmonary infection score.

CPIS: this has been shown to have a sensitivity of 72–89% and specificity of 17–85%.

3. What are the risk factors for VAP?
Patient risk factors include age >60 years, severe illness, chronic lung disease, hypoalbuminaemia, smoking, GCS <9, burns, head and neck trauma, immunodeficiency. Interventional risk factors include enteral feeding, reintubation, supine position, H_2 antagonists or proton pump inhibitors, excessive sedation, increasing ventilator days.

4. How might VAP be prevented?
- Reduce colonization—oral decontamination, selective decontamination of digestive tract, frequent changes of ventilator circuit, use of heat/moisture exchange (HME) filters.
- Prevent aspiration—avoid intubation where possible, 45° head-up, subglottic suctioning, maintaining adequate cuff pressures.
- Minimizing duration of ventilation—early tracheostomy, daily sedation holds.

5. What methods are there to obtain microbiology specimens from the lung? Which method is best?
Microbiological specimens can be obtained via endotracheal aspiration (ETA), protected specimen brush, bronchoalveolar lavage (BAL), or mini-BAL. ETA is associated with an over-diagnosis of VAP due to contaminants at sampling, yet invasive techniques do not provide a morbidity/mortality benefit but may increase the duration of ventilation. There is no evidence that any sampling technique is superior. Quantitative cultures are widely used with >10^4 cfu/ml generally considered the threshold with BAL.

6. How would you treat VAP?
Antibiotics for VAP are usually started before microbiology results are available (before VAP can be diagnosed via the CPIS criteria). Empirical therapy is initiated according to local policy (taking cultures first where possible). Narrow-spectrum antibiotics are substituted when the organism and sensitivity is known. 8 days of therapy is recommended (*Pseudomonas* requires 15). There is no benefit to combination antibiotic therapy.

7. What proportion of patients with VAP die? How does VAP affect overall ITU mortality?

Approximately 30% of patients with VAP will die. Despite this, VAP does not cause excess mortality in trauma or ARDS, with other patient groups difficult to quantify. VAP leads to significant morbidity, notably prolonged ITU stay and associated complications.

Further reading

Chandler, B. and Hunter, J. Ventilator-associated pneumonia; a concise review. *Journal of the Intensive Care Society* 2009; **10**:29–33.

Melsen, W.G., Rovers, M.M., and Bonten, M.J. Ventilator-associated pneumonia and mortality: a systematic review of observational studies. *Critical Care Medicine* 2009; **37**:2709–18.

Stewart, N.I. and Cuthbertson, B.H. The problems diagnosing ventilator-associated pneumonia. *Journal of the Intensive Care Society* 2009; **10**:266–72.

Wiener-Kronish, J.P. and Dorr, H.I. Ventilator-associated pneumonia: problems with diagnosis and therapy. *Best Practice & Research Clinical Anaesthesiology* 2008; **22**:437–49.

Clinical science

QUESTIONS

Anatomy: Vagus nerve and recurrent laryngeal nerve

1. Outline the origin, course, relations, and main branches of the vagus nerve.
2. What stimuli may increase vagal outflow? What effects might be seen?
3. How might different vagal nerve injuries affect the larynx?
4. A patient has stridor after thyroid surgery. What are the possible causes?

Physiology: Nutrition in a critically ill patient

1. Why do we feed critically ill patients?
2. How could you assess nutritional status?
3. What are the usual nutritional requirements in critical illness?
4. What other nutritional supplements may be beneficial?
5. Which route for nutrition is best—enteral or parenteral?

Pharmacology: Adrenaline

1. How is adrenaline synthesized and secreted *in vivo*?
2. What are the main actions of adrenaline?
3. How is adrenaline metabolized and excreted?
4. What are the clinical features of phaeochromocytomas?
5. How would you anaesthetize a phaeochromocytoma patient for adrenalectomy?

Physics and clinical measurements: Hagen–Poiseuille equation, Heliox

1. What is the Hagen–Poiseuille equation?
2. How does laminar flow differ from turbulent flow? What is Reynolds number?
3. What affects the rate of turbulent flow?
4. What is Heliox?
5. Why might Heliox be useful in upper airway obstruction?
6. What are the disadvantages of using Heliox?
7. Is Heliox useful in bronchospasm? Why/why not?

ANSWERS

Anatomy: Vagus nerve and recurrent laryngeal nerve

1. Outline the origin, course, relations, and main branches of the vagus nerve.

The vagus nerve (CN X) emerges from the upper medulla, arising from the dorsal nucleus of vagus, nucleus ambiguus, and nucleus of the tractus solitarius. Passing through the jugular foramen, it merges with the cranial part of the accessory nerve (CN XI) shortly after emergence. It descends within the carotid sheath (carotid artery anteromedial and internal jugular vein anterolateral). The cervical sympathetic chain is posterior (outside carotid sheath).

The left vagus nerve passes behind the brachiocephalic vein lying between the common carotid and subclavian arteries. It descends anterior to the aortic arch, moves inferiorly behind the left lung root, then crosses the diaphragm adjacent to the oesophagus (oesophageal hiatus) into the abdomen. The left recurrent laryngeal nerve passes under the aortic arch to ascend superiorly in the tracheo-oesophageal groove. The right vagus nerve has a similar course, but the right recurrent laryngeal nerve arches underneath the subclavian artery before ascending towards the larynx.

The superior laryngeal nerve emerges from the vagus within the neck. This forms an external branch (innervates cricothyroid) and an internal branch (sensory to mucosa above vocal cords and undersurface of epiglottis). The recurrent laryngeal nerve (left and right) innervates the intrinsic laryngeal muscles (not cricothyroid) and provides sensory supply below the cords.

Other important branches of the vagus nerve include pharyngeal (neck), pulmonary, pericardial, and oesophageal (thorax), gastric, hepatic, and coeliac (abdomen).

2. What stimuli may increase vagal outflow? What effects might be seen?

Whilst many surgical stimuli trigger vagal reflexes, stimulation of the anus or cervix (Brewer–Luckhardt reflex) and extraocular muscles (oculocardic reflex) may be particularly troublesome. Surgery affecting the mesentery, biliary tree, uterus, bladder, urethra, larynx, testes, glottis, bronchial tree, carotid sinus may increase vagal tone, as might laparoscopic surgery (any type) due to peritoneal distension.

Vagal reflexes commonly cause bradycardia, laryngospasm, and bronchospasm. Asystole may occur in severe cases.

3. How might different vagal nerve injuries affect the larynx?

Both the superior and recurrent laryngeal nerves may be damaged during thyroid or related surgery. Superior laryngeal nerve injuries denervate cricothyroid, reducing cord tension and causing hoarseness. This may be transient if unilateral as the opposite cricothyroid compensates.

Recurrent laryngeal nerve damage may also occur from tumours affecting the lung, oesophagus, or lymph nodes, or from dilation of the aortic arch or right atrium (Ortner's cardiovocal syndrome). Complete lesion of the recurrent laryngeal nerve results in a partially abducted cord. Bilateral complete lesions may lead to partial airway obstruction and stridor; unilateral lesions may be compensated for. Partial lesions predominantly affect cord abductors; the cord moves to the midline position. Bilateral partial lesions are potentially fatal, causing severe or complete airway obstruction.

4. A patient has stridor after thyroid surgery. What are the possible causes?

Differential diagnosis:
- Tracheomalacia—erosion of thyroid cartilages causing tracheal collapse.
- Bleeding causing extrinsic tracheal compression and obstruction.
- Recurrent laryngeal nerve injury (± laryngeal oedema).

Chapter 11

- Other respiratory disorders may result from phrenic nerve injury, pneumothorax, or tracheo-oesophageal fistula formation.

Further reading

Erdmann, A.G. *Concise Anatomy for Anaesthesia*. Cambridge: Cambridge University Press, 2011.

Hutton, P., Cooper, G., James, F.M., and Butterworth, J.F. *Fundamental Principles and Practice of Anaesthesia*. London: Dunitz, 2002.

Yentis, S.M., Hirsch, N.P., and Smith, G.S. *Anaesthesia and Intensive Care A–Z: An Encyclopaedia of Principles and Practice* 4th edn. Edinburgh: Churchill Livingstone, 2009.

Physiology: Nutrition in a critically ill patient

1. Why do we feed critically ill patients?

Critical illness triggers the inflammatory response leading to a hypermetabolic state. Skeletal muscle is lost as protein is disproportionately used as an energy source. Feeding critically ill patients reduces the rate of muscle loss. Many patients admitted to critical care have pre-existing malnutrition and are less able to tolerate further catabolism.

Starvation of <5 days is associated with increased infectious complications, and >5 days with increased mortality. Feeding is often started in patients who are not expected to resume a normal diet within 2 days, or in those already malnourished. Early feeding provides a safety margin against failed attempts.

2. How could you assess nutritional status?

General observation and examination of a patient for malnutrition is better than any specific test. The commonly employed measures outside intensive care are unreliable; oedema affects arm circumference and skin-fold thickness, sedated patients cannot always grip with their hands, laboratory tests are affected by critical illness.

3. What are the usual nutritional requirements in critical illness?

Both underfeeding and overfeeding can be harmful; however, calculation of energy requirement is frequently inaccurate. Most patients require 25 kCal/kg/day. Enteral feed commonly delivers this as 2/3 carbohydrate and 1/3 lipid. TPN can be similar or provide concentrated glucose with twice-weekly essential fatty acid supplements. Calculations of nitrogen balance are also unreliable. Most patients require 1–1.25 g/kg/day of protein. TPN delivers this as amino acids; enteral feeds may contain protein (requires digestion) or amino acids and peptides (suitable for malabsorption states, e.g. pancreatic insufficiency).

Water and electrolyte requirements vary widely between patients—regular assessment of hydration and correction of electrolytes is a fundamental aspect of critical care. Average daily requirements are:

- Water: 30 ml/kg
- Sodium: 1–2 mmol/kg
- Potassium: 0.7–1 mmol/kg
- Calcium: 0.1 mmol/kg
- Magnesium: 0.1 mmol/kg
- Phosphorous: 0.4 mmol/kg

4. What other nutritional supplements may be beneficial?

Glutamine is required for gut and immune function. Skeletal muscle releases glutamine in critical illness leading to depletion and the need for dietary intake. TPN has traditionally not contained glutamine due to problems with stability (now overcome). The evidence for glutamine supplementation is conflicting, but it is likely to be beneficial in patients receiving TPN for >10 days.

Selenium depletion is common and impairs the role of glutathione peroxidase as a free radical scavenger. There is growing evidence that selenium supplementation may be helpful in general ITU patients. Antioxidants vitamins (A/C/E) have also been investigated, but no convincing benefit has been shown.

Immunonutrition refers to omega-3 fatty acids, arginine, and nucleotides believed to enhance immune function. Reduced infection rates and length of stay have been reported, however increased mortality has been shown in several studies. Arginine is thought to be harmful to septic ITU patients.

5. Which route for nutrition is best—enteral or parenteral?

Enteral feeding is preferred where possible; it is cheaper and easier. Despite suggestions that enteral nutrition may reduce infectious complications, well-conducted studies have failed to show a consistent benefit. Furthermore, a meta-analysis has shown reduced mortality in patients fed parenterally. Nasogastric feeding is a known risk-factor for ventilator associated pneumonia. Where doubt exists over the ability to establish enteral feeding, it is better to start parenteral feeding early. Early nutrition is more important than the route.

Further reading

Bersten, A. and Soni, N (eds.). *Oh's Intensive Care Manual* 6th edn. Oxford: Butterworth Heinemann, 2009.

Edmondson, W.C. Nutritional support in critical care: an update. *Continuing Education in Anaesthesia Critical Care & Pain* 2007; **7**:199–202.

Evidence Based Decision Making [website]: http://www.evidencebased.net [Excellent Internet resource for critical care].

Martin, C.M., Doig, G.S., Heyland, D.K., et al. Multicentre, cluster-randomised clinical trial of algorithms for critical-care enteral and parenteral therapy (ACCEPT). *Canadian Medical Association Journal* 2004, **170**:197–204.

Simpson, F. and Doig, G.S. Parenteral vs. enteral nutrition in the critically ill patient: a meta-analysis of trials using the intention to treat principle. *Intensive Care Medicine* 2005, **31**:12–23.

Pharmacology: Adrenaline

1. How is adrenaline synthesized and secreted *in vivo*?

Adrenaline is synthesized and released from the adrenal medulla. Some is also produced within the CNS where it acts as a neurotransmitter. Phenylalanine is hydroxylated to tyrosine in the liver then concentrated within the adrenal gland. Tyrosine is further hydroxylated to DOPA, then decarboxylated to dopamine. This is taken into vesicles and hydroxylated to noradrenaline, then methylated to adrenaline.

Pre-ganglionic sympathetic neurons innervate the adrenal gland. Sympathetic stimulation leads to synaptic acetylcholine release and secretion of adrenaline by chromaffin cells into the systemic circulation.

2. What are the main actions of adrenaline?

The cardiovascular effects depend upon dose. Beta-effects occur at low dose with increased cardiac output, myocardial oxygen consumption, and coronary vasodilation; systemic vascular resistance falls, reducing diastolic BP (MAP slightly increased). At higher doses α–effects increase vascular resistance and blood pressure. Adrenaline is often used as a vasoconstrictor to prolong the effect of local anaesthetics.

Adrenaline is a bronchodilator and increases ventilation and pulmonary vascular resistance. It increases metabolism and blood glucose levels by increasing glycogenolysis. Lactate is increased. Adrenaline increases MAC and pain thresholds.

3. How is adrenaline metabolized and excreted?

Adrenaline is rapidly metabolized (half-life ≈ 2 min). It is metabolized by COMT then MAO to the inactive metabolite vanillylmandelic acid (VMA) which is excreted in the urine.

4. What are the clinical features of phaeochromocytomas?

Phaeochromocytomas are catecholamine secreting tumours of chromaffin cells. Most occur within the adrenal gland, but 10% occur at other sympathetic sites, 10% are bilateral, 10% malignant, and 10% familial. A minority are associated with multiple endocrine neoplasia, neurofibromatosis type I, or von Hippel–Lindau syndrome.

Classically, phaeochromocytomas present with episodic severe hypertension and headaches with drenching sweats, palpitations, anxiety, tremor, and chest pain. Sustained hypertension with other symptoms may be a more common presentation. Diagnosis is usually made via urinary VMA levels and plasma catecholamines, with later MRI scanning to guide treatment.

5. How would you anaesthetize a phaeochromocytoma patient for adrenalectomy?

Preoperative assessment should focus on the cardiovascular system—50% of patients will have catecholamine cardiomyopathy; many will have hypertensive complications. Hypertension is usually controlled preoperatively with alpha-blockers and beta-blockers; recently the sole use of selective alpha-1-blockers has been advocated (e.g. doxazosin).

Reliable large-bore IV access, invasive BP and CVP monitoring are essential. Events such as induction, intubation, tumour handling, and gas insufflation for laparoscopic approaches often precipitate cardiovascular instability. Rapid onset vasodilators and beta-blockers must be immediately available. Hypotension is common following tumour removal, often difficult to treat due to alpha-receptor downregulation. Angiotensin may be effective.

Postoperative high-dependency care with invasive cardiovascular monitoring is usual. Hypoglycaemia is common (symptoms masked by beta-blockade). Steroid replacement is often required.

Further reading

Pace, N. and Buttigieg, M. Phaeochromocytoma. *Continuing Education in Anaesthesia, Critical Care & Pain* 2003; 3:20–3.

Peck, T., Hill, S., and Williams, M. *Pharmacology for Anaesthesia and Intensive Care* 3rd edn. Cambridge: Cambridge University Press, 2008.

Yentis, S.M., Hirsch, N.P., and Smith, G.S. *Anaesthesia and Intensive Care A–Z: An Encyclopaedia of Principles and Practice* 4th edn. Edinburgh: Churchill Livingstone, 2009.

Physics and clinical measurements: Hagen–Poiseuille equation, Heliox

1. What is the Hagen-Poiseuille equation?
The Hagen–Poiseuille equation describes laminar flow:
$$Q = Pr^4\pi/8\eta L$$
where Q is flow, P is pressure gradient across vessel, r is radius of vessel, η is fluid viscosity, and L is vessel length.

2. How does laminar flow differ from turbulent flow? What is Reynolds number?
Laminar flow comprises layers (lamina) of fluid moving smoothly, with the central lamina flowing fastest and the outer lamina slowest. In contrast, turbulent flow consists of chaotic fluid motion with eddies. Reynolds number (Re) predicts whether flow will be laminar or turbulent. Re <2000 predicts laminar flow and >2000 turbulent flow.
$$Re = V\rho d/\eta$$
where V is fluid velocity, ρ is fluid density, d is vessel diameter, and η is fluid viscosity.

3. What affects the rate of turbulent flow?
No equation accurately describes turbulent flow, but certain factors are known:
- Flow $\propto r^2$ (square of the radius).
- Flow $\propto \sqrt{P}$ (square root of pressure gradient).
- Flow $\propto 1/L$ (inverse of vessel length).
- Flow $\propto 1/\rho$ (inverse of fluid density).

4. What is Heliox?
Heliox is a mixture of helium and oxygen, commonly produced as a 79:21% mixture in the UK, but available in other compositions elsewhere. The FiHe (and therefore FiO_2) can be adjusted via gas mixing devices. Heliox can also be delivered by mixing cylinder helium with oxygen.

Heliox is a low density gas as helium is a light atom (atomic number 2).

5. Why might Heliox be useful in upper airway obstruction?
Partial airway obstruction invariably leads to turbulent flow around the lesion. Heliox has a low density which increases flow (flow $\propto 1/\rho$) and also predisposes to laminar flow (reduces Reynolds number). Both factors increase flow through a narrowed airway, reducing work or breathing and fatigue whilst improving alveolar oxygenation.

6. What are the disadvantages of using Heliox?
The advantages of Heliox depend upon a high helium concentration, which necessarily limits the oxygen concentration delivered to the patient; however increasing the FiO_2 may decrease alveolar oxygenation by reducing oxygen flux to the lung. Voice changes with Heliox are temporary and harmless.

7. Is Heliox useful in bronchospasm? Why/why not?
Unlike upper airway obstruction, there is no strong evidence base to support the use of Heliox in bronchospasm. Bronchioles have narrower diameters and slower airflow velocities compared with upper airways. These differences may limit the impact of reduced gas density.

Further reading

Davis, P.D. and Kenny, G.N.C (eds.). *Basic Physics and Measurement in Anaesthesia* 5th edn. Oxford: Butterworth Heinemann, 2003.

Maloney, E. and Meakin, G.H. Acute stridor in children. *Continuing Education in Anaesthesia, Critical Care & Pain* 2007; **7**:183–6.

Stanley, D. and Tunnicliffe, W. Management of life-threatening asthma in adults. *Continuing Education in Anaesthesia, Critical Care & Pain* 2008; **8**:95–9.

Chapter 12

Clinical anaesthesia

Long case: A patient for dental clearance as day-case procedure   255
Short cases   261
   Questions   261
   Answers   263
      Short case 1: Tetanus   263
      Short case 2: Post-dural puncture headache   265
      Short case 3: Trauma patient with head injury   267

Clinical science

Questions   269
Answers   270
   Anatomy: Abdomen wall   270
   Physiology: Plasma proteins   273
   Pharmacology: Evidence-based medicine   275
   Physics and clinical measurement: Blood pressure measurement   277

Clinical anaesthesia

Long case: A patient for dental clearance as day-case procedure

A 39-year-old man presents for a full dental extraction. He is on lithium for manic depressive psychosis. He is a heavy smoker with a wheezy chest. He is on diuretics for hypertension, and has been investigated for polyuria over the past 2 months.
Other medications: flupenthixol, amitriptyline.

Clinical examination	Temperature: 38.2°C; weight: 95 kg; height: 160 cm			
	Pulse: 56/min, regular; BP: 150/85 mmHg; respiratory rate: 12/min			
	Chest: expiratory wheeze			
	Cardiovascular system: normal heart sound with no murmurs			
	Central nervous system: he has resting tremors; no neurological deficit			
	Ankle oedema			
Laboratory investigations	Hb	13.6 g/dL	Na	141 mEq/L
	MCV	89 fL	K	4.1 mEq/L
	WBC	12.1×10^9/L	Urea	10.3 mmol/L
	Platelets	236×10^9/L	Creatinine	150 μmol/L
			Lithium level	1.0 mmol/L

QUESTIONS

1. Summarize the case
2. What are the anaesthetic issues of concern in this patient?
3. What are the effects of smoking on the human body?
4. Discuss the X-ray.
5. Discuss the ECG findings.
6. Discuss the patient's current medications.
7. What are the causes of renal impairment in this patient?
8. What is the reason for polyuria in the patient?
9. What are the indications for lithium therapy?
10. Describe the effects of lithium?
11. Why should lithium levels be monitored?
12. What are the signs and symptoms of lithium toxicity?
13. What are the anaesthetic issues with lithium?
14. Would you stop lithium?
15. Would you anaesthetize this man? If not, why?
16. He is now optimized, how would you proceed?

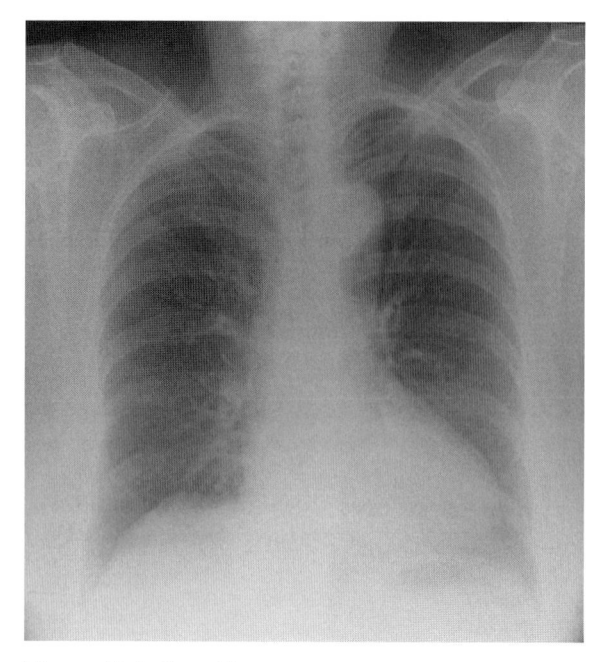

Structured Oral Examination Practice for the Final FRCA

Figure 12.1 Chest X-ray.

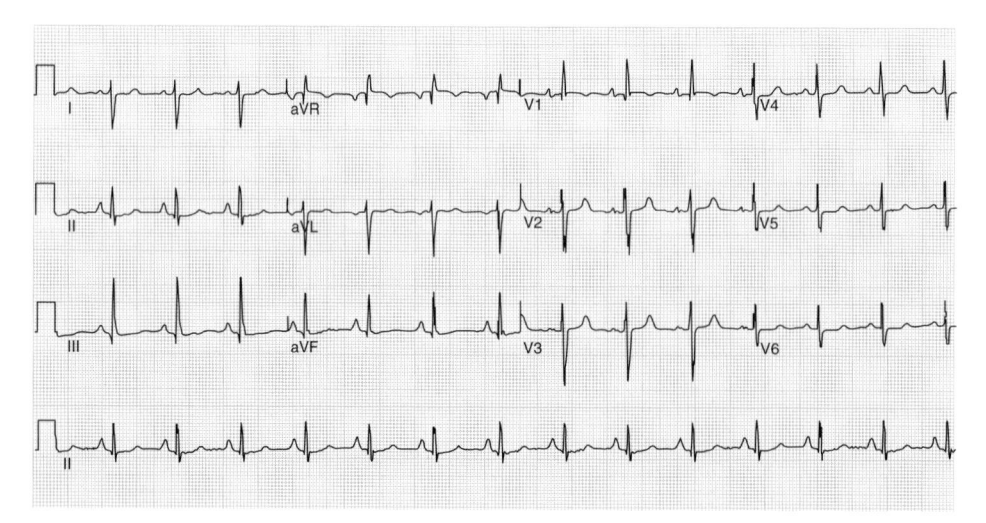

Figure 12.2 ECG.

ANSWERS

1. Summarize the case
We have a young psychiatric patient with associated hypertension who is a heavy smoker and has evidence of a wheeze.

2. What are the anaesthetic issues of concern in this patient?
My concerns regarding this patient are:
- Psychiatric disease
- Hypertension
- Renal impairment
- Medication of lithium
- Communication and capacity issues
- Postoperative pain relief and discharge

3. What are the effects of smoking on the human body?
- Cigarette smoking is highly addictive
- Respiratory tract mucous is produced in large quantities but mucociliary clearance is less efficient.
- Susceptible to infection due to postoperative atelectasis.
- Increased levels of carboxyhaemoglobin (COHb) may reach 5–15% causing reduced oxygen carriage by the blood.
- Increased airway irritability increases coughing, laryngospasm, and desaturation.

4. Discuss the chest X-ray.
Posterior–anterior chest X-ray. The heart is enlarged. The lungs and pleural spaces are clear.

5. Discuss the ECG findings.
The ECG shows sinus rhythm of 84 bpm with features of right ventricular hypertrophy. There is right axis deviation, dominant R wave in V1, and deep S wave in lateral leads (lead I). There are also abnormally tall P waves in inferior leads.

6. Discuss the patient's current medications.
- **Lithium carbonate**: this is a mood stabilizing drug which is mainly used for prophylaxis in patients with repeated episodes of mania and depression.
- **Flupenthixol**: antipsychotic drug for maintenance therapy of patients with chronic schizophrenia whose main manifestations do not include excitement, agitation, or hyperactivity.
- **Venlafaxine**: selective serotonin/noradrenaline reuptake inhibitor. SNRIs act upon and increase the levels of serotonin and noradrenaline (norepinephrine) neurotransmitters.

7. What are the causes of renal impairment in this patient?
The possible causes of renal impairment are:
- Chronic lithium therapy causes nephrogenic diabetes inspidus and reduced creatinine clearance.
- Long-term hypertension.

8. What is the reason for polyuria in the patient?
This patient is on lithium which may lead to increased volume of dilute urine known as diabetes inspidus. Lithium mimics sodium and reduces the sensitivity of renal tubules to antidiuretic hormone.

9. What are the indications for lithium therapy?

Lithium is a popular agent in the treatment of many psychiatric disorders. Lithium has a low therapeutic index with dose–non-dose related side effects. Hence patients receiving this medication can have problems that may complicate their anaesthetic course. Indications for lithium, usually given as lithium carbonate are:

- Acute treatment of mania and hypomania.
- Prophylaxis of chronic bipolar depression.
- Prophylaxis of recurrent depression.
- Prophylaxis of chronic cluster headache.

10. Describe the effects of lithium.

Lithium mimics sodium, hence in the cellular phase enters the cell via fast voltage gated channels but is not removed by the Na-K-ATPase. This leads to the intracellular accumulation of lithium.

Mechanism of action

The mechanism by which lithium has its therapeutic effect is complex and not fully elucidated.
- Increases the uptake of noradrenaline (norepinephrine) by the presynaptic membrane.
- Increases its subsequent metabolism by monoamine oxidases.
- Second messenger systems may be another target, lithium can inhibit adenylate cyclase, reducing cAMP signalling.

11. Why should lithium levels be monitored?

Lithium has a very narrow therapeutic window being clinically effective at 0.5–1.0 mmol/L but toxic over 1.5 mmol/L. Hence lithium should be stopped 24 hours prior to anaesthesia and the postoperative level should be monitored.

12. What are the signs and symptoms of lithium toxicity?

Lithium toxic level is when the serum level is above 1.5 mmol/L. The signs and symptoms of lithium toxicity are

- Nausea and vomiting
- Abdominal pain
- Diarrhoea
- Blurred vision
- Ataxia and tremor
- Dysrhythmia
- Nystagmus
- Hyper-reflexia
- Convulsions
- Coma
- Death when the level is >3 mmol/L

13. What are the anaesthetic issues with lithium?

Lithium administration prolongs both depolarizing and non-depolarizing neuromuscular block. All patients on lithium undergoing general anaesthesia with the use of neuromuscular blocking agents should receive appropriate neuromuscular monitoring.

Case reports have described a prolonged hypnotic effect in barbiturate-based anaesthesia in patients who are taking lithium, although in one report the plasma lithium level was above the normal therapeutic range.

Lithium has been associated with conduction defects and ST changes on ECG under anaesthesia.

Chapter 12

14. Would you stop lithium?

Yes, it is suggested that lithium be omitted in the 24 hours preceding general anaesthesia. The treatment should be restarted when patient is eating and drinking.

15. Would you anaesthetize this man? If not, why?

No, I will not go ahead and anaesthetize this patient. This patient:

- Is still on Lithium, he should have been off for 24 hours.
- Has chronic renal dysfunction.
- Has pyrexia.

The patient requires full preoperative assessment and a multidisciplinary team approach involving anaesthetist, psychiatrist, renal physician, pain team, and community nurse.

16. He is now optimized how would you proceed?

Preoperative assessment

- Full assessment of the patient
- To continue:
    - The antihypertensive medication.
    - Antidepressants
    - Stop lithium 24 hours prior
    - Pre-medication: anxiolytic prior to the surgery
- Serum lithium, urea, creatinine, TSH, and thyroxine level.

Monitoring

- Standard monitoring: oxygen saturation, ECG, NIBP, neuromuscular monitoring.

Induction and maintenance

- Pre-oxygenation and IV induction.
- Nasal intubation is required along with the throat pack.
- Maintenance with oxygen, air, and volatile agent.
- Restricted fluid administration in view of the renal impairment.
- Surgeon infiltrates lignocaine 2% with epinephrine 1:80,000. This is the time to look for any arrhythmias.

Recovery

Once the procedure is complete:

- The pack is removed.
- The oro-pharynx is suctioned.
- Reverse the neuromuscular blockade.
- Extubate when patient is awake.

Postoperative

- IV fentanyl should be prescribed if there is acute pain immediately.
- Regular paracetamol and codeine phosphate.
- Non-steroidal anti-inflammatory drugs should be avoided.

Further reading

Allman, K.G. and Wilson, I.H. *Oxford Handbook of Anaesthesia*, 2nd edn. Chapter 12: Psychiatric disorder and drugs, see p. 276. Oxford: Oxford University Press, 2006.

Flood, S. and Bodenham, A. Lithium: mimicry, mania, and muscle relaxants. *Continuing Education in Anaesthesia, Critical Care & Pain* 2010; **10**:77–80.

Chapter 12

Short cases

QUESTIONS

Short case 1: Tetanus

A 28-year-old male farmer presents to the A&E with a 2-day history of difficulty in mouth opening, dysphagia, and neck stiffness. He had a laceration of his right arm a week ago. As the ICU registrar on call, you are called down to A&E as the patient is having muscle spasms and there are concerns about his airway/breathing.

1. What are the causes of such a presentation (differential diagnosis)?
2. What is tetanus?
3. Briefly explain the pathophysiology of tetanus.
4. How would you go ahead and manage this case?
5. How is circulating toxin which is present in the body outside CNS neutralized?
6. How do you prevent the toxin release?
7. How do we suppress the effects of tetanospasmin?
8. What are the complications of tetanus and what is the prevention?

Short case 2: Post-dural-puncture headache

On your visit to the postnatal ward you are asked to review a lady who had an epidural yesterday in the early hours of the morning. She is now complaining of headache.

1. What are you going to do?
2. What are the possible causes of headache?
3. What is the pathophysiology of this headache?
4. What is the incidence of headache following an epidural?
5. What are the clinical features of a post-dural puncture headache (PDPH)?
6. How would you diagnose a PDPH?
7. What are the complications of a PDPH?
8. How would you manage the diagnosed PDPH?

Short case 3: Trauma patient with head injury

You are called by the orthopaedic registrar in the middle of the night for a 19-year-old male involved in a road traffic accident. He has a compound tibial fracture with GCS 13 and linear skull fracture on plain X-ray. He is haemodynamically stable. His right foot is cool and dusky and the orthopaedic registrar wants to take him to theatre immediately to do an open reduction and internal fixation (ORIF) for the fracture. Answer the following questions.

1. What do you think is going on?
2. Will you anaesthetize this patient in his present condition? If not, why?
3. Is the fall in GCS significant? What could be the possible causes for this deterioration?
4. What are the indications for ICP monitoring following head injury?

Structured Oral Examination Practice for the Final FRCA

5. How will you assess integrity of his cervical spine?
6. What more information do you need about the patient and the circumstances of the accident?
7. What anaesthetic technique would you use to anaesthetize this patient for ORIF of the tibial fracture?

Chapter 12

ANSWERS

Short case 1: Tetanus

1. What are the causes of such a presentation (differential diagnosis)?

The differential diagnosis can be:
- Tetanus
- Meningitis, tumours
- Dental abscess
- Local temporomandibular and oral disease
- Dystonic reaction to tricyclic antidepressants
- Strychnine poisoning
- Psychiatric disorders
- Epilepsy

2. What is tetanus?

Tetanus is caused by a Gram-positive bacillus, *Clostridium tetani*, which is commonly found in soil, but may also be isolated from animal or human faeces. It is a motile, spore-forming, obligate anaerobe. Spores are not destroyed by boiling but are eliminated by autoclaving at 120°C for 15 min (at one atmosphere pressure). Tetanus is usually diagnosed clinically as the bacterium is rarely cultured.

3. Briefly explain the pathophysiology of tetanus.

Under the anaerobic conditions found in infected or necrotic tissue, the bacillus secretes two toxins: tetanolysin and tetanospasmin.
- Tetanolysin damages the surrounding viable tissue and optimizes conditions for bacterial multiplication.
- Tetanospasmin causes the clinical syndrome of tetanus, by entering peripheral nerves and travelling via axonal retrograde transport to the CNS. Tetanospasmin disables release of neurotransmitter from presynaptic vesicles (particularly the inhibitory neurotransmitters GABA and glycine). The result is disinhibition of motor and autonomic neurons, causing rigidity, muscle spasms, and autonomic dysfunction. A relative deficiency of synaptic acetylcholine causes flaccid paralysis that is clinically mild in humans.
- High toxin load results in diffusion of toxin via the blood to nerves throughout the body.

4. How would you go ahead and manage this case?

The aim of management of a case requires a multidisciplinary mode of approach involving critical care, microbiologist, and surgeons
- Assess the patient's ABC.
- Neutralize circulating toxin: passive immunization.
- Eradicate the source of the toxin: extensive debridement, antibiotics.
- Minimize effects of bound toxins.
- General supportive care.

5. How is circulating toxin which is present in the body outside CNS neutralized?

The circulating toxins are neutralized by administering human tetanus immunoglobulin (Ig) 150 units/kg IM into different sites within 24 hours of diagnosis. An IV preparation may be available in some centres (5000–10,000 IU).

6. How do you prevent the toxin release?

The toxin release is prevented by:
- Wound care.
- Surgical debridement of wounds, repeated as necessary.
- IV antibiotic:
    - Metronidazole 500mg IV 8-hourly is the antibiotic of choice.
    - Benzylpenicillin 1MU IV 6-hourly is an alternative (but is a GABA antagonist). Erythromycin, tetracycline, chloramphenicol, and clindamycin are acceptable choices.

7. How do we suppress the effects of tetanospasmin?

Control rigidity and spasms with sedation, give respiratory support where necessary, and control autonomic dysfunction.
- If muscle spasms are present: urgently secure the airway with endotracheal intubation and provide ventilatory support.
- Autonomic dysfunction is managed with:
    - Deep sedation.
    - Magnesium.
    - Clonidine.
    - Combination of alpha and beta blockers.

8. What are the complications of tetanus and what is the prevention?

Common complications
- Cardiovascular: cardiac arrhythmias, cardiac failure, hypertensive crises, pulmonary oedema.
- Complications of mechanical ventilation.
- Syndrome of inappropriate antidiuretic hormone secretion (SIADH).
- Bedsores.
- Bone fractures.
- DVT.

Prevention
- All patients with tetanus require active immunization with tetanus toxoid, as infection does not confer immunity.
- In the UK, a course of five injections is recommended: a primary course at the age of 2, 3, 4 months and boosters at 5 and 15 years. All patients with tetanus require active immunization with tetanus toxoid, as infection does not confer immunity.

Further reading

Beeching, N.J. and Crowcroft, N.S. Tetanus in injecting drug users. *British Medical Journal* 2005; **330**:208–9.
Cook, T.M., Protheroe, R.T., and Handel, J.M. Tetanus: a review of the literature. *British Journal of Anaesthesia* 2001; **87**:477–87.
Towey, R. Tetanus: a review. *Update in Anaesthesia* 2005; **19**: Article 17.

Chapter 12

Short case 2: Post-dural puncture headache

1. What are you going to do?

My immediate action would be to reassure the patient and take full history and examination which will include:

- The timing of the headache in relation to the neuraxial procedure.
- The nature of the headache as well as other symptoms and signs.
- Considering an unrecognized dural puncture with an epidural needle or catheter, I will take the details of the epidural insertion by reviewing the notes including the difficulty of the procedure and number of attempts.
- I will try to diagnose the cause of headache and explain the modalities of the treatment available. I will provide a information leaflet about PDPH.

2. What are the possible causes of headache?

The differential diagnosis of PDPH includes:

- Pre-eclamptia and eclamptia
- Migraine
- Tension headache
- Meningitis
- Pneumocephalus
- Cortical vein and sagittal sinus thrombosis
- Subdural haematoma
- Hypertensive encephalopathy

3. What is the pathophysiology of this headache?

There are a number of theories regarding the cause of PDPH. The most commonly held belief is that it is due to the CSF leaking through the dural puncture site, leading to intracranial hypotension. This causes settling of the brain and stretching of intracranial nerves, meninges, and blood vessels. This theory is supported by the fact that the headache improves upon adoption of the supine position and by the decreased incidence of PDPH with the use of smaller needles with atraumatic points.

4. What is the incidence of headache following an epidural?

The incidence of PDPH is estimated to be between 30–50% following diagnostic or therapeutic lumbar puncture. In a pregnant patient the risk of dural puncture with the epidural needle is 1.5% out of these 52.1% of patients with dural puncture will experience PDPH. The incidence of PDPH following spinal anaesthesia ranges from 1.5 to 11.2% depending on the size of the spinal needle. PDPH commonly occurs at a rate of about 1% following epidural placement.

5. What are the clinical features of a post-dural puncture headache (PDPH)?

The classic features of the headache caused by dural puncture are

- Headache is often frontal-occipital. Most headaches do not develop immediately after dural puncture but 24–48 hours after the procedure with 90% of headaches presenting within 3 days.
- The headache is worse in the upright position and eases when supine.
- Pressure over the abdomen with the woman in the upright position may give transient relief to the headache by raising intracranial pressure secondary to a rise in intra-abdominal pressure (Gutsche sign).
- Other associated symptoms may be nausea, vomiting, neck stiffness, photophobia, vertigo, diplopia (due to traction on the 6th cranial nerve), hearing loss, and tinnitus. Other, more serious, signs have been described, such as convulsions and visual field defects.

6. How would you diagnose a PDPH?

The diagnosis of PDPH is based on
- A history of neuraxial blockade and the timing of the dural puncture.
- Clinical features of a typical headache along with the associated symptoms.
- Examination findings supporting the diagnosis and excluding other differentials.
- In cases of extreme headaches, head CT and MRI to exclude serious pathology.

7. What are the complications of a PDPH?

Neglected dural leak may lead to a chronic headache or more seriously, it may lead to a number of neurological complications such as a cranial nerve palsy. Rarely, it may lead to subdural haematoma, or even coning and death.

8. How would you manage the diagnosed PDPH?

- **Conservative:**
    - Encourage oral fluids and/or IV hydration.
    - Reassurance.
    - Bed rest will not fix the CSF leak but it relieves the headache symptom. Despite this, the Cochrane review concludes that bed rest should be abandoned.
- **Pharmacological:**
    - Caffeine – either IV (e.g. 500 mg caffeine in 1 L of saline) or orally.
    - Synacthen (synthetic ACTH).
    - Regular analgesia: paracetamol, diclofenac, etc.
    - Other drugs with insufficient evidence in the literature are:
        - 5-HT agonists (e.g. sumatriptan).
        - Gabapentin, DDAVP.
        - Theophylline.
        - Hydrocortisone.
- **Interventional:**
    - Immediate:
        - Insertion of long-term intrathecal catheter placement (15%) and epidural saline bolus (13%).
        - Epidural morphine
    - Epidural blood patch: this involves injecting approximately 20 ml of the patient's own fresh blood (taken in a strict sterile fashion) into the epidural space near the site of the suspected puncture. It is successful in the majority of cases and the onset of relief from headache may be immediate (but occasionally takes up to 24 hours). In patients in whom a blood patch is not successful, or where relief is temporary, it may be repeated, although the likelihood of improvement is reduced.

Further reading

Apfel, C.C. Prevention of postdural puncture headache after accidental dural puncture: a quantitative systematic review. *British Journal of Anaesthesia* 2010; **105**:255–63.

Halker, R.B., Demaerschalk, B.M., Wellik, K.E., et al. Caffeine for the prevention and treatment of postdural puncture headache: Debunking the myth. *Neurologist* 2007; **13**:323–7.

Paech, M.J. Epidural blood patch, myths and legends. *Canadian Journal of Anaesthesia* 2005; **52**(Supp 1):R12.

Segal, S. and Arendt, K.W. A retrospective effectiveness study of loss of resistance to air or saline for identification of the epidural space. *Anesthesia & Analgesia* 2010; **110**:558–63.

Sudlow, C.L.M. and Warlow, C.P. Posture and fluids for preventing post-dural puncture headache. *Cochrane Database of Systematic Reviews* 2001; **2**:CD001790. Available at: http://www2.cochrane.org/reviews/en/ab001790.html

Short case 3: Trauma patient with head injury

1. What do you think is going on?
Here is a young patient involved in a road traffic accident with falling Glasgow Coma Scale and open compound fracture which require surgery. He requires full trauma survey with examination and investigation to find the cause of falling GCS.

2. Will you anaesthetize this patient in his present condition? If not, why?
I will not anaesthetize this patient because:
- This patient needs primary survey (airway with cervical spine, breathing, circulation, disability, and exposure) and
- Resuscitation followed by secondary survey as per ATLS protocol.

3. Is the fall in GCS significant? What could be the possible causes for this deterioration?
The fall in GCS is significant as this could suggest a rise in intracranial pressure (ICP). The rise in ICP could be due to:
- Cerebral oedema (vasogenic, cytotoxic, interstitial).
- Blood (extradural, subdural, subarachnoid, intracerebral).
- CSF (outflow obstruction due to subarachnoid haemorrhage).

4. What are the indications for ICP monitoring following head injury?
The indication for intracranial pressure monitoring is when GCS is <8 with an abnormal CT scan.
Normal CT scan but 2 or more of the following factors:
- Age >40 years
- Hypotension
- Unilateral/bilateral posturing

5. How will you assess integrity of his cervical spine?
The best method is by clinical assessment but this may not be possible in this patient. He should have AP and lateral cervical spine radiographs. Helical CT scans with 3D reconstruction will provide adequate radiological 'evidence' to clear the cervical spine in the majority of comatose patients.

6. What more information do you need about the patient and the circumstances of the accident?
- History of transient loss of consciousness, convulsions, vomiting following the accident.
- CSF/ blood discharge from nose, ears.
- Previous anaesthetics, allergies, time of last oral intake.
- Drugs administered by the paramedics (morphine etc.).

7. What anaesthetic technique would you use to anaesthetize this patient for ORIF of the tibial fracture?
My main aim is to prevent secondary brain damage and maintain the cerebral perfusion. I will use general anaesthesia with rapid sequence induction technique with IPPV which would be a good anaesthetic for this patient as it would prevent increase in ICP due to rise in $PaCO_2$ which is possible during spontaneous ventilation. Furthermore, there is a potential for aspiration because of his depressed neurological status. I will take care during intubation to prevent a surge in ICP.

Further reading

American College of Surgeons. *Advanced Trauma Life Support for Doctors Student Course Manual*. Chicago, IL: American College of Surgeons, 2001.

Harrison, P. and Cairns, C. Clearing the cervical spine in the unconscious patient. *Continuing Education in Anaesthesia, Critical Care & Pain* 2008; **8**:117–20.

Clinical science

QUESTIONS

Anatomy: Abdomen wall

1. What are the layers of the abdominal wall (from superficial to deep)?
2. Describe the muscles of the abdominal wall (muscle, origin, insertion action, and innervation).
3. What is transversus abdominis plane (TAP) block?
4. What are the indications of TAP block?
5. How would you perform an ultrasound-guided TAP-block?
6. What are the complications?

Physiology: Plasma proteins

1. What are the main serum proteins?
2. Which is the most important?
3. What is the normal plasma concentration of these proteins?
4. Where is albumin produced?
5. What are the main functions of plasma proteins and albumin?
6. What are the causes of decreased plasma albumin?
7. If a critically ill patient has low albumin should hypoalbuminaemia be corrected?

Pharmacology: Evidence-based medicine

1. What do you understand by evidence-based medicine (EBM)?
2. What are the steps in the EBM process?
3. What is best available clinical evidence?
4. What are the levels of evidences?
5. How would you assess quality of evidence?
6. How would you grade strength of recommendations?
7. What is meta-analysis?
8. What are the criticisms of EBM?

Physics and clinical measurement: Blood pressure measurement

1. Define pressure and what is the SI unit to measure blood pressure?
2. What is blood pressure, pulse pressure, and mean arterial blood pressure?
3. Why do you need to measure blood pressure? How do you measure it?

Structured Oral Examination Practice for the Final FRCA

4. What are the components required to measure blood pressure and enumerate the techniques for measuring non-invasive blood pressure?
5. How does the continuous automated non-invasive blood pressure device work?
6. What are the causes of inaccuracies with automated non-invasive BP device?
7. What is continuous non-invasive blood pressure measurement? How does it work?

ANSWERS

Anatomy: Abdomen wall

1. What are the layers of the abdominal wall (from superficial to deep)?
- Skin
- Fascia:
  - Camper's fascia—fatty superficial layer
  - Scarpa's fascia—deep fibrous layer
- Muscle:
  - Rectus abdominis
  - External oblique muscle
  - Internal oblique muscle
  - Transverse abdominal muscle
- Fascia transversalis
- Peritoneum

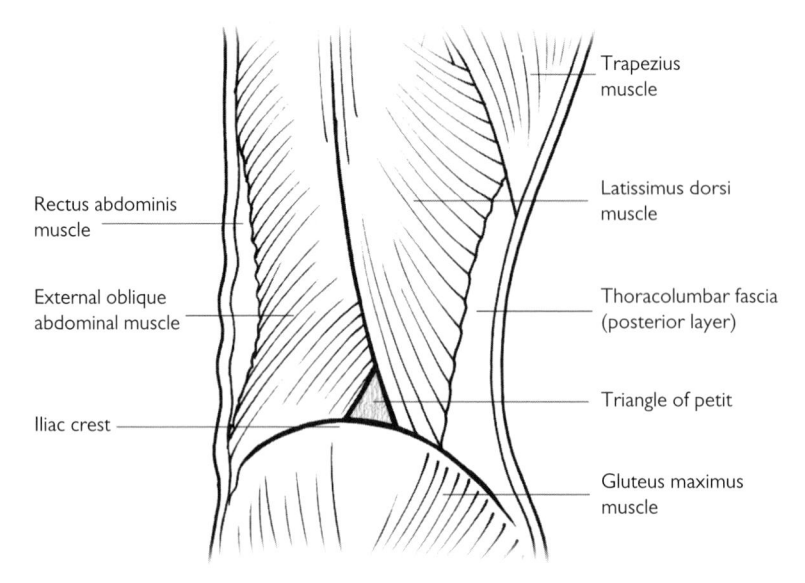

Figure 12.3 Muscle layers of the abdominal wall.
Reproduced with permission from the British Journal of Anaesthesia (Yarwood, J. and Berrill, A. Nerve blocks of the anterior abdominal wall. *Continuing Education in Anaesthesia Critical Care & Pain* 2010; **10**:182–6.)

2. Describe the muscles of the abdominal wall (muscle, origin, insertion action, and innervation).

Muscles of abdominal wall

Muscle	Origin	Insertion	Action	Innervation
Rectus abdominis	Pubis and the pubic symphysis	Xiphoid process of the sternum and costal cartilages 5–7	Flexes the trunk	Intercostal nerves 7–11 and subcostal nerve
External abdominal oblique	Lower 8 ribs	Linea alba, pubic crest and tubercle, anterior superior iliac spine and anterior half of iliac crest	Flexes and laterally bends the trunk	Intercostal nerves 7–11, subcostal, iliohypogastric and ilioinguinal nerves
Internal abdominal oblique	Thoracolumbar fascia, anterior 2/3 of the iliac crest, lateral 2/3 of the inguinal ligament	Lower 3 or 4 ribs, linea alba, pubic crest	Flexes and laterally bends the trunk	Intercostal nerves 7–11, subcostal, iliohypogastric and ilioinguinal nerves
Transversus abdominis	Lower 6 ribs, thoracolumbar fascia, anterior 3/4 of the iliac crest, lateral 1/3	Linea alba, pubic crest and pecten of the pubis	Compresses the abdomen	Intercostal nerves 7–11, subcostal, iliohypogastric and ilioinguinal nerves

3. What is transversus abdominis plane (TAP) block?

The TAP block was first described as a landmark-guided technique involving needle insertion at the triangle of Petit. This provides access to number of abdominal wall nerves hence providing more widespread analgesia.

4. What are the indications of TAP block?

This block is indicated for any lower abdominal surgery including appendectomy, hernia repair, Caesarean section, abdominal hysterectomy, and prostatectomy. Efficacy in laparoscopic surgery has also been demonstrated. Bilateral blocks can be given for midline incisions or laparoscopic surgery.

Applied anatomy

The triangle of Petit is an area bounded by:

- The latissimus dorsi muscle posteriorly.
- The external oblique muscle anteriorly.
- The iliac crest inferiorly (the base of the triangle).

Nerve supply

Innervation of the anterolateral abdominal wall arises from the anterior rami of spinal nerves T7 to L1. These include the intercostal nerves (T7–T11), the subcostal nerve (T12), and the iliohypogastric and ilioinguinal nerves (L1).

The aim of a TAP block is to deposit local anaesthetic in the plane between the internal oblique and transversus abdominis muscles targeting the spinal nerves in this plane. The innervation to abdominal skin, muscles, and parietal peritoneum will be interrupted.

Structured Oral Examination Practice for the Final FRCA

Blind TAP

The point of entry is the lumbar triangle of Petit which is situated between the lower costal margin and iliac crest. It is bound anteriorly by the external oblique muscle and posteriorly by the latissimus dorsi. This technique relies on feeling double pops as the needle traverses the external oblique and internal oblique muscles. A blunt needle will make the loss of resistance more appreciable.

Ultrasound-guided TAP

The ultrasound probe is placed in a transverse plane to the lateral abdominal wall in the mid-axillary line, between the lower costal margin and iliac crest. The use of ultrasound allows for accurate deposition of the local anaesthetic in the correct neurovascular plane.

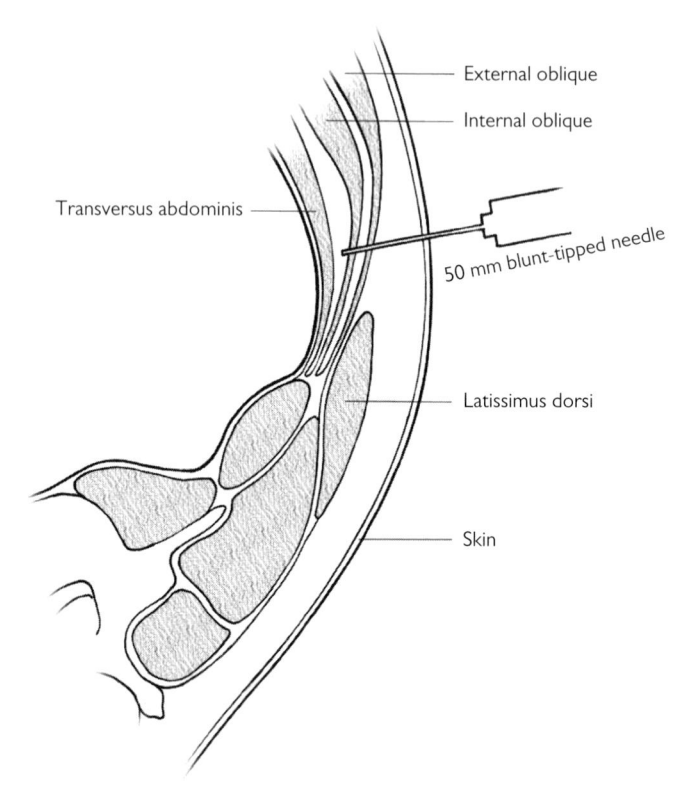

Figure 12.4 Placement of a TAP block.
Reproduced with permission from the British Journal of Anaesthesia (Yarwood, J. and Berrill, A. Nerve blocks of the anterior abdominal wall. *Continuing Education in Anaesthesia Critical Care & Pain* 2010; **10**:182–6.)

5. How would you perform the ultrasound-guided block?

- The patient is placed in a supine position and the abdomen is exposed between the costal margin and the iliac crest.
- Ultrasound machine with a high frequency probe (10–15 MHz).
- Ultrasound probe cover.
- Antiseptic for skin disinfection.

- Identify the fascial plane between the internal oblique and transversus abdominis. muscles. Sterile ultrasound gel.
- Needle: 50-mm or 80-mm needle.
- 20-ml needle and injection tubing.
- 20–30 ml local anaesthetic (any local anaesthetic concentration, this block relies on local anaesthetic spread rather than concentration, i.e. is volume dependant).

6. What are the complications?

There have been no reported complications to date with the ultrasound-guided technique. A few complications have been reported with blind TAP block, the most significant of which was a case report of intrahepatic injection. Other complications include: intraperitoneal injection, bowel haematoma, and transient femoral nerve palsy. Local anaesthetic toxicity could also occur due to the large volumes required to perform this block especially if it was done bilaterally. As with any regional technique, careful aspiration will help avoid intravascular injections.

Further reading

Aveline, C., Le Hetet, H., Vautier, P., et al. Comparison between ultrasound-guided transversus abdominis plane and conventional ilioinguinal/iliohypogastric nerve blocks for day-case open inguinal hernia repair. *British Journal of Anaesthesia* 2011; **106**:380–6.

McDonnell, J.G., O'Donnell, B., and Curley, G. The analgesic efficacy of transversus abdominis plane block after abdominal surgery: a prospective randomized controlled trial. *Anesthesia & Analgesia* 2007; **104**:193–7.

Mukhtar, K. Transversus abdominis plane (TAP) block. *Journal of The New York School of Regional Anesthesia* 2009; **12**:28–33.

Yarwood, J. and Berrill, A. Nerve blocks of the anterior abdominal wall. *Continuing Education in Anaesthesia Critical Care & Pain* 2010; **10**:182–6.

Physiology: Plasma proteins

1. What are the main serum proteins?

The main serum proteins are albumin, globulin (alpha-1 acid glycoprotein, alpha-2 beta and gamma globulins), and fibrinogen.

2. Which is the most important?

Albumin is the most important.

3. What is the normal plasma concentration of these proteins?

The serum concentration is 50–80 g/L. The concentration of albumin is 45 g/L, globulin 25 g/L, and fibrinogen 3 g/L.

4. Where is albumin produced?

Albumin is produced by liver at a rate of 9–12 g per day and released in the circulation. Albumin has a strong negative charge. There is no storage of albumin and it is not metabolized during a catabolic state. The rate of production depends on the colloid osmotic pressure and osmolality of extravascular space.

The total extravascular albumin actually exceeds the total intravascular amount by 30%. The ratio of albumin to water is, however, higher in the intravascular space (the extracellular fluid is 2/3 interstitial and 1/3 intravascular), hence the colloidal effect. Albumin cyclically leaves the circulation, through the endothelial barrier at the level of the capillaries, passes into the interstitium and returns to the bloodstream through the lymph system via the thoracic duct. The circulation half time for this process is 16–18 hours. 4–5% of total intravascular albumin extravascates in this way per hour: this rate of movement is known as the transcapillary escape rate (TER). The concentration of albumin in lymph protein content is approximately 80% that of plasma.

5. What are the main functions of plasma proteins and albumin?

The major function of plasma proteins are:
- Binding and transport (endogenous e.g. bilirubin, and exogenous, e.g. drugs).
- Maintenance of colloid osmotic pressure: albumin is responsible for 75% of osmotic pressure.
- Free radical scavenging: albumin is a major source of SH-groups 'thiols' which scavenge free radicals (nitrogen and oxygen species). Albumin may be an important free radical scavenger in sepsis.
- Proteolytic system:
    - Complement function.
    - Kinin system.
    - Coagulation system.
    - Fibrinolytic system.
- Acid–base balance.
- Immune response.
- Enzyme activity.

The main functions of albumin are oncotic pressure and transport functions.

6. What are the causes of decreased plasma albumin?
- Decreased synthesis.
- Increased catabolism.
- Increased loss: nephrotic syndrome, exudative loss in burns, haemorrhage, gut loss.
- Redistribution: haemodilution, increased capillary permeability (increased interstitial albumin), decreased lymph clearance.

7. If a critically ill patient has low albumin should hypoalbuminaemia be corrected?

The low serum albumin concentration is a consequence of a disease process and successful treatment of the underlying disease would gradually return to the normal albumin concentrations. This is suggested by the evidence from the Cochrane group's 'meta' analysis and SAFE study reveals that correcting hypoalbuminaemia in critically ill patient is not beneficial.

Further reading

A comparison of albumin and saline for fluid resuscitation in the intensive care unit. *New England Journal of Medicine* 2004; **350**:2247–56.

Pharmacology: Evidence-based medicine

1. What do you understand by evidence-based medicine (EBM)?

'Evidence based medicine is the conscientious, explicit, and judicious use of current best evidence in making decisions about the care of individual patients. The practice of evidence based medicine means integrating individual clinical expertise with the best available external clinical evidence from systematic research.' (Sackett et al. 1996.)

EBM is the integration of best research evidence with clinical expertise and patient values.

2. What are the steps in the EBM process?

EBM forms part of the **multifaceted process** of assuring clinical effectiveness, the main elements of which are:

- Production of evidence through research and scientific review.
- Production and dissemination of evidence-based clinical guidelines.
- Implementation of evidence-based, cost-effective practice through education and management of change.
- Evaluation of compliance with agreed practice guidance through clinical audit and outcomes-focused incentives.

3. What is best available clinical evidence?

Best research evidence may come from basic medical sciences, but more often it arises from patient-centred clinical research. Clinicians may often seek evidence for the efficacy and safety of therapeutic, rehabilitative, and preventive regimens, but evidence may also relate to the accuracy and precision of diagnostic tests or the power of prognostic markers.

- Therapy: double-blind, placebo-controlled, randomized clinical trial.
- Diagnosis: independent, blind comparison with a reference standard.
- Prognosis: representative and well-defined prospective cohort of patients at a similar point in the course of disease.

4. What are the levels of evidences?

The Oxford Centre for Evidence-based Medicine suggests levels of evidence (LOE) according to the study designs and critical appraisal of prevention, diagnosis, prognosis, therapy, and harm studies:

- Level A: Consistent Randomized Controlled Clinical Trial, cohort study, all or none, clinical decision rule validated in different populations.
- Level B: Consistent Retrospective Cohort, Exploratory Cohort, Ecological Study, Outcomes Research, case–control study; or extrapolations from level A studies.
- Level C: Case-series study or extrapolations from level B studies.
- Level D: Expert opinion without explicit critical appraisal, or based on physiology, bench research or first principles.

The US Preventive Services Task Force for ranking evidence about the effectiveness of treatments or screening:

- Level I: evidence obtained from at least one properly designed randomized controlled trial.
- Level II-1: evidence obtained from well-designed controlled trials without randomization.
- Level II-2: evidence obtained from well-designed cohort or case–control analytic studies, preferably from more than one centre or research group.
- Level II-3: evidence obtained from multiple time series with or without the intervention. Dramatic results in uncontrolled trials might also be regarded as this type of evidence.

- Level III: opinions of respected authorities, based on clinical experience, descriptive studies, or reports of expert committees.

5. How would you assess quality of evidence?
- Assessing for importance of outcomes:
  - Identifying critical outcomes.
  - Identifying important but not critical outcomes.
  - Identifying unimportant outcomes that can be ignored.
- Key components: study design, study quality, consistency, directness.
- Other factors affecting quality of evidence:
  - Imprecise or sparse data.
  - Reporting bias.
  - Strength of association.
  - Evidence of a dose–response gradient.
- Grading the overall quality of evidence: based on the lowest quality of evidence across the critical outcomes.

6. How would you grade strength of recommendations?
- Obtaining the quality of evidence.
- Assessing trade-offs: balance of benefits and risks and balance of net benefits and costs.
- Applicability: translation of the evidence into practice in a specific setting.
- Uncertainty about baseline risk for the study population:
  - A. Consistent with level I studies.
  - B. Consistent level II or III studies or expectations from level I studies.
  - C. Level IV studies or expectations from Level II or III studies.
  - D. Level V evidence or inconsistent or inconclusive studies of any level.

7. What is meta-analysis?
Meta-analysis is a statistical technique for combining the findings from independent studies. Meta-analysis is most often used to assess the clinical effectiveness of healthcare interventions; it does this by combining data from two or more randomized control trials (RCTs). Meta-analysis of trials provides a precise estimate of treatment effect, giving due weight to the size of the different studies included. The validity of the meta-analysis depends on the quality of the systematic review on which it is based.

Good meta-analyses aim for complete coverage of all relevant studies, look for the presence of heterogeneity, and explore the robustness of the main findings using sensitivity analysis.

8. What are the criticisms of EBM?
- RCTs do not guarantee the absence of bias; clinicians need to develop new skills in searching the literature, critically appraising and grading all the available evidence.
- 'Cookbook' medicine; guidelines and recommendations appear to promote 'cook book' medicine, suppressing clinical freedom and expertise.
- RCTs cannot provide appropriate evidence for most clinical situations; although at the top of the evidence hierarchy, RCT methodology is superfluous in many clinical situations, for example, when presented with a patient with tension pneumothorax. However, EBM urges one to use the best available evidence.
- Shortage of coherent, consistent, and valid information.
- Difficulties in applying evidence to the care of individual patients.
- Other barriers to the practice of high quality medicine.

Further reading

Belsey, J. What is evidence-based medicine? http://www.whatisseries.co.uk
Sackett, D.L., Rosenberg, W.M.C., Muir-Gray, J.A., et al. Evidence-based medicine: What it is and what it isn't (Editorial). *British Medical Journal* 1996; **312**:71–2.

Physics and clinical measurement: Blood pressure measurement

1. Define pressure and what is the SI unit to measure blood pressure?

Pressure is defined as force exerted per unit area The SI unit of pressure is the pascal (Pa). But the most widely used unit to measure blood pressure is millimetres of mercury (mmHg).

2. What is blood pressure, pulse pressure, and mean arterial blood pressure?

The rhythmic contraction of the left ventricle, ejecting blood into the vascular system, results in pulsatile arterial pressures. The peak pressure generated during systolic contraction is the systolic arterial blood pressure (SBP); the trough pressure during diastolic relaxation is the diastolic arterial blood pressure (DBP).

Pulse pressure is the difference between the systolic and diastolic pressures.

The time-weighted average of arterial pressures during a pulse cycle is the mean arterial pressure (MAP).

$$\text{Mean BP} = \frac{\text{SBP} + (2 \times \text{DBP})}{3}$$

3. Why do you need to measure blood pressure? How do you measure it?

BP is one of the minimum standards of patient monitoring required during anaesthesia. The measure of BP, oxygen saturation, and capnography in combination will detect most of the adverse events under anaesthesia. The common method of measuring BP are the non invasive and invasive direct arterial (gold standards).

4. What are the components required to measure blood pressure and enumerate the techniques for measuring non-invasive blood pressure?

The intermittent, non-invasive BP systems require three key components:

- Inflatable cuff for occluding the arterial supply to the distal limb.
- Method for determining the point of systolic and diastolic BPs.
- Method for measuring pressure.

The cuff is inflated to a pressure above that of the arterial systolic pressure. At this point, the walls of the artery are opposed, preventing blood flow. The cuff is then deflated below systolic pressure allowing blood flow to resume; this flow can then be detected using various means.

- Palpation (classical)
- Doppler
- Auscultation
- Oscillotonometry: the Von Recklinghausen oscillotonometer
- Liquid manometers

- Aneroid gauge
- Electronic systems

5. How does the continuous automated non-invasive blood pressure device works?

- A microprocessor controls the sequence of inflation and deflation of the cuff.
- The cuff is inflated to a pressure above the previous systolic pressure; it is then deflated incrementally. A transducer senses the pressure changes, which are processed by the microprocessor. This has an accuracy of ± 2%.
- The mean arterial pressure (MAP) corresponds to the maximum oscillation at the lowest cuff pressure. The systolic pressure corresponds to the onset of rapidly increasing oscillations. Diastolic pressure corresponds to the onset of rapidly decreasing oscillations. It is also calculated from the systolic and MAP (MAP = diastolic + one-third pulse pressure).

6. What are the causes of inaccuracies with automated non-invasive BP device?

- Relies on a pulse of regular rate and rhythm for accurate measurement with no arrhythmias.
- Appropriately sized cuff should be used. The cuff should cover two-third of the upper arm or be 20% larger than the diameter of the extremity being used. Too small a cuff leads to over-estimation of BP.
- Accidental movement of the limb will impair measurement. Limb should be level with heart.
- The cuff should not be compressed external, i.e. it should not be placed on the lower limb when the patient is placed in the lateral position.
- It is not possible to measure very low pressures accurately.
- Requires an artery to be compressed. Non-compliant vessels, e.g. calcified will alter measured BP.
- Tissues, including nerves, can be damaged due to compression.
- Often painful for the awake patient. The initial reading requires especially high inflation pressures.

7. What is continuous non-invasive blood pressure measurement? How does it work?

The Finapres (Finapres Medical Systems) arterial tonometry is a non-invasive technique that offers the clinician a beat-to-beat BP waveform along with numeric values for systolic, mean, diastolic pressures, as well as pulse rate.

The Penaz principle which states 'a force exerted by a body can be determined by measuring an opposing force that prevents physical disruption'.

A small cuff is placed around a finger. A light emitting diode within the cuff shines light through the finger and is detected on the other side. The amount of light absorbed by the tissues is proportional to the volume of tissue through which it passes. With each cardiac cycle, the volume of blood within the finger varies and with it, the amount of light absorbed. In order to keep the amount of light absorbed constant, the volume must also be kept constant and so pressure is applied to the finger. The applied pressure waveform correlates to the pressure waveform of the arterial supply to the finger. The information can be displayed as a real time waveform and as a trend. The system requires calibration using an arm cuff.

Further reading

Davis, P.D. and Kenny, G.N.C (eds.). *Basic Physics and Measurement in Anaesthesia* 5th edn. Oxford: Butterworth Heinemann, 2003.

Ward, M. and Langton, J.A. Blood pressure measurement. *Continuing Education in Anaesthesia, Critical Care & Pain* 2007; **7**:122–6.

Wesseling, K.H. A century of non-invasive arterial pressure measurement: from Marey to Penaz and Finapres. *Homeostasis* 1995; **36**:50–66.

Chapter 13

Clinical anaesthesia

Long case: A patient for major cancer surgery   281

Short cases   287

   Questions   287

   Answers   288

      Short case 1: Patient with HIV   288

      Short case 2: Aortic stenosis   290

      Short case 3: Anaesthesia for ECT   292

Clinical science

Questions   295

Answers   296

   Anatomy: Pituitary gland   296

   Physiology: Coagulation   297

   Pharmacology: Gabapentin   299

   Physics and clinical measurements: Invasive pressure monitoring   301

Clinical anaesthesia

Long case: A patient for major cancer surgery

A 42-year-old female is posted for an Ivor Lewis oesophagectomy. She suffers from scleroderma with Raynaud's disease affecting upper limbs. She also has active acid reflux. She is hypertensive and gets breathless with minimal exertion. She has limited mouth opening of 2 cm and limited neck extension.

Medications
- Prednisolone 10mg once a day
- Enalapril 5mg once a day
- Sildenafil
- Prostacyclin infusion twice a month

Clinical examination				

Clinical examination	Temperature: 38.2°C; weight: 85 kg; height: 160 cm
	Pulse: 85/min, regular; BP: 170/80 mmHg; respiratory rate: 12/min
	Chest: decreased air entry bilateral bases, vesicular breath sound, fine inspiratory crepitations on auscultation
	Cardiovascular system: normal heart sound with no murmurs
	Central nervous system: no neurological deficit
Laboratory investigations	Hb — 12.2 g/dL — Na — 141 mEq/L
	MCV — 94 fL — K — 4.8 mEq/L
	WBC — 8.5 × 10^9/L — Urea — 12 mmol/L
	Platelets — 351 × 10^9/L — Creatinine — 180 μmol/L
	CRP — 110 — Glucose — 6 mmol/L
Pulmonary function tests	FEV$_1$ — 50% predicted — TLCO 50%
	FVC — 50% predicted
	FEV$_1$/FVC — Normal

QUESTIONS

1. Summarize the case.
2. Comment on the investigations.
3. Why do you get raised renal parameters in scleroderma?
4. Why is the glomerular filtration rate (GFR) decreased in this condition?
5. Comment on the pulmonary function tests.
6. Comment on the chest-X ray and ECG.
7. What is scleroderma?
8. Why is she on steroids?
9. What problems do you expect in patients on steroids?
10. What is sildenafil? Why is the patient on this treatment?
11. What other investigations can you do? Explain them.
12. Comment on the perioperative supplementation of steroids.
13. What will be your airway management plan in this case?

Structured Oral Examination Practice for the Final FRCA

14. What manoeuvres do you do once the DLT is inserted? How do you confirm the position of left-sided DLT?
15. What are the intraoperative problems with DLT?
16. What is your plan for postoperative analgesia?
17. Should this patient undergo postoperative ventilation? What are the implications?
18. How do you manage postoperative hypertension—pulmonary and systemic?

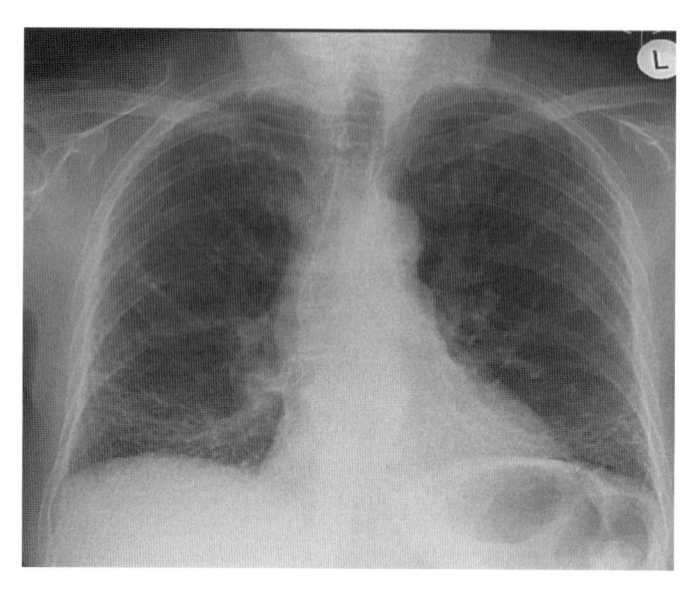

Figure 13.1 Chest X-ray.

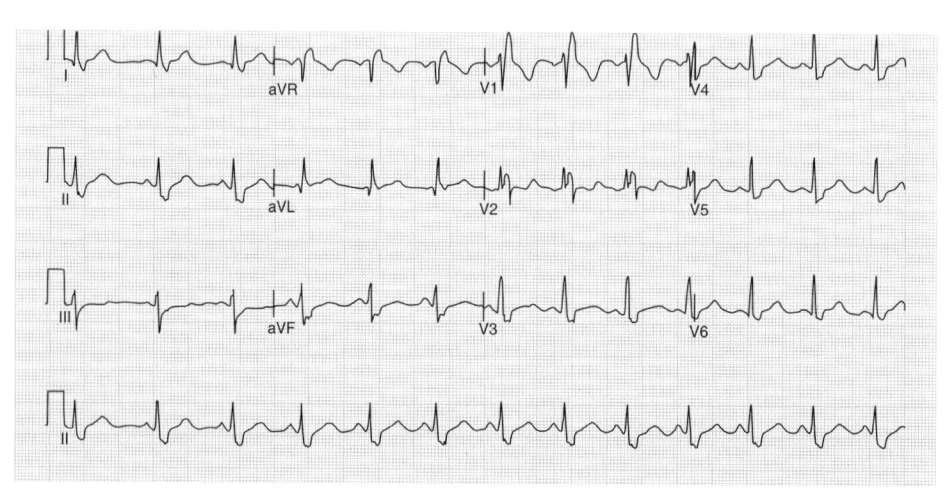

Figure 13.2 ECG.

Chapter 13

ANSWERS

1. Summarize the case.

We have a young female patient with an autoimmune connective tissue disease. She is listed as urgent for major upper GI surgery for malignancy. She has multisystem compromise with significant respiratory compromise and a potentially difficult airway. She will require a thorough preoperative assessment and careful and diligent intraoperative and postoperative management.

2. Comment on the investigations.

- Haematology is within normal limits.
- Urea and creatinine are raised—indicative of impaired renal function.

3. Why do you get raised renal parameters in scleroderma?

The cause of impaired renal function in scleroderma is secondary to the pathological changes in renal vasculature just like in skin. Renal crisis can develop due to malignant hypertension causing acute renal failure. ACE inhibitors like enalapril are used for the treatment of renal dysfunction and hypertension.

4. Why is the glomerular filtration rate (GFR) decreased in this condition?

Renal vascular changes cause a decreased GFR. GFR is a marker of the degree of renal dysfunction and changes much earlier than serum creatinine levels.

5. Comment on the pulmonary function tests.

The PFT shows reduction in both FEV1 and FVC but the ratio is normal, which is characteristic of restrictive lung disease. The PFTs also show impaired oxygenation (decreased TLCO) which may occur in scleroderma from pulmonary fibrosis.

6. Comment on the chest X-ray and ECG.

Chest X-ray: anterior-posterior chest-X ray showing bilateral mid and lower zone reticular shadowing. The appearances are in keeping with established fibrosis. The heart size is normal. No focal bone abnormality. No evidence of a dilated oesophagus.

ECG: Heart rate of 75 beats/min with sinus rhythm. The broad QRS complex (>0.12s) suggests either a ventricular rhythm or conduction delay such as bundle branch block. There is slurred S wave in lead I, RSR' in V1–RBBB. There is a premature atrial contraction (PAC) as well. My impression is of sinus rate with right bundle branch block with occasional premature atrial contraction.

7. What is scleroderma?

Scleroderma is a chronic autoimmune collagen vascular disease causing widespread fibrosis of vascular endothelium resulting in end-organ damage. It mainly involves skin, lungs, heart, kidneys, and oesophagus. The prognosis is related to the number of viscera involved and is poor in case of multivisceral involvement.

8. Why is she on steroids?

The pathophysiology of scleroderma involves an autoimmune process with inflammatory narrowing of arteries. Steroids work by their anti-inflammatory and immunosuppressant effect.

9. What problems do you expect in patients on steroids?

Patients on long-term steroids are likely to show some side-effects
- General:
  - Skin changes
  - Easy bruising

- ◆ Immunosuppression
- ◆ Increase risk of infection
- ◆ Cataracts
- ◆ Central obesity
- ◆ Osteoporosis
- CVS: hypertension
- GI: peptic ulcers

10. What is sildenafil? Why is the patient on this treatment?

Sildenafil is a selective inhibitor of phosphodiesterase type 5 (PDE5) which is widely present in the body and is found in high concentration in the lungs. Inhibition of PDE5 enhances the vasodilatory effects of nitric oxide in pulmonary hypertension by preventing the degradation of cyclic guanosine monophosphate (cGMP), which promotes relaxation of vascular smooth muscle and increases blood flow. Therefore it is used in scleroderma for the treatment of severe pulmonary hypertension.

11. What other investigations can you do? Explain them.

I would further investigate the patient using:

- **Echocardiography:** ECHO is useful to quantify the degree of myocardial dysfunction and rule out any structural or valvular problems. It will also help to estimate the pulmonary pressure although you need right heart catheterization for more accurate estimate of the pulmonary pressures.
- **Cardiopulmonary exercise** (CPX) testing will help you to calculate the anaerobic threshold (AT), oxygen uptake (VO_2) and also look for any ischaemic changes on the ECG during the CPX. Ischaemic changes or severe arrhythmias occurring at AT <11 ml/kg/min will indicate a poor prognosis in which case the surgery may not be advisable.

12. Comment on the perioperative supplementation of steroids.

Endogenous cortisol production is in the range of 25 to 30 mg/24 hr. Under the stress of major operation the cortisol production increases to 75 to 100 mg/day.

- If a patient is on <10 mg prednisolone there is little danger of hypothalmo–pituitary–adrenal (HPA) axis suppression.
- On the other hand if the patient is on >10 mg of prednisolone for over 2 weeks they risk HPA suppression. For major surgery it is required to supplement exogenous steroids in a dose of 25 mg IV at induction then followed by 6 hourly doses for 48–72 hr.

13. What will be your airway management plan in this case?

The patient presents a unique challenge of difficult airway but also needing lung isolation for operative access during oesophagectomy. The safest option will be awake fibreoptic intubation with the patient slightly sitting up. For lung isolation we can use a left-sided double lumen tube (DLT). However, if the mouth opening is very limited even for a DLT insertion or there is a plan/possibility for elective postoperative ventilation, we should use a single lumen tube with a selective bronchial blocker.

14. What manoeuvres do you do once the DLT is inserted? How do you confirm the position of left-sided DLT?

First connect the DLT to the breathing system using a double catheter mount, each lumen is connected via a capped angle connector.

Cuff inflation

The tracheal cuff is inflated first and ventilates through both lumens. There should be no air leak and both lungs should have good air entry.

The catheter mount to the tracheal lumen is then clamped and the trachea is opened to air by taking the cap off the angle connector. The lung is then inflated via the bronchial lumen and air filled in the bronchial cuff slowly until there is no leak of air through the tracheal lumen open to air.

There should be air entry in the lung on the bronchial lumen side and no air entry on the tracheal lumen side. The tracheal lumen is then unclamped and the cap closed. The air entry should be back to normal on both sides.

Best way to confirm the correct position is by fibreoptic scope. Put the scope down the tracheal lumen and you should be able to see the carina distal to the opening and the right main bronchus branching out. The blue cuff of the bronchial lumen may be just visible going into the left main bronchus. Then put the scope down the bronchial lumen and you should be able to see the left upper lobe bronchus distal to the tube tip.

Clinical assessment is not very reliable therefore fibreoptic confirmation of tube position is essential.

15. What are the intraoperative problems with DLT?

The double lumen endotracheal tubes are semi-rigid tubes and can cause:

- Trauma: to oral, dental, or pharyngeal structures during intubation especially in scleroderma. In difficult airway they can be more difficult to insert and also traumatize the cords or trachea.
- Malposition: the DLT can move during lateral positioning. This malpositioning can result in failure of lung isolation or, occasionally, difficulty with ventilation.

16. What is your plan for postoperative analgesia?

The postoperative analgesia can be provided as multimodal analgesia regimen by:

- Regional anaesthesia:
    - Thoracic epidural (T6–T7) will cover for the laprotomy and thoracotomy pain.
    - Paravertebral blocks where the paravertebral catheters are directly sited by surgeons are supported by evidence of good pain relief and are better than epidurals for thoracotomies. However, they don't cover laparotomy pain.
- IV opioid if regional anaesthesia is contraindicated:
    - Parenteral opioid: morphine continuous infusion or patient controlled PCA—morphine.
    - Regional techniques like paravertebral blocks, intercostal blocks, intrapleural catheter. These other regional techniques won't provide complete analgesia so they will need to be supplemented with parenteral drugs like IV PCA morphine and IV paracetamol.
    - We should avoid NSAIDs in this case.

17. Should this patient undergo postoperative elective ventilation? What are the implications?

The pulmonary hypertension demands avoidance of hypoxia, hypercapnia, acidosis, and sympathetic activity. This is best achieved by elective ventilation. This necessitates the need to change from DLT to a single lumen tube at the end of surgery. This can be done with the help of a long bougie like the Cook's airway exchange catheter but has to be done very carefully. To avoid the risk of further airway management at the end of the operation, a single lumen endotracheal tube with the bronchial blocker should be used at the beginning of the operation.

18. How do you manage postoperative hypertension—pulmonary and systemic?

Postoperative hypertension is usually because of pain and needs to be managed with good balanced analgesia. Other pharmacological treatments include GTN infusion, esmolol infusion, labetalol, or hydralazine. To avoid pulmonary hypertension we have to avoid hypercapnia, hypoxia, acidosis, and other causes of sympathetic activity.

Further reading

Allman, K.G. and Wilson, I.H. *Oxford Handbook of Anaesthesia*, 2nd edn. Chapter 15: Thoracic surgery; Oesophagectomy, pp. 351–84; Chapter 36: Airway assessment and management; Awake fibre-optic intubation, pp. 917–953. Oxford: Oxford University Press, 2006.

Ovassapian, A., Krejcie T. C., Yelich, S. J. and Dykes, M. H. M. Awake fibreoptic intubation in the patient at high risk of aspiration. *Br. J. Anaesth.* (1989) **62**(1): 13–16.

Popat, M. *Practical Fibre-optic Intubation*. Oxford:Butterworth Heinemann, 2001.

Yentis, S.M., Hirsch, N.P., and Smith, G.S. One-lung ventilation. In *Anaesthesia and Intensive Care A–Z: An Encyclopaedia of Principles and Practice* 4th edn., p. 397. Edinburgh: Churchill Livingstone, 2009.

Chapter 13

Short cases

QUESTIONS

Short case 1: Patient with HIV

You have a patient on your list for incision and drainage of abscess on her right arm. She is an intravenous drug abuser and the nurse says she has a blood-borne infection.

1. What are the issues surrounding this patient?
2. What is the pathophysiology of HIV?
3. What are the modes of transmission in a case of HIV?
4. How is HIV infection diagnosed?
5. What are the causes of respiratory infections in a patient with HIV infection?
6. What type of cardiovascular pathologies can occur in a patient with HIV?
7. What are the implications of HIV in pregnancy and obstetric anaesthesia?
8. What are the common drugs and the side effects of drug therapy in HIV patients?
9. What are the implications of a patient with HIV for healthcare workers?
10. What precautions are you going to take for anaesthetic procedures in patients with HIV?

Short case 2: Aortic stenosis

A 75-year-old lady is coming for an elective total knee replacement. On her pre-assessment visit, she says she gets occasional chest pain and shortness of breath on exertion. On examination you hear a loud ejection systolic murmur.

1. What are the causes of ejection systolic murmur?
2. What is the pathophysiology of aortic stenosis?
3. How would you proceed with this case?
4. How do you propose to assess the cardiac lesion?
5. Why would you do echocardiography?
6. How do you grade the severity of aortic stenosis?
7. When would you consider replacing the valve before surgery?
8. How would you anaesthetize the patient if she did not have her valve replaced before surgery?

Short case 3: Anaesthesia for ECT

1. What can you tell us about electroconvulsive therapy?
2. What are the indications for electroconvulsive therapy?
3. How would assess a patient who is for ECT?
4. What would be your anaesthetic management?
5. What are the effects of electroconvulsive therapy?
6. What induction agent would you use?
7. Why should you add muscle relaxant?

ANSWERS

Short case 1: Patient with HIV

1. What are the issues surrounding this patient?

This patient is a known intravenous drug user and is likely to have difficult venous access. The other issues related to blood-borne infection are:

- Immunocompromised patient
- Health risk to staff
- Cross contamination
- Associated comorbid conditions

2. What is the pathophysiology of HIV?

HIV is caused by a human retrovirus in the subfamily of lentiviruses. Retroviruses contain the enzyme reverse transcriptase that allows viral RNA to be transcribed into DNA, which is then incorporated into the host cell genome. The virus preferentially infects T-helper lymphocytes (T cells) and progressively destroys them, leading to increased susceptibility to opportunistic infections and malignancies.

3. What are the modes of transmission in a case of HIV?

- Sexual intercourse (vaginal and anal)
- Mother to child (during pregnancy, labour and breastfeeding)
- Contaminated blood, blood products, and organ donations
- Contaminated needles

4. How is HIV infection diagnosed?

The diagnosis is made by a highly sensitive initial screening test for detection of anti-HIV IgG antibodies which is called enzyme-linked immunosorbent assay (ELISA). This test may not be positive during the initial window period in which case, the test will have to be repeated in 3–6 months. However, if ELISA is positive, an antigen-based confirmatory test is performed, called a western blot test, which is highly specific.

5. What are the causes of respiratory infections in a patient with HIV infection?

The dominant respiratory complications in HIV/AIDS are as a result of opportunistic infections This includes *Pneumocystis jiroveci* pneumonia (PCP), aspergillosis, herpetic infections, oral and pharyngeal candidiasis and cytomegaloviral (CMV) pneumonia. Mycobacterial infections (*Mycobacterium tuberculosis* and atypical organisms, e.g. *M. avium intracellulare*) have reached epidemic proportions, especially in some African countries. Bacterial pneumonia (*Streptococcus pneumoniae, Haemophilus influenzae, Staphylococcus aureus* and *Psudomonas aeuruginosa*) may progress to acute respiratory failure.

6. What type of cardiovascular pathologies can occur in a patient with HIV?

The cardiovascular involvement is about 25–75%, seen in an autopsy series. HIV is associated with:

- Cardiomyopathy
- Pericardial effusion—TB, Kaposi's sarcoma, lymphoma, cryptococcal infection
- Endocarditis

7. What are the implications of HIV in pregnancy and obstetric anaesthesia?

The incidence is approximately 2.1 million children under 15 infected worldwide as a result of mother-to-child transmission (MTCT).

Without intervention:

- 15–30% of mothers will transmit HIV during pregnancy and delivery.
- 10–20% through breast milk.

Vertical transmission is dramatically reduced by antiretroviral therapy:

- Nevirapine is given to the mother at delivery and the neonate within 72 hours of delivery to prevent mother-to-child transmission.
- Caesarean section independently to reduce the vertical transmission and, when combined with antiretroviral therapy (ART), the rate of transmission falls to 2%.
- Regional anaesthesia is not contraindicated:
  - Epidural blood patch for PDPH appears to be safe, but other analgesic techniques should be tried first.

8. What are the common drugs and side effects of the therapy in HIV patients?

The common drugs are:

- **Reverse transcriptase inhibitors**:
  - Zidovudine, lamivudine, stavudine, Zalcitabine
  - Side effects: skin rashes, anaemia, granulocytopenia, pancreatitis, hepatomegaly with steatosis, peripheral neuropathy, lactic acidosis
- **Protease inhibitors**:
  - Saquinavir, ritonavir, indinavir
  - Side effects: lipodystrophy—fat redistribution resulting in a cushingoid appearance, hypercholesterolaemia, hyperglycaemia

9. What are the implications of a patient with HIV for healthcare workers?

- In-hospital transmission of HIV in anaesthetic practice may occur from patient to anaesthetist, from patient to patient, or from anaesthetist to patient.
- HIV can be transmitted to the anaesthetist via:
  - Sharps injury.
  - Splashing of a mucosal surface or broken skin by body fluid:
    - Incidence about 0.09%.
    - Incidence of percutaneous exposure to HIV infected blood is about 0.3 % (more with hollow needles than suture needles).
    - Factors increasing the risk of transmission following needle stick injury are the volume of blood inoculated (e.g. hollow needle injuries) and deep punctures. The cumulative risk over an anaesthetic career may be as high as 4.5%.
  - Contamination of anaesthetic equipment is a potential route for patient-to-patient transmission.

10. What precautions are you going to take for anaesthetic procedures in patients with HIV?

Carrying out procedures in an operating theatre does not pose a lower risk of infection than other hospital locations and the risk of infection depends on the procedure and on the level of barrier protection rather than the surrounding environment.

Universal precautions

- Maximal barrier precautions to prevent transmission via skin and mucous membrane:
    - Full hand washing.
    - Wearing of sterile gloves and gown, a cap, mask, plastic gown, and protective eye shields.
    - The use of a large sterile drape.
    - The skin entry site should be cleaned with an alcoholic chlorhexidine gluconate solution or alcoholic povidone–iodine-iodine solution. The antiseptic should be allowed to dry before proceeding.
- Careful handling of sharp objects, avoid recapping needles.
- Disposable equipment should be used where available.
- If a heat- and moisture-exchange filter is used with each patient, it is unnecessary to change the breathing circuit.
- Healthcare workers with exudative lesions should avoid direct patient contact.
- Use CPR equipment that obviates the need for mouth to mouth resuscitation.
- Spills should be immediately disinfected with bleach.

Further reading

Fletcher, S.J. and Bodenham, A.R. Catheter-related sepsis: an overview. *British Journal of Intensive Care* 1999; **9**: 74–80.

Maki D.G., Ringer, M., and Alvacado, C.J. Prospective randomised trial of providone-iodine, alcohol, and chlorhexidine for prevention of infection associated with central venous and arterial catheters. *Lancet* 1991; **338**:339–43.

Prout, J. and Agarwal, B. Anaesthesia and critical care for patients with HIV infection. *Continuing Education in Anaesthesia, Critical Care & Pain* 2005; **5**:153–6.

Thomas, I. and Carter, J.A. Occupational hazards of anaesthesia. *Continuing Education in Anaesthesia, Critical Care & Pain* 2006; **6**:182–7.

Short case 2: Aortic stenosis

1. What are the causes of ejection systolic murmur?

Ejection systolic murmurs or midsystolic murmurs are due to turbulent forward flow across the right and left ventricular outflow tract, aortic or pulmonary valve, or through the aorta or pulmonary artery. They are due to supravalvular aortic stenosis or outflow obstruction, VSD and pulmonary stenosis.

2. What is the pathophysiology of aortic stenosis?

Aortic stenosisis a fixed outlet obstruction to left ventricular ejection. Anatomical obstruction to left ventricular ejection leads to concentric hypertrophy of the left ventricular heart muscle. This reduces the compliance of the left ventricular chamber making it difficult to fill. Contractility and ejection fraction are usually maintained until late stages. Atrial contraction accounts for up to 40% of ventricular filling.

There is a high risk of myocardial ischaemia due to increased oxygen demand and wall tension in the hypertrophied left ventricle. 30% of patients who have aortic stenosis with normal coronary arteries have angina.

3. How would you go ahead with this case?

Valvular heart disease is found in 4% of patients over the age of 65 in the developed world.

Chapter 13

These patients have a fixed cardiac output and are unable to compensate for the reduction in systemic vascular resistance caused by the vasodilating effect of a general anaesthetic which could have disastrous consequences.

In this case my aim is to:

- Assess the significance of the cardiac lesion for the proposed TKR surgery.
- Plan anaesthesia according to the haemodynamic parameters.
- Antibiotic prophylaxis is no longer routinely recommended by NICE.

4. How do you propose to assess the cardiac lesion?

I will take a full history including the exercise tolerance and examination of the patient.

- History:
    - Angina.
    - Syncope and pre-syncope.
    - Dyspnoea.
- Examination:
    - Slow rising, low volume pulse.
    - Ejection systolic murmur with radiation to the carotids.
- Investigations:
    - Echocardiography—left ventricular contractility and the gradient across valve or valve area commonly measured.
    - ECG: LVH.
    - Cardiac catheterization to estimate the gradient across the valve.

5. Why would you do echocardiography?

The Doppler echocardiography is the standard test which identifies increased velocity of flow across stenotic valves from which pressure gradients and severity of a stenosed valve may be estimated. Doppler flow imaging can also provide estimates of the severity of regurgitant valve disease.

6. How do you grade the severity of aortic stenosis?

The severity is based of the aortic surface area and left ventricle–aortic gradient

Aortic valve area	LV-aortic gradient
Normal 2.6–3.5 cm^2	Mild 12–25 mmHg
Mild 1.2–1.8 cm^2	Moderate 25–40 mmHg
Moderate: 0.8–1.2 cm^2	Significant 40–50 mmHg
Significant: 0.6–0.8 cm^2	Critical >50 mmHg
Critical: <0.6 cm^2	

7. When would you consider replacing the valve before surgery?

This is a major case and considering the pathophysiology of the disease it would involve a multidisciplinary approach which includes orthopaedics, cardiologist, anaesthetist, and critical care.

- If the patient is symptomatic for elective surgery I would consider aortic valve replacement first as they are at great risk of sudden death perioperatively (untreated severe symptomatic stenosis has a 50% 1-year survival).
- Asymptomatic patients for TKR are associated with marked fluid shifts and with gradients across the valve >50 mmHg should have valve replacement considered prior to surgery.

8. How would you anaesthetize the patient if she did not have her valve replaced before surgery?

My aim for haemodynamic goals would be:
- (Low) normal heart rate.
- Maintain sinus rhythm.
- Adequate volume loading.
- High normal systemic vascular resistance.

To proceed with the surgery I would have a:
- Senior experienced anaesthetist.
- Senior orthopaedic surgeon.
- Full risk assessment with MDT and involvement of the family.
- Critical care bed booked for enhanced recovery in HDU/ITU postoperatively.
- Monitoring:
    - Full anaesthetic monitoring.
    - Invasive monitoring:
        - Arterial line before induction.
        - Central venous access.
- My technique of anaesthesia would be:
    - Perform awake ultrasound-guided femoral nerve block with nerve block catheter.
    - General anaesthesia with ETT.
    - A variety of techniques are possible, as long as care is taken to maintain haemodynamic parameters as close to baseline as possible
- Postoperative plan:
    - Fast track or enhanced recovery with full monitoring.
    - Acute Pain Team involvement for regional anaesthetic techniques
    - PCA morphine for additional analgesia (femoral block does not cover the entire knee joint).

Further reading

Allman, K.G. and Wilson, I.H. *Oxford Handbook of Anaesthesia*, 2nd edn. Chapter 14: Cardiac Surgery, see pp. 332–3. Oxford: Oxford University Press, 2006.

Brown, J. and Morgan-Hughes, N.J. Aortic stenosis and non-cardiac surgery. *Continuing Education in Anaesthesia Critical Care & Pain* 2005; **5**:1–4.

Short case 3: Anaesthesia for ECT

1. What can you tell us about electroconvulsive therapy?

Electroconvulsive therapy (ECT) is most commonly used to treat severe or medication resistant depression, although it can also be beneficial in mania and catatonia. ECT induces a generalized, tonic–clonic epileptic seizure.

2. What is the aim of electroconvulsive therapy?

The aim of ECT is to induce a therapeutic clonic seizure (a seizure where the person loses consciousness and has convulsions) lasting for at least 15 seconds.

The usual course of 6–12 treatments administered 2 or 3 times a week.

Chapter 13

3. How would you proceed with assessment of this patient?

The patients require full preoperative assessment which includes history and examination especially cardiopulmonary and central nervous system. History should rule out reflux and airway evaluation is important. If there is any history of coronary artery disease or raised intracranial pressure further investigation would be required.

4. What are the effects of electroconvulsive therapy?

The physiological and physical responses to ECT are:
- CVS:
  - This is secondary to activation of the autonomic nervous system. This starts with the electrical stimulus, there is an initial parasympathetic discharge lasting 10–15 sec. This can result in bradycardia, hypotension, or even asystole.
  - This is followed by sympathetic response which may have cardiac arrhythmias.
  - With pre-existing disease myocardial ischaemia and infarction can occur.
- CNS:
  - Cerebral oxygen consumption, blood flow, and intracranial pressure all increase.
  - There have been reports of transient ischaemic deficits, intracranial haemorrhage, and cortical blindness.
  - Intraocular and intragastric pressure increases.
- General effects:
  - Inadequate sedation with no muscle relaxant can result in fractures and dislocations.
  - Headaches, myalgia (either from the seizure or suxamethonium), drowsiness, weakness, nausea, and anorexia may all occur but symptoms are usually mild.
  - Increased salivation.
  - Dental damage, tongue, and oral cavity lacerations.

5. What would be your anaesthetic management?

I will follow The Royal College of Anaesthetists' guidelines for ECT provision at remote sites. I will assess the patient as for any other preoperative assessment with informed consent. Of course, the Association of Anaesthetists of Great Britain and Ireland's standards for monitoring, trained assistance, and recovery facilities should be made available along with full resuscitation equipment and drugs.

- I will pre-oxygenate the patient and after induction, ventilation can be gently assisted with a face mask.
- Inserting a bite block protects the patient's teeth, lips, and tongue.
- Postoperative considerations:
  - Standard monitoring should be applied during recovery and oxygen supplementation continued until oxygen saturations are adequate on air.
  - Most patients recover quickly and can be discharged according to the standard criteria.

6. What induction agent would you use?

I would use propofol (0.75–2.5 mg/kg.) as used commonly. There is better CVS stability; less PONV; quicker emergence.

A recent systematic review concluded that all currently available induction agents are suitable for ECT and the small variations in emergence and recovery times should not govern drug choice.

The other drugs used are:

- Methohexital: 0.5–1.5 mg/kg.
- Etomidate: 0.15–0.3mg/kg.
- Thiopental: 2–5 mg/kg.

7. Why should you add muscle relaxant?

There is violent muscular contraction due to induced seizure which may lead to skeletal injury. The use of neuromuscular blocking agents reduce muscular convulsions and decrease the risk of serious injury. Succinylcholine (0.5 mg/kg) is most commonly used.

Further reading

Hooten, W.M. and Rasmussen, K.G. Jr. Effects of general anesthetic agents in adults receiving electro convulsive therapy: a systematic review. *Journal of Electroconvulsive Therapy* 2008; **24**:208–23.

Uppal, V., Dourish, J., and Macfarlane, A. Anaesthesia for electroconvulsive therapy. *Continuing Education in Anaesthesia Critical Care & Pain* 2010; **10**:192–6.

Clinical science

QUESTIONS

Anatomy: Pituitary gland

1. Tell me about the pituitary gland.
2. What are the structures of the anterior pituitary?
3. What hormones are secreted by the anterior pituitary?
4. What are the hormones secreted by the posterior pituitary?
5. What is the influence of hypothalamus on the pituitary gland?
6. What are the functions of the pituitary gland?

Physiology: Coagulation

1. Tell me about the haemostasis mechanism in the body.
2. Outline the coagulation process.
3. How is a clot formed at an injury site?
4. Why does blood not clot when a tourniquet is inflated during total knee replacement in that limb?
5. What other mechanism prevents the clotting process?

Pharmacology: Gabapentin

1. What can you tell us about gabapentin?
2. What are the indications for use of gabapentin?
3. Is there any role of gabapentin in acute pain?
4. What is the mechanism of action of gabapentin?
5. How would you prescribe gabapentin?
6. What are the side effects of this drug?

Physics and clinical measurements: Invasive pressure monitoring

1. When would you consider invasive blood pressure monitoring in a patient?
2. How do you invasively measure the blood pressure?
3. Which artery is used and why?
4. What cannula would you use?
5. What is the significance of the fluid-filled tubing?
6. What is a transducer? Give examples.
7. What are the problems of invasive blood pressure measurement?
8. What is damping? What is its effect?

ANSWERS

Anatomy: Pituitary gland

1. Tell me about the pituitary gland.

The pituitary gland is an endocrine gland which is about the size of a pea and weighing 100 g. The gland is centrally located at the base of the brain in the sella turcica within the sphenoid bone. It is attached to the hypothalamus by the pituitary stalk and a fine vascular network.

The pituitary gland consists of the anterior lobe (adenohypophysis), the posterior lobe (neurohypophysis), and an intermediate zone.

2. What are the structures of the anterior pituitary?

The anterior pituitary gland has three parts:
- Pars tuberalis
- Pars intermedius
- Pars distalis

3. What hormones are secreted by the anterior pituitary?

Pars diatalis produces most of the hormones. All the hormones are the trophic hormones which have a growth promoting action.

The following hormones are produced by anterior pituitary:
- **Polypetides:**
  - ACTH, adrenocorticotropic hormone
  - MSH, melanocyte-stimulating hormone
- **Gycoproteins:**
  - FSH, follicle-stimulating hormone
  - LH, luteinizing hormone
  - TSH, thyrotropic hormone
- **Protein:**
  - GH, growth hormone;
  - PRL, prolactin

4. What are the hormones secreted by the posterior pituitary?

Posterior pituitary (neurohypophysis) produces oxytocin and antidiuretic hormone (ADH). These are both produced in the hypothalamus.

5. What is the influence of the hypothalamus on the pituitary gland?

The secretion of the anterior pituitary hormones is under regulation exerted by hypothalamic peptides and, with the exception of prolactin, by the negative feedback of hormones from the target glands. The hypothalamic peptides are secreted in the median eminence and are transferred to the anterior pituitary gland via the hypothalamic–pituitary portal system.

6. What are the functions of the pituitary gland?

The hormones secreted from the pituitary gland help control the following body processes:
- Growth.
- Blood pressure.

- Some aspects of pregnancy and childbirth including stimulation of uterine contractions during childbirth.
- Breast milk production.
- Sex organ functions in both men and women.
- Thyroid gland function.
- The conversion of food into energy (metabolism).
- Water and osmolarity regulation in the body.
- Secretes ADH to control the absorption of water into the kidneys.
- Temperature regulation.

Physiology: Coagulation

1. Tell me about the haemostasis mechanism in your body.

Haemostasis is a mechanism by which blood is able to remain in liquid form in the vasculature system but when there is injury to a vessel, minimizes the blood loss by coagulation of the blood.

2. Outline the coagulation process.

Coagulation can be explained by a cell-based model of haemostasis which replaces the classical model of the coagulation cascade.

- The first phase, or initiation, occurs on a tissue factor (TF)-bearing cell.
- In the amplification phase, platelets and co-factors are activated in order to prepare for large-scale thrombin generation.

Coagulation cascade

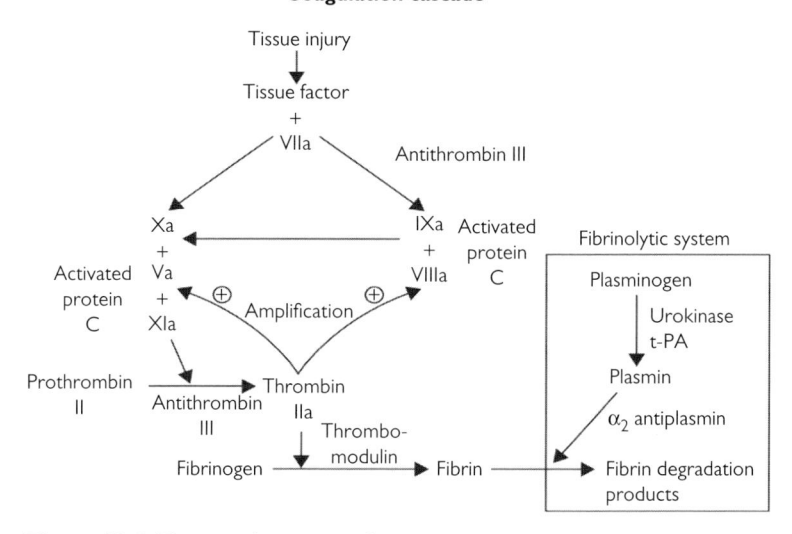

Figure 13.3 The coagulation cascade.
Reproduced with permission from Allman, K.G. and Wilson, I.H.
Oxford Handbook of Anaesthesia, 2nd edn. Oxford: Oxford University Press, 2006.

- Finally, propagation occurs on the surface of platelets, and results in the propagation of large amounts of thrombin.

3. How is a clot formed at the injury site?
The clot formation can be explained using a cell-based model.

During the first phase or initiation phase there is
- Injury of vessels wall leading to contact between blood and subendothelial cells.
- Tissue factor is exposed and binds to Factor VII.
- Factor VII is subsequently converted to Factor VIIa.
- The complex between Tissue Factor and Factor VIIa activates Factor IX and X.
- Factor Xa binds to Factor Va on the cell surface.

The second stage of amplification
- The Factor Xa–Factor Va complex converts small amounts of prothrombin into thrombin.
- The small amount of thrombin generated activates Factors VIII, V, XI and platelets locally.
- Factor XIa converts Factor IX to Factor IXa.
- Activated platelets bind Factors Va, VIIIa, and FIXa.

The final stage of coagulation
The final phase occurs on the surface of platelets
- The Factor VIIIa–IXa complex activates Factor X.
- Factor Xa in association with Factor Va converts large amounts of prothrombin into thrombin creating a 'thrombin burst'.
- The 'thrombin burst' leads to the formation of a stable fibrin clot.

4. Why does blood not get clotted when a tourniquet is inflated on total knee replacement in that limb?
The haemostasis mechanism has two important functions: one is to prevent blood loss from an injured vessel and the second is to maintain the liquid state in order to deliver the blood to tissues. The method by which blood does not clot in intact blood vessels is:
- Intact endothelium:
  - Prevents exposure to exposed collagen and tissue thromboplastin.
  - The endothelium has a glycocalyx layer which make the surface smooth.
  - Endothelium produces prostacyclin and results in vasodilatation.
  - Endothelium produces thrombomodulin and heparan sulphate.
- Coagulation factors are in active state.
- Blood washes and dilutes the active mediators.
- Inhibitory substances are present in plasma.

5. What other mechanism prevent clotting process?
Blood and plasma contains proteins which prevent or inhibits coagulation. Five mechanisms keep platelet activation and the coagulation cascade in check. Abnormalities can lead to an increased tendency toward thrombosis:
- **Protein C** is a major physiological anticoagulant. Protein C is activated by binding of Protein C and thrombin to a cell surface protein thrombomodulin. The activated form, along with protein S and a phospholipid as cofactors, degrades FVa and FVIIIa. The deficiency of either may lead to thrombophilia. Impaired action of Protein C, for example, by having the 'Leiden' variant of Factor V or high levels of FVIII also may lead to a thrombotic tendency.

- **Antithrombin** is a serine protease inhibitor (srpin) that degrades the serine proteases: thrombin, FIXa, FXa, FXIa, and FXIIa. It is constantly active, but its adhesion to these factors is increased by the presence of heparan sulphate. Deficiency of antithrombin (inborn or acquired, e.g. in proteinuria) leads to thrombophilia.
- **Tissue factor pathway inhibitor** (TFPI) limits the action of tissue factor (TF).
- **Plasmin** is generated by proteolytic cleavage of plasminogen, a plasma protein synthesized in the liver. This cleavage is catalysed by tissue plasminogen activator (t-PA), which is synthesized and secreted by endothelium. Plasmin proteolytically cleaves fibrin into fibrin degradation products that inhibit excessive fibrin formation.
- **Prostacyclin** (PGI$_2$) is released by endothelium and activates platelet G$_s$ protein-linked receptors. This, in turn, activates adenylyl cyclase, which synthesizes cAMP. cAMP inhibits platelet activation by decreasing cytosolic levels of calcium and, by doing so, inhibits the release of granules that would lead to activation of additional platelets and the coagulation cascade.

Further reading

Allman, K.G. and Wilson, I.H. *Oxford Handbook of Anaesthesia*, 2nd edn. Chapter 10: Haematological disorders, pp. 197–228. Oxford: Oxford University Press, 2006.

Hoffman, M. and Monroe, D.M. 3rd. A cell-based model of hemostasis. *Thrombosis and Haemostasis* 2001; **85**(6):958–65.

Hoffman, M. A cell-base model of coagulation and the role of factor VIIa. *Blood Reviews* 2003; **17**(Suppl 1): S1–S5.

Pharmacology: Gabapentin

1. What can you tell us about gabapentin?

Gabapentin (1–[aminomethyl] cyclohexane-acetic acid) was introduced in 1993 as an antiepileptic drug and is approved for treatment of partial seizures but is currently used to manage pain.

2. What are the indications for use of gabapentin?

Recently, its efficacy in the treatment of various neuropathic pain states has been reported, such as:
- Complex regional pain syndrome
- Deafferentation neuropathy of the face
- Post-herpetic neuralgia
- Sciatic-type pain
- HIV-related neuropathy

3. Is there any role for gabapentin in acute pain?

Recently there has been use of gabapentin in acute pain. There is considerable overlap in the pathophysiology of neuropathic and acute pain. Allodynia and hyperalgesia are cardinal signs and symptoms of neuropathic pain but they are also often present after trauma and surgery. Sensitization of neurons in the dorsal horns, a mechanism in neuropathic pain, has been demonstrated in acute pain models. The persistence of this mechanism may be responsible for the increasingly recognized problem of chronic pain after surgery.

4. What is the mechanism of action of gabapentin?

- Gabapentin has a high binding affinity for the $\alpha_2\delta$ subunit of the presynaptic voltage-gated calcium channels which inhibits calcium influx and subsequent release of excitatory neurotransmitters in the pain pathways.
- It reduces the membrane voltage-gated Ca currents (VGCC channels) in dorsal horn ganglion neurons.
- It has high affinity for the subunit of the pre-synaptic VGCC channels which inhibit calcium influx and subsequent release of excitatory neurotransmitters by sensory neurons.
- It increases serotonin concentration in brain.
- Gabapentin does not affect nociceptive thresholds but has a selective effect on nociceptive process involving central sensitization. Central sensitization plays an important role in amplification of postoperative pain. Only few data in literature are available regarding the effect of gabapentin on CVS. 1200 mg administered orally 1 hour before surgery has no effect on the mean BP and HR of patient 0–24 hours after operation.
- As well as a direct analgesic effect, gabapentin may prevent and/or reverse opioid tolerance.

5. How would you prescribe gabapentin?

- The recommended starting dose of gabapentin for neuropathic pain is 300 mg on day 300 mg twice daily on day 2 and then 300 mg three times daily thereafter.
- This dose is often insufficient and doses of up to 1800 mg may be required.
- The practice of administering a first dose of 1200 mg immediately before anaesthesia and surgery is clearly in contravention to this recommendation. The potential for dizziness and drowsiness has been discussed but, as yet, no serious side effects have been reported in the acute pain studies.
- Significant reductions in postoperative analgesic requirements 24 hours after surgery were found in six studies (abdominal hysterectomy, spinal surgery, vaginal hysterectomy, radical mastectomy and laparoscopic cholecystectomy). Gabapentin also has anxiolytic properties.

6. What are the side effects of this drug?

It is a well tolerated drug with a favourable side effect profile.

Side effects include:

- Dizziness (10.9%)
- Somnolence (15.2%)
- Nausea (3.2%)
- Ataxia (2.6%)
- Tremor
- Asthenia (6%)
- Weight gain (2.6%)
- Amblyopia (2.1%). These effects usually are mild to moderate in severity but resolve within 2 weeks of onset during continued treatment.

Further reading

Rowbotham, D.J., Editorial II: Gabapentin: a new drug for postoperative pain? *British Journal of Anaesthesia* 2006; **96**:152–5.

Lascelles, B.D.X., Waterman, A.E., Cripps, P.J., et al. Central sensitization as a result of surgical pain: investigation of the effect of the pre-emptive value of pethidine for ovariohysterctomy in the rat. *Pain* 1995; **62**:201–12.

Perkins, F.M. and Kehlet, H. Chronic pain as an outcome of surgery. A review of predictive factors. *Anesthesiology* 2000; **93**:1123–33.

Physics and clinical measurements: Invasive pressure monitoring

1. When would you consider invasive blood pressure monitoring in a patient?

The gold standard of BP measurement giving accurate beat-to-beat information.

- It is useful when rapid changes in BP are anticipated:
  - Due to cardiovascular instability
  - Large fluid shifts—major laparotomy.
  - Hypotensive anaesthesia—pharmacological effects.
- When non-invasive BP monitoring is not possible or likely to be inaccurate:
  - Arrhythmias such as atrial fibrillation.
  - Obesity.
  - Non-pulsatile blood flow during cardiopulmonary bypass.
- It is also used for long-term measurement in sick patients in critical care:
  - Monitoring and management.
  - For repeated sampling for blood gases and laboratory analysis.

2. How do you invasively measure the blood pressure?

The continuous invasive BP monitors display the information both numerically and graphically. The basic principle is to provide a solid column of liquid connecting arterial blood to a pressure transducer (hydraulic coupling) and requires the following components:

- Intra-arterial cannula
- Tubing (incorporating an infusion system)
- Transducer
- Microprocessor and display screen
- Mechanism for zeroing and calibration

3. Which artery is used and why?

Preferably, a non-end artery, such as radial or dorsalis pedis is cannulated. Should thrombosis of the artery occur, arterial sufficiency is maintained via a collateral supply. The collateral supply to the hand can be assessed using Allen's test although this is not 100% reliable. If cannulation of those arteries is not possible, end arteries such as brachial or femoral may be used with due care to distal arterial sufficiency.

4. What cannula would you use?

The intra-arterial cannula should be a short, parallel-sided cannula made of Teflon or polyurethane which is inserted into an artery. The arterial cannula should be short and wide as a wide cannula has less effect on the natural frequency of the transducer system and less effect on damping. Normally, a 20-G cannula is used.

5. What is the significance of the fluid-filled tubing?

The cannula is connected to a disposable tubing system, which delivers a constant infusion of plain or heparinized 0.9% saline, delivered at a rate of 2–4 ml/hour. This helps prevent occlusion of the cannula by thrombus. The infusion fluid is kept pressurized to ensure a constant flow into the arterial system. The tubing should be stiff and not contain any bubbles in order to minimize resonance and damping.

6. What is a transducer? Give examples.

A device that converts one form of energy to another.

Transducers can be classified into two types:

- **Passive**: involving changes in:
    - Resistance, e.g. strain gauge, thermistor, photoresistor
    - Inductance, e.g. pressure transducers
    - Capacitance
- **Active**: involving generation of potentials:
    - Piezoelectric effect—generation of voltage across the faces of a quartz crystal when deformed, e.g. ultrasound probe
    - Thermocouple
    - Electrode potentials, e.g. pH electrode

7. What are the problems of invasive blood pressure measurement?

Improper *damping, calibration, and resonance* account for a large percentage of the errors in direct arterial pressure monitoring.

The problems of invasive BP systems include:

- System must be zeroed
- Transducer must be level with heart
- Complication of arterial cannulation:
    - Infection
    - Damage to local structures, e.g. nerves
    - Thrombosis
    - Air embolus
    - Infarction of distal limb
    - Haemorrhage
    - Inadvertent arterial injection of drugs

8. What is damping? What is its effect?

Damping is progressive diminution of amplitude of oscillations in a resonant system, caused by dissipation of stored energy. Damping results from friction of the fluid moving within the tubing which tends to extinguish any oscillations and decrease the frequency response of the transducer system. Excessive damping causes loss of detail in the waveform and underestimation of pressures. *Air bubbles in the system, clotting or kinking in the cannula and arterial spasm increase damping.* The use of relatively wide-bore cannulae and minimizing stopcocks improves the frequency response of the system.

The amount of damping in a system is assessed by snapping the flush valve and observing the response. The degree of damping is described by the damping factor (D):

- **Optimally damped**: the system responds rapidly to a change in signal by allowing a small amount of overshoot (D = 0.7). This produces fastest response without many oscillations.
- **Critically damped**: no overshooting occurs but the system may be too slow (D = 1.0).
- **Under-damped**: resonance occurs causing the signal to oscillate and overshoot (D = 0.7). There is marked overshoot followed by many oscillations.
- **Over-damped**: this may be due to soft tubing, a bubble, or a constriction. The signal takes a long time to reach equilibrium but will not overshoot. It may not reach equilibrium in time for a true reading to be given.

Further reading

Davis, P.D. and Kenny, G.N.C (eds.). *Basic Physics and Measurement in Anaesthesia* 5th edn. Oxford: Butterworth Heinemann, 2003.

Ward, M. and Langton, J.A. Blood pressure measurement. *Continuing Education in Anaesthesia, Critical Care & Pain* 2007; **7**:122–6.

Wesseling, K.H. A century of non-invasive arterial pressure measurement: from Marey to Penaz and Finapres. *Homeostasis* 1995; **36**:50–66.

Chapter 14

Clinical anaesthesia

Long case: A patient with epilepsy on emergency operating list *307*
Short cases *313*
   Questions *313*
   Answers *314*
      Short case 1: Patient with jaundice *314*
      Short case 2: Patient with anticoagulants *315*
      Short case 3: Cardiac tamponade *316*

Clinical science

Questions *319*
Answers *320*
   Anatomy: Diaphragm *320*
   Physiology: Placenta *321*
   Pharmacology: Tranexamic acid *323*
   Physics and clinical measurements: Humidity *324*

Clinical anaesthesia

Long case: A patient with epilepsy on emergency operating list

On your emergency list you have a 32-year-old man with poorly controlled epilepsy, and mental retardation. He had a fall at the residential home and sustained penetrating eye injury. His carer says he snores at night and smokes at least 20 cigarettes a day. His BMI is 44 kg/m².

Clinical examination	**Temperature: 38.2°C; weight: 127 kg; height: 170 cm**
	Pulse: 92/min, regular; BP: 130/80 mmHg; respiratory rate: 12/min; BMI: 44; SaO_2: 95%
	Airway: Mallampati of grade III, reduced mouth opening
	Chest: clear, no added sound
	Cardiovascular system: normal heart sound with no murmurs
	Central nervous system: no neurological deficit
Laboratory investigations	Hb 17.2 g/dL Na 141 mEq/L
	MCV 94 fL K 4.8 mEq/L
	WBC 8.5×10^9/L Urea 12 mmol/L
	Platelets 351×10^9/L Creatinine 180 μmol/L
	CRP 110 Glucose 6 mmol/L
ABGs	pH: 7.35 PaO_2: 9.8 kPa pCO_2: 4.6 kPa HCO_3^-: 26 mEq/L BE: 4
Sleep studies	Showed apnoea hypopnoea index 79

QUESTIONS

1. Summarize the case.
2. Outline the problems in this case
3. How do you assess preoperatively?
4. What can you see in the blood investigations?
5. Interpret the chest X-ray and ECG provided.
6. Is there anything else you would like to know?
7. What are the problems of epilepsy with anaesthesia in this case?
8. Is open eye injury a surgical emergency?
9. How do you manage the airway?
10. Will you do awake fibreoptic airway? Why/why not?
11. What induction drugs will you use for rapid sequence? Why not thiopentone?
12. Will you use suxamethonium? What are the problems with it? How do you minimize?
13. What is an alternative to suxamethonium?
14. What monitoring will you use? Why do you want a nerve stimulator?
15. How will you extubate this patient?

Structured Oral Examination Practice for the Final FRCA

16. After extubation patient is confused in recovery. What are the possible causes? How do you manage?
17. What is your postoperative plan?
18. In recovery patient has status epilepticus. How would you manage?

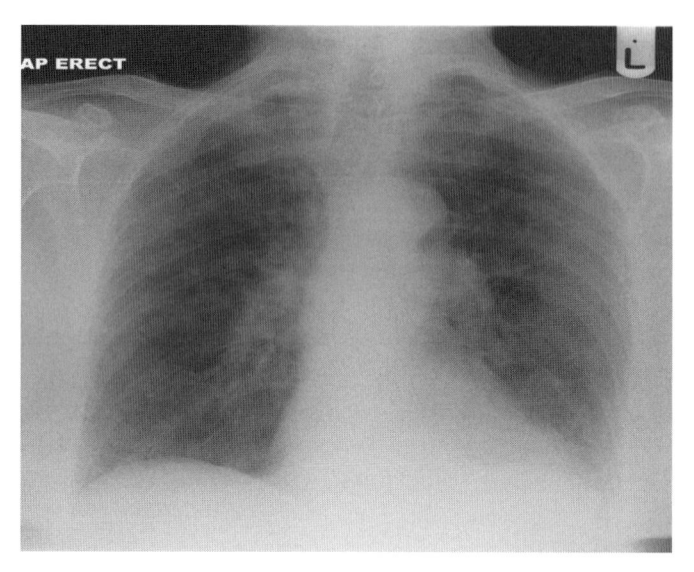

Figure 14.1 Chest X-ray.

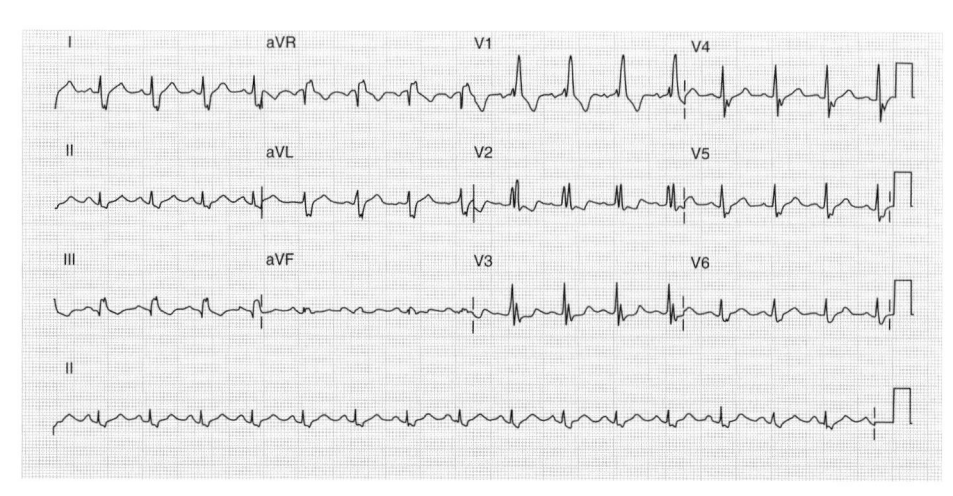

Figure 14.2 ECG.

Chapter 14

ANSWERS

1. Summarize the case.

This is a young man with complex medical problems presenting with a penetrating eye injury for surgical repair. He has intractable epilepsy, mental retardation, and morbid obesity with obstructive sleep apnoea. He also has a potentially difficult airway.

2. Outline the problems in this case.

- Penetrating eye injury with full stomach.
- Morbid obesity and difficult airway with restricted mouth opening.
- Mental retardation—unlikely to give any good history or cooperate with examination or pre-oxygenation.
- Poor controlled epilepsy—prone for recurrence of seizures. Also epilepsy medications may interact with anaesthetic drugs.
- Heavy smoker—likely to have an irritable and reactive airway and possible COPD. Risk of respiratory complications and coughing at extubation.
- Higher risk of respiratory complications because of above.
- Polycythaemia with risk of thrombotic complications.

3. How do you assess preoperatively?

Proper preoperative assessment will consist of history, examination, and investigations. Detailed history obtained from past medical records and patient's carers about his coexisting medical problems and the degree of severity of these problems.

General physical examination should be done with emphasis on airway assessment and chest examination.

Arterial blood gas analysis is the only urgent bedside investigation needed.

4. What can you see in the blood investigations?

- Full Blood count shows polycythemia
- Urea Creatinine and electrolyte are raised signifies renal dysfunction
- Blood gas shows compensated respiratory alkalosis

5. Interpret the chest X-ray and ECG provided.

Chest X-ray: anterior–posterior chest X-ray. Disorganized pulmonary architecture with small bulla in keeping with COPD. Heart size normal.

ECG: the ECG is in sinus rhythm with heart rate of 100/min. QRS > 0.12 sec—ventricular beat or bundle branch block. There is slurred S wave in lead I, no q waves in I and V6, RSR pattern in V1, V2, hence left bundle branch block, and left axis deviation considering the vectors in lead I and lead aVF. My impression is rhythm with left bundle branch block and left axis deviation.

6. Is there anything else you would like to know?

This is a difficult case with penetrating eye injury and mental retardation. I would like to know about the urgency of the surgery from the surgeon. I would like to delay the surgery in order to allow time for gastric emptying and have senior anaesthetic help to outline the plan for anaesthetic management.

7. What are the problems of epilepsy with anaesthesia in this case?

The problems in this case with regards to epilepsy are:
- Poorly controlled epilepsy can precipitate perioperative seizures.
- Together with full stomach and open eye injury there is risk of aspiration, epilepsy, drug, or any manoeuvre can increase the intra-ocular pressure, which can cause extrusion of vitreous humour and loss of vision.
- Most of the drugs used for epilepsy induce liver enzymes causing rapid metabolism of anaesthetic drugs.

8. Is open eye injury a surgical emergency?

The urgency of the surgery depends on the viability of vision in the injured eye and the risk of sympathetic ophthalmitis to the other eye. The decision should be made by a team discussion. In most of the cases, surgery is not required immediately and time can be taken for proper preparation of the patient. The surgery should be performed within 12 hours to minimize the possibility of infection.

9. How do you mange the airway?

The plan for induction would be rapid sequence induction with cricoid pressure. The patient needs to be pre-oxygenated in a semi-sitting position to improve FRC and decrease aspiration risk. The failed intubation algorithm should be clearly in place with the difficult airway trolley readily available. It is also useful to have an ENT surgeon on stand-by for emergency surgical airway.

10. Will you do awake fibreoptic airway? Why/why not?

Awake fibreoptic will be difficult as the patient has mental retardation and is unlikely to be cooperative. Also, there is a likelihood of coughing at the time of intubation, which can cause extrusion of the globe contents. However, in experienced hands, awake fibreoptic (with remifantanil sedation) and good topical anaesthesia can be a good option.

11. What induction drugs will you use for rapid sequence? Why thiopentone?

Thiopentone is the induction agent of choice for this patient for a number of reasons. It is a potent anticonvulsant therefore is the drug of choice for poorly controlled epileptics. It has more predictable dose response especially in morbidly obese patients and also suppresses the rise in intra-ocular pressure (IOP) during intubation.

12. Will you use suxamethonium? What are the problems with it? How do you minimize the risk associated with its use?

The use of suxamethonium is controversial. It can causes transient increase in IOP and if possible, should be avoided in open eye injuries.

However, suxamethonium should be used as part of a conventional rapid sequence induction, particularly if there are any concerns about the airway. There have actually been no well-documented reports describing vitreous extrusion following the administration of suxamethonium. Premature attempts at intubation provokes coughing which significantly raises IOP and therefore should be avoided and a nerve stimulator is helpful in indicating when full relaxation has occurred.

13. What is an alternative to suxamethonium?

An excellent alternative is rocuronium in the dose of 1mg/kg provided sugammadex is available for immediate reversal.

If suxamethonium is the only drug available, its effects can be minimized by giving a small defasciculating dose of non-depolarizing agent like vecuronium or by a generous dose of induction agent which negates the rise in IOP.

Chapter 14

14. What monitoring will you use? Why do you want a nerve stimulator?

In addition to standard monitoring of ECG, NIBP, SpO_2, $ETCO_2$, FiO_2 and end-tidal anaesthetic gases, neuromuscular junction monitoring is also essential to keep the patient adequately paralysed so they don't cough during surgery. It also helps to ensure complete reversal of the muscle relaxant, which is quite important in morbid obesity.

15. How will you extubate this patient?

Before extubation:

- Empty the stomach before reversing the muscle relaxant.
- Suction of pharynx.
- IV antiemetic.
- The patient should be sitting up once awake and able to maintain his airway.
- The patient should have a smooth extubation to avoiding coughing and bucking to avoid rise in IOP.
- Extubating an obese patient in the sitting up position improves FRC, prevents airway obstruction due to tongue falling back, and makes diaphragmatic movement easier. Therefore it is easier to maintain good oxygenation and ventilation.

16. After extubation patient is confused in recovery. What are the possible causes? How do you manage?

Possible causes of confusion in recovery:

- Hypoxia or hypercarbia.
- Residual effect of anaesthetic drugs or inhalational agent.
- Cerebral hypoperfusion due to hypotension.
- Metabolic causes like hypoglycaemia, dyselectrolytaemia.
- CVA.

Managing the confused patient is along the same lines as any sick patient—ABCDE approach:

- A. Make sure airway is clear, give oxygen.
- B. Prop up the patient to help with breathing. May need help with breathing like CPAP/NIV.
- C. Ensure of good haemodynamic parameters.
- D. Check GCS and do blood sugar/ABG and treat accordingly.

17. What is your postoperative plan?

The patient needs to go to HDU postoperatively as he will need close monitoring and care in view of his medical problems. He is at high risk of postoperative respiratory complications and may require some ventilatory support like CPAP or NIV due to his sleep apnoea symptoms. He may also need regular arterial blood gas analysis.

18. In recovery patient has status epilepticus. How would you manage?

Status epilepticus is continuous seizure activity lasting >30 min or intermittent seizure activity lasting >30 min during which consciousness is not regained.

My emergency management plan would be:

- ABC:
    - Airway.
    - Breathing—100% O_2.
    - Circulation—IV access with fluid resuscitation to maintain adequate systemic BP and cerebral perfusion pressure.
    - Check blood glucose level and correct hypoglycaemia.

- First-line therapy: IV benzodiazepines - lorazepam (0.1 mg/kg) or diazepam (0.1 mg/kg).
- Second-line therapy if seizures not terminated within 10 min: IV phenytoin (15–17 mg/kg) by slow infusion (rate <50 mg/min).
- Intubation and ventilation to maintain normal PaO_2 and $PaCO_2$: rapid sequence induction should be performed.
- If seizures are not controlled after 30 min with second-line therapy, consider propofol or low-dose thiopentone infusion anaesthesia preferably under EEG control. Alternatives include phenobarbitone and paraldehyde.
- Consider muscle relaxants stop the seizure movements, but not the abnormal cerebral activity, therefore in the paralysed patient, anticonvulsants are also essential.

Further reading

Allman, K.G., McIndoe, A.K., and Wilson, I.H. *Emergencies in Anaesthesia*. Oxford: Oxford University Press, 2005.

Sander, J.W. The incidence and prevalence of epilepsy. Library of articles. http://www.e-epilepsy.org.uk September 2003.

Vachon, C.A., Warner, D.O., and Bacon, D.R. Succinylcholine and the open globe: tracing the teaching. *Anesthesiology* 2003; **99**:220–3.

Chapter 14

Short cases

QUESTIONS

Short case 1: Patient with jaundice

A 45-year-old female patient with history of episodic colicky right upper abdominal pain and jaundice is coming for urgent laparoscopic cholecystectomy.

1. How would you define jaundice?
2. What are the different types of jaundice you know?
3. What are the causes of jaundice?
4. Describe the pathway of bilirubin formation.
5. Describe the problems associated with severely jaundiced patients.

Short case 2: Patient with anticoagulants

A 70-year-old patient had hip replacement 2 weeks ago and has dislocated his hip. He is on the trauma list. He is on ramipril, simvastatin, aspirin, and rivaroxaban.

1. What is rivaroxaban?
2. What are the other common anticoagulants used clinically for DVT prophylaxis?
3. What are the mechanism of action of each?
4. What clinical parameter would you use to monitor the effects?
5. When can you do central neuraxial block on these patients?

Short case 3: Cardiac tamponade

You are called by a nurse in cardiac intensive care to review a patient who is still hypotensive and tachycardic after fluid challenge but the CVP is 25.

1. What could be the causes of such a clinical situation?
2. What is the pathophysiology of cardiac tamponade?
3. If this situation is of cardiac tamponade what signs would you see?
4. How do you diagnose?
5. Outline the management plan of cardiac tamponade.

ANSWERS

Short case 1: Patient with jaundice

1. How would you define jaundice?
Jaundice is the yellowish discoloration of skin and mucous membranes caused by excessive levels of bilirubin in the blood. The serum bilirubin level needs to be >35 micromoles/L for jaundice to be clinically apparent. The most obvious site of the discoloration is the conjunctival mucous membrane (not the sclera). Jaundice is a sign of a disease and not a disease in itself.

2. What are the different types of jaundice you know?
Jaundice is classified as conjugated hyperbilirubinaemia and unconjugated hyperbilirubinaemia. This is based on the type of bilirubin but it is also classified on the basis of its aetiology.

3. What are the causes of jaundice?
The different causes of jaundice can be classified as:
- **Pre-hepatic:** this is caused by increased haemolysis and jaundice is unconjugated type.
    - Due to acquired cause: malaria, transfusion reaction, extracorporeal circulation
    - Due to genetic conditions such as: sickle cell anaemia, G6PD deficiency, hereditary spherocytosis, etc.
- **Hepatocellular:** this is due to liver parenchymal disease.
    - It usually presents as mixed hyperbilirubinaemia depending upon whether the bilirubin metabolism is affected more or its excretion within the liver is affected.
    - Some of the acquired causes are alcoholic cirrhosis, hepatitis, acute hepatic failure.
    - Genetic causes include Gilbert's syndrome, primary biliary cirrhosis, Crigler–Najjar syndrome
- **Post-hepatic:** predominantly conjugated hyperbilirubinaemia.
    - Caused by obstruction to the hepatic duct, common bile duct, or the sphincter of Oddi.
    - The usual causes of obstruction are gall stones, malignancy, and inflammation.

4. Describe the pathway of bilirubin formation.
- Bilirubin is the breakdown product of haem proteins, mainly haemoglobin, but also myoglobin and cytochromes. The haemoglobin from RBCs is broken down in the macrophages into haem and globin. The haem moiety is oxidized by haem oxygenase to form biliverdin, which is then reduced by enzyme biliverdin reductase to bilirubin. This bilirubin is then released in circulation, mainly bound to albumin and forms the water-insoluble unconjugated fraction, which is transported to liver.
- In the liver, bilirubin is combined with glucoronic acid by the enzyme UDP glucoronyl transferase to form conjugated bilirubin which is water soluble and is excreted into the biliary and cystic ducts and finally in the intestine. Intestinal bacteria convert bilirubin into urobilinogen some of which forms stercobilinogen and then gets oxidized to stercoblin which gives faeces its colour. The rest is absorbed into the bloodstream and excreted via urine as urobilin.

5. Describe the problems associated with severely jaundiced patients.
Since jaundice is a sign and not a disease, the anaesthetic implications depend on the severity of the underlying disease. Most common cause is hepatic therefore the implications are same as that for hepatic failure.
- Acute oliguric renal failure due to acute tubular necrosis. Prevention of hypovolaemia, maintain urine output (1–2 ml/kg) and use mannitol.

Chapter 14

Renal failure can also occur due to hepato-renal syndrome resulting from hepatic failure.
- Coagulopathy: vitamin K-dependent factor 2, 7.9 and 10 are reduced with raised PT.
- Altered drug metabolism for drug excreted by liver.
- Stress ulcer may lead to upper GI bleed.

Further reading:
Allman, K.G. and Wilson, I.H. *Oxford Handbook of Anaesthesia*, 2nd edn. Chapter 7: Hepatic disease, pp. 133–148. Oxford: Oxford University Press, 2006.

Short case 2: Patient with anticoagulants

1. What is rivaroxaban?
It is a new oral anticoagulant approved by NICE for thromboprophylaxis after hip or knee joint replacement surgeries. Usual dose is 10mg once a day. It works by inhibiting activated Factor X (FXa).

2. What are the other common anticoagulants used clinically for DVT prophylaxis?
The commonly used anticoagulants for DVT prophylaxis are:
- Unfractionated heparin—used as IV infusion and subcutaneous dose 6-hourly.
- Low molecular weight heparins (LMWH)—enoxaparin, tinzaparin, dalteparin. Given as once a day subcutaneous dose.
- Fondaparinux—used once a day subcutaneous dose.
- Dabigatran—orally active once a day dose.

3. What are the mechanism of action of each?
- **Heparin**: this works by activating a natural anticoagulant present in blood called antithrombin 3 (AT3), increasing its efficacy almost 1000 times which then inactivates thrombin, factor Xa and factor IXa. It also inhibits platelets at higher doses.
- **LMWH**: this also work by activating AT-3 but has more effect on Factor Xa and less on thrombin.
- **Rivaroxaban and fondaparinux**: these work by specifically inhibiting Factor Xa
- **Dabigatran:** This is a direct thrombin inhibitor.

4. What clinical parameter would you use to monitor the effects?
The clinical parameter required for:
- **Heparin** is APTT
- **LMWH and fondaparinux** do not need monitoring but if needed can be monitored by anti-factor Xa assay
- **Rivaroxaban and dabigatran** don't need monitoring.

5. When can you do central neuraxial block on these patients?
Central neuraxial procedure should be delayed by at least 2 half-lives of these anticoagulant drugs. The minimum time interval mentioned below for any invasive procedure including central blocks is applicable for prophylactic dose only.

- IV heparin: wait for 3–4 hours after last dose. Next dose to be given after at least 1 hr of the procedure
- LMWH: wait for at least 12 hours after last dose. Next dose given after 4 hours.
- Rivaroxaban: wait for at least 20 hours after last dose. Next dose after 6 hours.
- Dabigatran: wait for at least 36 hours after last dose. Next dose after 12 hours
- Fondaparinux: 36 hours.

Further reading
NICE. *Venous throembolism – rivaroxaban* (NICE guidelines TA 170). London: NICE, 2009.
Rosencher, N., Bonnet, M.-P., and Sessler, D.I. Selected new antithrombotic agents and neuraxial anaesthesia for major orthopaedic surgery: management strategies *Anaesthesia* 2007; **62**:1154–60.

Short case 3: Cardiac tamponade

1. What could be the causes of such a clinical situation?
The causes of obstructive shock (obstructions to venous return):
- **Cardiac tamponade**/pericardial effusion:
    - Chest trauma (both blunt and penetrating)
    - Myocardial rupture
    - Cancer
    - Uraemia
    - Pericarditis
    - Cardiac surgery
- Tension pneumothorax
- High levels of PEEP or intrinsic PEEP
- Massive pleural effusion
- Abdominal tamponade
- Venous occlusion (clot, air, tumour, pregnancy)
- Atrial occlusion (clot, air, tumour)
- A similar picture can also be seen in cases of massive myocardial infarction with congestive cardiac failure and should be ruled out by ECG and troponin investigation. Echocardiography will be able to differentiate between the two.

2. What is the pathophysiology of cardiac tamponade?
Cardiac tamponade results from accumulation of excess fluid in the pericardial space. This excess fluid volume accumulated in pericardial space leads to increased pressure throughout the cardiac cycle resulting in impaired cardiac filling and emptying. During inspiration, as right ventricle volume increases, the right ventricle is unable to expand into the maximally stretched pericardium. This leads to the interventricular septum bulges to the left, decreasing LVEDV and thereby decreasing cardiac output, causing a decrease in SBP during inspiration. The end result is ineffective pumping of blood, shock, and often death.

3. If this situation is of cardiac tamponade what signs would you see?

The classical signs of cardiac tamponade are: hypotension, rising CVP, and muffled heart sounds (Beck's triad). Hypotension occurs because of decreased stroke volume, jugular–venous distension due to impaired venous return to the heart, and muffled heart sounds due to fluid inside the pericardium.

4. How do you diagnose?

Initial diagnosis can be challenging, as there are a number of differential diagnoses, including tension pneumothorax, and acute heart failure.

In a trauma patient presenting with PEA (pulseless electrical activity) in the absence of hypovolaemia and tension pneumothorax, the most likely diagnosis is cardiac tamponade. There are no specific laboratory tests that diagnose tamponade. Echocardiogram is typically used to help establish the diagnosis.

Signs
- BP may fall (pulsus paradoxical) when the person inhales deeply.
- Breathing may be rapid (faster than 12 breaths in an adult per minute).
- Heart rate may be over 100 (normal is 60–100 bpm).
- Heart sounds are faint during examination with a stethoscope.
- Neck veins may be abnormally extended (distended) but the BP may be low.
- Peripheral pulses may be weak or absent.

Other tests may include:
- Chest CT or MRI of chest
- Chest X-ray
- Coronary angiography
- ECG
- Echocardiography

5. Outline your management plan of cardiac tamponade.

Cardiac tamponade is an emergency condition.

Approach is Airway, Breathing, Circulation, and the fluid around the heart must be drained.

- When clinical signs suggest a haemodynamically significant effusion, treatment should begin immediately with expansion of intravascular volume and inotropic support if the patient is hypotensive (sometimes brings out tamponade physiology and physical signs).
- The patient should be given oxygen. This reduces the workload on the heart by decreasing tissue demands for blood flow.
- Ultrasound-guided pericardiocentesis is a procedure of choice that uses a needle to remove fluid from the pericardial sac, the tissue that surrounds the heart.
- In profoundly compromised patients, pericardiocentesis should be performed 'on site' in those with impending or manifest cardiovascular 'collapse' (SBP <70 mmHg with signs of cerebral hypoperfusion); or done blindly if necessary even without echocardiographic monitoring.
    - Pericardiocentesis: paraxiphoid (left), needle at 15° angle to skin, toward left shoulder, with patient sitting forward.
- A procedure to cut and remove part of the pericardium (surgical pericardiectomy or pericardial window) can also be done.
- The patient should be continued to be in care of HDU/critical care.

Further reading

Schiller, N.B. and Foster, E. Echocardiographic evaluation of the pericardium. *UptoDate 2004*, v 11.3
Spodick, D.H. Acute cardiac tamponade. *New England Journal of Medicine* 2003; **349**:684–90.

Clinical science

QUESTIONS

Anatomy: Diaphragm

1. Describe the anatomy of the diaphragm.
2. What are the openings in the diaphragm and what structures pass through them?
3. What is the nerve supply of the diaphragm?
4. What are the differentials for a uni/bilateral raised hemidiaphragm?
5. What are the effects of anaesthesia on the tone of the diaphragm?
6. If there is a patient with blunt trauma how would you rule out diaphragmatic rupture?

Physiology: Placenta

1. What are the functions of the placenta?
2. How do the placenta and the lungs compare as gas exchanging units?
3. As the fetus grows it requires an increasing oxygen supply. How is this increased oxygen demand met?
4. What is the 'double Bohr effect'?
5. What is the uterine blood flow at term? Is it autoregulated?
6. What are the special factors which assist carbon dioxide transfer across the placenta?
7. What is the special feature of fetal haemoglobin? How does it assist the fetus?
8. Why does fetal haemoglobin have such a low P50?

Pharmacology: Tranexamic acid

1. What is tranexamic acid?
2. How does tranexamic acid act?
3. What are the indications for the use of tranexamic acid?
4. What are the recommended dosages?
5. What are the common side effects?
6. What other drugs can you use for antifibrinolytic activity?

Physics and clinical measurements: Humidity

1. What do you understand by the terms absolute and relative humidity?
2. What are the relations between absolute and relative humidity with temperature?
3. What are the instruments used to measure humidity?
4. How is humidity measured?

5. What are the adverse effects of using dry gases for ventilation in the perioperative period?
6. How does use of dry gases for ventilation cause heat loss?
7. How can you ensure humidification in theatre and intensive care?
8. What can you tell us about heat/moisture exchange (HME) filters?

ANSWERS

Anatomy: Diaphragm

1. Describe the anatomy of the diaphragm.

The diaphragm is a dome-shaped musculofibrous septum which separates the thoracic cavity from the abdominal cavity, its convex upper surface forming the floor of the former, and its concave undersurface the roof of the latter. Its peripheral part consists of muscular fibres which originate from the circumference of the thoracic outlet and converge to be inserted into a central tendon. The muscular fibres may be grouped according to their origins into three parts:

- **Sternal**: two fleshy slips from the back of the xiphoid process.
- **Costal**: the inner surfaces of the cartilages and adjacent portions of the lower six ribs on either side, interdigitating with the transversus abdominis.
- **Lumbar**: aponeurotic arches, named the lumbocostal arches, and from the lumbar vertebrae by two pillars or crura.

2. What are the openings in the diaphragm and what structures pass through them?

- **Caval opening**: T8, inferior vena cava, and some branches of the right phrenic nerve.
- **Oesophageal hiatus**: T10, oesophagus, the vagus nerves, and some small oesophageal arteries.
- **Aortic hiatus**: T12, the aorta, the azygos vein, and the thoracic duct.
- Two lesser apertures of right crus: greater and lesser right splanchnic nerves.
- Three lesser apertures of left crus: greater and lesser left splanchnic nerves and the hemiazygos vein.
- Behind the diaphragm, under the medial lumbocostal arches: ganglionated trunks of the sympathetic system.

3. What is the nerve supply of the diaphragm?

- **Motor:** phrenic nerve (from C_4—with contribution from C_3 and C_5).
- **Sensory:** sensory afferents of phrenic nerve. The peripheral area is innervated by the lower intercostal nerves.

4. What are the differentials for a uni/bilateral raised hemidiaphragm?

- Phrenic nerve palsy (unilateral hemidiaphragm)
- Pregnancy
- Ascites
- Obesity
- Intra-abdominal tumours

Chapter 14

5. What are the effects of anaesthesia on the tone of the diaphragm?

Mechanical ventilation decreases the inspiratory displacement of the dependent part of the muscle. This minor movement of the diaphragm may play an additional role in atelectasis formation.

- **Spontaneous breathing during anaesthesia**: movement of dependent diaphragm regions is greater than that of non-dependent regions.
- **Following paralysis**: reduced diaphragmatic movement on IPPV—most motion occurs in the nondependent regions.

6. If there is a patient with blunt trauma how would you rule out diaphragmatic rupture?

Diaphragmatic rupture can result from blunt or penetrating trauma and occurs in about 5% of cases of severe blunt trauma to the trunk. Diagnosis is often difficult because signs may not show up on X-ray, or signs that do show up appear similar to other conditions.

Signs and symptoms (depends on the intestinal contents in the thorax):

- Chest and abdominal pain.
- Difficulty breathing, and decreased lung sounds. When a tear is discovered, surgery is needed to repair it.
- Diaphragmatic rupture is more commonly diagnosed on the left side as the right side it is covered by liver.

Diagnostic techniques

- Radiology: chest X-ray and CT would confirm the rupture.
- Surgical: diagnostic laparotomy.

Treatment

- Resuscitation.
- Surgical repair is a major procedure which will be required once the patient is stable.

Further reading

Nolan, J.P. Major trauma. In Adams, A.P., Cashman, J.N., and Grounds, R.M. (eds.) *Recent Advances in Anaesthesia and Intensive Care: Volume 22*, p. 182. London: Greenwich Medical Media, 2002.

Physiology: Placenta

1. What are the functions of the placenta?

- Gas exchange.
- Nutrient exchange: energy substrates, water, minerals, electrolytes.
- Hormonal synthesis and release: chorionic gonadotropin, oestrogens, progesterone, rennin, pregnenolone.

2. How do the placenta and the lungs compare as gas exchanging units?

As compared to the adult lung, the placenta is inefficient at gas exchange because of larger diffusion distance and lower gas permeability.

3. As the fetus grows it requires an increasing oxygen supply. How is this increased oxygen demand met?

The increase in demand is met by:
- Maternal uterine blood flow is increased 20-fold during pregnancy.
- Increased blood supply to placenta.
- Presence of fetal haemoglobin (HbF) with increased affinity to oxygen compared to adult HbA.
- Higher haemoglobin concentration in the fetus (40% higher than in adult).
- The double Bohr effect.

4. What is the 'double Bohr effect'?

The term double Bohr effect refers to the situation in the placenta where the Bohr effect is operative in both the maternal and fetal circulations. The increase in pCO_2 in the maternal intervillous sinuses assists oxygen unloading. The decrease in pCO_2 on the fetal side of the circulation assists oxygen uptake. The Bohr effect facilitates the reciprocal exchange of oxygen for carbon dioxide. The double Bohr effect means that the oxygen dissociation curves for maternal HbA and fetal HbF move apart (i.e. in opposite directions) ultimately resulting in improved oxygen transfer from maternal to fetal blood.

5. What is the uterine blood flow of gravid uterus? Is it autoregulated?

The uterine blood flow is about 500–750 ml/min and 85% of this goes to the placenta. The uterine supply to the placenta is not autoregulated and flow is directly related to mean uterine artery perfusion pressure and inversely related to uterine vascular resistance.

UBF can be reduced by:
- Maternal hypotension
- Hyperventilation
- Stress
- Vasopressor drugs

6. What are the special factors which assist carbon dioxide transfer across the placenta?

Maternal hyperventilation results in a low maternal pCO_2 which increases the gradient favouring CO_2 transfer. A double Haldane effect occurs and this is unique to the placenta.

7. What is the special feature of fetal haemoglobin? How does it assist the fetus?

Lower P50 (18–20 mmHg) than adult Hb (26.6 mmHg). This means fetal haemoglobin has a higher oxygen affinity and this assists it to load oxygen in the placenta while maternal haemoglobin is unloading oxygen. It has a higher saturation at a given pO_2 than adult haemoglobin, e.g. fetal Hb has a saturation of 80% at a pO_2 of 30 mmHg.

8. Why does fetal haemoglobin have such a low P50?

The higher P50 of adult haemoglobin in red cells is due to the right shift that occurs in the presence of high levels of 2,3 DPG in the red cell. The 2,3 DPG binds to the beta-chains of HbA (especially deoxy HbA) to cause this effect. There are no beta-chains, so HbF is insensitive to a shift due to 2,3 DPG binding.

Pharmacology: Tranexamic acid

1. What is tranexamic acid ?
Tranexamic acid is an antifibrinolytic agent used to prevent excessive bleeding during surgery or trauma caused by excessive fibrinolysis.

2. How does tranexamic acid act?
Tranexamic acid is a synthetic derivative of the amino acid lysine. It has a very high affinity for the lysine binding sites of plasminogen. Human plasminogen is converted into its active form plasmin, by the plasminogen activator (t-PA). Lysine-binding sites bind plasmin to the surface of the fibrin, to cause fibrinolysis.

Tranexamic acid blocks these sites and prevents activation of plasminogen to plasmin thus exerting its antifibrinolytic effect.

Fibrin is the basic framework for the formation of a blood clot in haemostasis.

3. What are the indications for the use of tranexamic acid?
Tranexamic acid is used for conditions in which there is bleeding or risk of bleeding due to increased fibrinolysis. The usual indications are:
- Coronary artery bypass surgeries
- Prostatectomy
- Major bladder surgeries
- Spine surgeries
- Revision joint replacement surgeries
- High-risk tooth extractions in haemophiliacs
- It has been investigated and found useful in bleeding trauma patients (CRASH-2 Trials)
- Thromboelastogram can be a useful tool in the diagnosis of fibrinolysis and can help guide antithrombolytic therapy

4. What are the recommended dosages?
The recommended dosage are
- Oral dose is 15–25 mg/kg three times a day.
- Parenteral dose is 0.5–1 g slow IV three times a day.

5. What are the common side effects?
- The common side effects are nausea, vomiting, diarrhoea.
- Rarely, thromboembolic events, allergic reactions, and hypotension by rapid IV injection.

6. What other drugs can you use for antifibrinolytic activity?
Aprotinin is another fibrinolytic which was previously used but is no longer licensed because of increased incidence of renal failure.

Further reading
British Medical Association and the Royal Pharmaceutical Society of Great Britain. *British National Formulary* 61st edn. London: BMJ Publishing Group, 2011.

CRASH-2 trial collaborators. Effects of tranexamic acid on death, vascular occlusive events, and blood transfusion in trauma patients with significant haemorrhage (CRASH-2): a randomized, placebo-controlled trial. *Lancet* 2010; **376**: 23–32.

Physics and clinical measurements: Humidity

1. What do you understand by the terms absolute and relative humidity?

Absolute humidity: the amount of water vapour per unit volume of gas at given temperature and pressure. The SI unit is g/m^{-3}.

Relative humidity: the absolute humidity divided by the amount present in the gas expressed as a percentage of amount of water vapour that would be present if the gas was saturated with water vapour. Expressed as a percentage.

2. What are the relations between absolute and relative humidity with temperature?

The absolute humidity is independent of temperature. The relative humidity is temperature dependent. Increase in temperature decreases relative humidity provided the total water vapour content remains constant. This is because the SVP of water is temperature dependent.

3. What is the instrument used to measure humidity?

This is called a hygrometer.

4. How is humidity measured?

- **Hair hygrometer:** increase in hair length as humidity increases. Calibrated scale to read relative humidity with a range of 5–85%. Suitable for operating theatre environment.
- **Wet and dry bulb hygrometer:** the difference in temperature readings between two thermometers due to the effect of humidity is used to calculate relative humidity.
- **Regnault's hygrometer:** a silver tube containing ether is cooled by blowing air through it. The temperature at which water from atmosphere condenses on the outside of the tube is the dew point. Relative humidity is SVP at dew point divided by SVP at room temperature.
- **Humidity transducers:** changes in resistance or capacitance in an electric circuit due to the addition of a water absorbing substance (usually lithium chloride).
- **Weighing:** impractical.
- **Mass spectrometer:** measurement by breath measurement is possible but this is very expensive.

5. What are the adverse effects of using dry gases for ventilation in the perioperative period?

The adverse effects are:

- Drying of respiratory mucosa with reduced ciliary activity.
- Keratinization and ulceration of respiratory mucosa.
- Increased tenacity of mucus with plugging of airways, atelectasis, reduced gas exchange— decreased compliance and functional residual capacity of the lungs.
- Heat loss.
- Equipment contamination and colonization of bacteria.

6. How does use of dry gases for ventilation cause heat loss?

When the dry gases in anaesthesia and intensive care for ventilation they bypass the upper airways and use the latent heat of vaporization to humidify the gases which is about 10–15% of total basal heat loss and warming of gases leads to 2% of total basal heat loss.

7. How can you ensure humidification of your patients in theatre and intensive care?

Heat and moisture exchangers and breathing system filters are commonly used in breathing systems to conserver moisture and heat lost from the patient in expired gases.

There is a recommendation for their use when the upper airways are bypassed during anaesthesia and intensive care. Their efficiency is about 70%.

8. What can you tell us about heat moisture exchange (HME) filters?

Heat and moisture exchangers and breathing system filters are passive devices which conserve heat and moisture. They have a condensing filter, hygroscopic material (paper coated with calcium chloride) or hydrophobic material (ceramic fibres).

Principle: expired gases (saturated with water vapour) pass through the device so that water is retained in the filter and this condensation causes a further increase in heat which helps to moisten and heat the inhaled gases. It is made of material which has low thermal conductivity.

Disadvantage: increased dead space, increased flow resistance, water accumulation in filter and breathing circuits and decreased efficiency with larger tidal volumes.

Further reading

British Standards Institution. *Breathing System Filters for Anaesthetic and Respiratory Use – Part 1: Salt Test Method to Assess Filtration Performance* (BS EN ISO 23328-1:2008). London: British Standards Institution, 2008.

Wilkes, A.R. Review Article; Heat and moisture exchangers and breathing system filters: their use in anaesthesia and intensive care. Part 1 – history, principles and efficiency. *Anaesthesia* 2011; **66**:31–9.

Chapter 15

Hot topics for the final FRCA

A child with upper respiratory tract infection   *329*

Anaesthetic management of a patient with severe sepsis   *331*

Smoking and drinking alcohol and anaesthesia   *334*

Fast tracking in anaesthesia   *336*

What is ziconotide?   *337*

What is dabigatran?   *338*

What is sugammadex?   *339*

Applications of transdermal drug delivery   *340*

Role of cell salvage in anaesthesia   *342*

Sedation in children and young people: current recommendations   *344*

Failed spinal anaesthesia: mechanisms, management, and prevention   *347*

Ultrasound-guided or peripheral nerve stimulation for peripheral nerve blocks   *349*

Rapid sequence induction and intubation: current controversy   *351*

The current findings of The Centre for Maternal and Child Enquiries (CMACE)   *354*

A child with upper respiratory tract infection

The decision to proceed with anaesthesia and surgery in a child with upper respiratory tract infection (URTI) is bound to produce mixed reactions from most anaesthetists. Although it is much easier to cancel a proposed elective procedure in a child with systemic illness it is much more difficult to delay or advance the procedure in the other subset of children with milder URTI.

Problems

- Anaesthesia in the presence of URTI is associated with a higher risk of complications in younger children. There is an increased incidence of excess secretions, airway obstruction, laryngospasm, and bronchoconstriction. This risk is increased fivefold using an LMA and by a factor of 10 if the child is intubated.
- Emergency procedure: history of URTI is important for the anaesthetist to prepare and anticipate for any perioperative respiratory complications and also to alter the anaesthetic to try and prevent respiratory complications.
- Elective procedure with a URTI will need careful preoperative assessment:
  - History of the illness with reference to duration of symptoms like fever, dyspnoea, productive cough, sputum production, nasal congestion, lethargy, and wheezing is elicited.
  - Targeted physical examination is performed to look for lower respiratory tract involvement—wheeze, crepitations.

Options

- In general, if a child with URTI is afebrile, systemically well, and with absent lower respiratory signs you should proceed with elective surgery.
- If a child with URTI presents with productive cough, mucopurulent secretions, fever >38°C, with lower respiratory tract signs, surgery should be postponed for at least 4 weeks.
- The risk:benefit analysis is important before the decision to proceed in a child with URTI. As URTIs common in children you should also consider the symptoms and presentation of the child, age of the child, proposed procedure, urgency, and comorbid conditions of the child (asthma, cardiac disease).
- Laboratory tests such as:
  - White cell count, chest x-ray, or nasopharyngeal swabs usually add little to the process or they are too cumbersome in present day practice.
  - The duration of postponement of the proposed operation is generally considered based on the hyper-reactivity of the airways and it is considered to be hyper-reactive for about 4–6 weeks.

Anaesthetic management

Meticulous patient assessment:
- If URTI present:
  - Full explanation to patient and family.
  - Reschedule the procedure after the symptoms are settled (4–6 weeks).
- If URTI with no fever:
  - Aim should be to minimize secretions and avoid stimulating the potentially irritable airway.
  - Avoid ETT if possible—use LMA.
  - Airway suctioning under deep anaesthesia may help.
  - Improved hydration—systemic and airway (humidification).

- Anticholinergics to reduce secretions—this is of questionable value.
- Awake vs deep extubation—depending on clinician's experience.

Further reading

Tait, A.R. and Malviya, S. Anesthesia for the child with an upper respiratory tract infection: still a dilemma? *Anesthesia & Analgesia* 2005; **100**:59–65.

Anaesthetic management of a patient with severe sepsis

Severe sepsis is seen in 1–2% of admissions to hospital and in up to 25% of ICU bed utilization. Sepsis is also a major cause of death in ICUs worldwide and despite the improved care the mortality has remained high over the last decade. Systemic inflammatory response syndrome (SIRS) describes the systemic response to a wide variety of insults, many of which do not have an infectious aetiology (e.g. pancreatitis, burns). SIRS is characterized by two or more of the following:
- Body temperature >38°C or <36°C.
- Heart rate >90 bpm.
- Respiratory rate >20 bpm, or requiring mechanical ventilation.
- White cell count of >12,000 cells per mm^3 or <4000 cells per mm^3 or >10% immature neutrophils.

Systemic inflammatory response syndrome (SIRS) can be caused by:

- Infective (bacterial, viral, fungal): in CNS, CVS respiratory, renal, GIT, bone and joints.
- Non-infective:
  - Trauma, haemorrhage, pancreatitis.
  - Cardiac tamponade or myocardial infarction or pulmonary embolism.
  - Subarachnoid haemorrhage.
  - Burns.

Management goals

In view of these patients' haemodynamic status and the procedure:
- Preoperative optimization and early resuscitation is vital:
  - Central venous pressure: 8–12 mmHg.
  - Mean arterial pressure: >65 mmHg.
  - Urine output: >0.5 ml/kg/hour.
  - Central venous oxygen saturation: >70%.
- Antimicrobial therapy as early as possible.
- Intraoperative resuscitation during surgical interventions.
- Anaesthesia is hazardous in these cardiovascularly unstable patients and care is needed to manage intraoperative and postoperative stages.

Preoperative assessment

Targeted history and focussed examination for source of infective focus, severity of sepsis/shock, intravascular hydration, evaluation of major organ dysfunction, and adequacy of haemodynamic resuscitation.

Antibiotic therapy: early antimicrobial therapy should be initiated with the involvement of microbiologist which should be based on clinical history, likely source of infection, optimal penetration and local sensitivity pattern of the pathogens. Before antimicrobials are started it is imperative to take samples for culture.

Haemodynamic resuscitation: aim is to restore adequate tissue perfusion and oxygen delivery.
- Invasive monitoring.
- Infusion of inotropes administered centrally with aim to maintain MAP >65 mmHg.
- Planned admission to intensive care if patient is haemodynamically unstable.

- Aim for fluid resuscitation to achieve the following:
  - Central venous pressure: 8–12 mmHg.
  - Mean arterial pressure: 65–90 mmHg.
  - Central venous oxygen saturation in >70%.
  - Urine output: 0.5 ml/kg/hour.
  - Haematocrit: about 30.
  - Fluid resuscitation, vasopressors with noradrenaline and/or vasopressin, and inotropes like dobutamine/adrenaline are added as appropriate.

Diagnostic imaging: helpful to identify source of infection, to rule out alternate or additional pathology, and guide in radiological or surgical source control.

Source control: debridement or drainage of infectious source with correction of ongoing contamination will reduce the inflammatory response and with least physiological embarrassment.

Intraoperative management

Primary aim should be to provide safe and optimal care for the critically ill, prevent any further major organ dysfunction, and optimize fluid resuscitation.

Preoperative stage

- To continue antibiotic therapy of antimicrobial therapy.
- Invasive monitoring.
- Blood gas and lactate monitoring with continued resuscitation.

Induction

- Anaesthetic dose of the drugs need to be titrated with the haemodynamic status.
- Pre-oxygenation with cardiostable induction using midazolam, ketamine, or etomidate has been advocated.
- Short-acting opioids, like remifentanil or alfentanil is suggested.
- Use of modified rapid sequence would be preferred instead of suxamethonium.
- Use of vasopressors for both short-term (ephedrine, metaraminol, and phenylephrine) or longer-term (noradrenaline) is suggested.

Maintenance of anaesthesia

- There is no difference in TIVA vs. inhalational anaesthetic technique.
- Adequate oxygenation (PaO_2 12 kPa) and permissive hypercapnia is accepted as a part of lung protection strategy.
- Global oxygen delivery is assessed by:
  - Serum lactate levels <2 mmol/L, and
  - Mixed venous oxygen saturations of 70%.

End of procedure

- Continue appropriate antimicrobial agents.
- Adequacy of fluid resuscitation.
- Replacement of blood loss.
- Continuing sedation and ventilation in CCU.
- A focused handover in the ITU is essential for the continuity of care.

Postoperative management

- Resuscitation to continue based on the intravascular volume.
- Haemodynamic support with appropriate inotropic and vasopressor drug.
- Ventilation with lung protection strategies with target tidal volume 6 ml/kg.
- Continuation of the antimicrobial therapy.
- Nutrition with adequate glycaemic control.
- Short-term steroid therapy.
- Multimodal postoperative pain relief.
- Adequate sedatives.

These patients are, by definition, high risk, require multiple supports, and require experienced and skilful decision-making to optimize the chances of a favourable outcome. The initial hours ('golden hours') of clinical management of severe sepsis represent an important opportunity to reduce morbidity and mortality.

Further reading

Eissa, D., Carton, E.G., and Buggy, D.J. Anaesthetic management of patients with severe sepsis. *British Journal of Anaesthesia* 2010; **105**:734–43.

Smoking and drinking alcohol and anaesthesia

The evidence suggest the complications after surgery increases with both smoking and hazardous drinking. The underlying pathophysiological mechanisms include organic dysfunctions that can recover with abstinence.

Abstinence starting 3–8 weeks before surgery will significantly reduce the incidence of several serious postoperative complications, such as wound and cardiopulmonary complications and infections.

Side effects of smoking

Oxygen carriage
Carboxyhaemoglobin half-life about 4 hours:
- Impedes release of oxygen to tissues, leading to increased frequency of cardiac arrhythmias.
- Impedes release of oxygen to tissues, so impairing oxygen supply/demand ratio.

Respiratory function
- Induces inflammatory state in lung:
  - Increase in macrophages.
  - Increase in neutrophil numbers.
  - Impaired function of macrophage.
- Induces goblet cell hyperplasia.
- Decreases mucociliary clearance.
- Increases airway smooth muscle and fibrosis.
- Increases airway reactivity and increased risk of laryngospasm in recovery.
- Accelerates age-related decline in FEV_1.
- Increases closing capacity.
- Postoperative chest infection.

Cardiovascular
Nicotine (has direct peripheral effects and increases sympathetic activity):
- Increases heart rate, BP, and contractility.
- Increases in concentration of circulating catecholamine.
- Half-life about 1 hour.

Altered pharmacokinetics
- Increased opiate requirements.
- Decreased potency aminosteroidal muscle relaxants.
- Induction of CYP1 A2 enzyme.

Wound and bone healing
- Increased incidence of wound dehiscence and infection (especially in face-lifts!).
- Increased incidence of non-union and delayed healing of fractures. The mechanisms are unknown (?impaired nitric-oxide release in microvessels).
- Postoperative abstinence is more important than preoperative abstinence for effects on bone healing (unaffected by nicotine replacement therapy (NRT)).
- Incidence of wound complications normalized if 4-week preoperative abstinence.

Abstinence from smoking

- Abstinence for >3 months decreases overall perioperative cardiovascular risk by 33%.
- Acute preoperative abstinence (e.g. 12 hours) theoretically should decrease perioperative ischaemia risk (unproven).
- Sustained postoperative abstinence decreases long-term mortality after CABG.

Nicotine replacement therapy
- Use of NRT decreases overall cardiovascular risk in patients with ischaemic heart disease because:
    - Other components of smoke are damaging.
    - Serum concentration of nicotine less than peak concentration produced by cigarettes.
- NRT given to healthy patients does not increase their perioperative cardiovascular risk.
- Smokers receiving NRT preoperatively have exaggerated tachycardia after intubation.

Intervention programmes for perioperative abstinence
- Mucociliary clearance (partially) improves after >1 week.
- Airway reactivity normalizes after few days.
- Alveolar macrophage number and function improves only after 6 months.
- Symptoms of cough and wheezing improve after many weeks/months.
- At least 12 weeks of abstinence needed to ensure that risk of postoperative respiratory problem requiring intervention is reduced to normal.

Alcohol and anaesthesia

A daily intake of more than 2–3 drinks produces a reduction in the immune capacity in most patients or volunteers. The effect is most marked on the cellular element, which can be measured by a significant suppression of delayed type hypersensitivity:

- Increased endocrine response to surgery.
- Subclinical cardiac insufficiency and arrhythmias.
- Prolonged bleeding time.
- Cardiopulmonary complications.

Intervention programmes for preoperative abstinence
- All complications reduced by a period of abstinence prior to surgery.
- Identify at-risk patients.
- Intervention programmes.

Clinical expertise
Risk reduction including preoperative smoking and alcohol cessation intervention programmes requires competent and dedicated health professionals.

Further reading

Tønnesen, R. Smoking and alcohol intervention before surgery: evidence for best practice. *British Journal of Anaesthesia* 2009; **102**:297–306.

Warner, D.O. Perioperative abstinence from cigarettes: Physiologic and clinical consequences. *Anesthesiology* 2006; **104**:356–67.

Fast tracking in anaesthesia

'Fast tracking' or 'enhanced recovery' is the term used for the concept of early extubation, early mobilization, and early hospital discharge to reduce perioperative morbidity and costs.

Major surgery induces profound physiological responses in a patient leading to issues of pain management, postoperative nausea, ileus, and increased demand on the heart and respiratory functions. These complications can lead to delayed mobilization of patient, prolonged hospitalization, with risk of acquired infection.

Hence a multidisciplinary mode of management is designed which includes an effective multidisciplinary patient management strategy involving preanaesthetic assessments, modification of anaesthetic techniques, minimally invasive procedures, multimodal analgesic techniques, enhanced recovery based on evidence, involvement of nurses, and also physiotherapists.

Preanaesthetic assessment

- Protocol-based preoperative assessment and investigation allows:
    - Risk assessment.
    - Pre-optimization of physiological status of the patient before surgery.
- Education of patient regarding the course of treatment and benefits of fast tracking.
- Communication to patient to motivate them for the recovery:
    - Operative outcomes and convalescence.
    - The preoperative fasting.
    - To continue cardiac medications changes.

Anaesthetic techniques

- Adaptation of techniques with fast onset and offset drugs which allow early safe extubation.
- Utilization of the multimodal analgesic methods and develop procedure-specific pain management.
- Use of regional anaesthesia if possible to reduce surgical stress and avoid long-acting opioid.
- Goal-directed fluid therapy for optimization of fluid status (use of oesophageal Doppler).
- Preoperative carbohydrate administration may also help in enhanced recovery.

Potential benefits of fast tracking

- Early mobilization.
- Reduced requirement of sedatives or opioid, hence reduced side effects.
- Decreased ventilator-associated complications like mucous plugging, laryngotracheal trauma, ventilator-associated infections, and atelectasis, barotraumas, etc.
- Decreased length of hospital stay.
- Reduced costs.

Further reading

Kehlet, H. Fast-track colorectal surgery. *Lancet* 2008; **371**:791–3.
Kitching, A.J. and O'Neill, S.S. Fast-track surgery and anaesthesia. *Continuing Education in Anaesthesia, Critical Care & Pain* 2009; **9**:39–43.

What is ziconotide?

Ziconotide is a secretory peptide neurotoxin derived from a snail (fish hunting snail) which is a non-opioid analgesic administered as an intrathecal infusion. The pharmacological management of severe chronic pain is difficult to achieve with currently available analgesic drug; this new drug, the synthetic peptide ziconotide has been approved by the US Food and Drug Administration and the European Medicines Agency for intrathecal treatment of patients with severe chronic pain that is refractory to other treatment modalities.

Mechanism of action

- Blocks the N-type calcium channels which are predominantly situated on presynaptic areas of nerve fibres.
- The blockade of the calcium channels in the dorsal horn of spinal cord results in non-/decreased release of excitatory neurotransmitters and thus reduces the conduction of pain above it.
- It has additive or synergistic antinociceptive actions when combined with morphine, clonidine, or baclofen.

Pharmacokinetics

- It is administered as an intrathecal infusion for its action in the spinal cord but has to be absorbed into systemic circulation to be metabolized by peptidases.
- The metabolized products are neither active nor toxic.
- There is limited information from studies about the drug interaction which is minimal.
- The dose of ziconotide does not need to decrease in renal or hepatic dysfunction.

Side effects

Ziconotide has a narrow therapeutic window because of substantial CNS side effects, and thus treatment with ziconotide is appropriate for only a small subset of patients with severe chronic pain.

- Low doses with slow titration results in increased incidence of dizziness, confusion, abnormal gait, memory impairment, nystagmus, hallucinations, and vertigo.
- Nausea and vomiting also occur.
- Occasional myopathy has been noted.
- Intrathecal delivery pumps are associated with infection as well as other complications.
- Caution has been recommended in patients with a history of psychiatric illness.
- Monitor serum creatinine kinase levels, signs and symptoms of meningitis (intrathecal pump), and signs and symptoms of rhabdomyolysis.

Uses

Severe chronic pain inadequately controlled or intolerant to systemic or intrathecal analgesics or both.

Dosage

Due to high incidence of side effects from oral administration intrathecal administration is used starting from 0.1 mcg/hour to 2.4 mcg/hour.

Further reading

Schmidko, A., Lötsch, J., Freynhagen, R., et al. Ziconotide for treatment of severe chronic pain. *Lancet* 2010; **375**:1569–77.

Wallace, M.S., Rauck, R.L., and Deer, T. Ziconotide combination intrathecal therapy: rationale and evidence. *Clinical Journal of Pain* 2010; **26**:635–44.

What is dabigatran?

Dabigatran is a new oral anticoagulant for prevention of venous thromboembolism (VTE). This drug is a specific, competitive, and reversible thrombin inhibitor.

Mechanism of action

- It is a direct thrombin inhibitor.
- Used as pro-drug dabigatran etexilate.
- It is metabolized by plasma esterases into active drug—dabigatran.
- It prolongs APTT, PT, and TT.

Advantages

- The real advantage of the drug is it does not need routine coagulation monitoring. It does not have a specific antidote.
- It has a dose proportional increase in plasma concentrations and effects on APTT, PT, INR, and TT.

Absorption, distribution, metabolism, and excretion

- Dabigatran etexilate has oral bioavailability of about 7%.
- It is metabolized completely to dabigatran, which is the active form.
- Has low protein binding and hence is dialysable in emergency situations.
- Half-life of 12–14 hours and predominantly (80%) excreted unchanged in urine.

Contraindications

Active bleeding, impaired haemostasis, and hepatic impairment.

Toxicity/side effects

- In pooled analyses of the trials the most common side effects were bleeding from the wound and anaemia.
- The incidence of major or minor bleeding events was similar when compared to enoxaparin sodium in studies.
- Caution is advised with rifampicin, verapamil, and amiodarone.
- There is no major drug interactions with atorvastatin or proton pump inhibitors.

Dose

110 mg 1–4 hours after surgery, then 220 mg once daily for 9 days.

Uses

It is currently licensed in the European Union for VTE prevention in patients undergoing total knee and hip replacement. It is being studied for VTE prophylaxis in AF patients.

Further reading

Briish Medical Association and the Royal Pharmaceutical Society of Great Britain. *British National Formulary* 61st edn. London: BMJ Publishing Group, 2011.

Eisert, W.G., Hauel, N., Stangier, J., et al. Dabigatran: an oral novel potent reversible nonpeptide inhibitor of thrombin. *Arteriosclerosis, Thrombosis and Vascular Biology* 2010; **30**:1885–9.

Sanford, M. and Plosker, G.L. Dabigatran etexilate. *Drugs* 2008, **68**:1699–709.

What is sugammadex?

Sugammadex is the first selective relaxant binding agent to reverse neuromuscular blockade. It is a gamma cyclodextrin that forms a tight one-to-one complex with rocuronium (vecuronium to a lesser extent), reducing the plasma concentration of the neuromuscular blocking agents and rapidly reversing their effects.

Mechanism of action

- Sugammadex is unique in the way in which it works.
- It encapsulates and inactivates rocuronium.
- The inactive complex follows the elimination kinetics of sugammadex.

Routes of administration/doses

- The recommended dose for reversal after 3–5 min after an intubating dose of rocuronium is 16 mg/kg.
- Three trials indicated that sugammadex 2 to 4 mg/kg produces more rapid recovery from moderate (profound) neuromuscular block than neostigmine/glycopyrrolate.
- For more moderate blocks a dose of 2–4 mg/kg is recommended.

Toxicity/side effects

- Generally well tolerated in surgical patients including elderly and paediatric group.
- Most commonly reported adverse events were procedural pain, nausea, and vomiting.
- Uncommon adverse events include anaesthetic complications and dysgeusia.
- There have been reports of QT_C interval prolongation.

Pharmacokinetics

- Post-IV administration, sugammadex demonstrates the linear pharmacokinetics.
- The inactive complex of rocuronium and sugammadex do not bind to plasma proteins and are primarily excreted in urine unchanged.
- The elimination half-life is 1.8 hours. Renal impairment delays the elimination of sugammadex and its complex with rocuronium.

Uses

- Licensed to use in adults to reverse muscle relaxant effects of rocuronium and vecuronium.
- Also can be used in paediatric patients (2–16 years) for moderate muscle relaxation.
- The evidence suggests that there are potential benefits of sugammadex in terms of increased patient safety, increased predictability of recovery from NMB, and more efficient use of theatre time and staff.

Further reading

Naguib M. Sugammadex: another milestone in clinical neuromuscular pharmacology. *Anesthesia & Analgesia* 2007; **104**:575–81.

Paton F *et al*. Sugammadex compared with neostigmine/glycopyrrolate for routine reversal of neuromuscular block: a systematic review and economic evaluation. *British Journal of Anaesthesia* 2010; **105**:558–67.

Applications of transdermal drug delivery

The application of medications to the skin to ease ailments is an age-old practice that includes the application of gels, ointments, creams, and pastes. Initially these applications were primarily intended for a local effect. The important area of pharmaceutical research and development over the last few decades has lead to the current use as adhesive skin patches to deliver drugs systemically. There are pharmacological advantages over the oral route and improved patient acceptability and compliance.

Drug transport occurs by diffusion through the stratum corneum via the lipid rich intercellular pathway and to a lesser extent through the hair follicles and sweat ducts. There are various factors which influence the diffusion such as thickness of the stratum corneum, skin hydration, underlying skin diseases or injuries, ethnic differences, and body temperature.

Transdermal drug delivery pharmacokinetics

Step I: the drug is stored as an application to skin where there is a drug concentration gradient which drives the drug into stratum corneum.

Step II: the drug gets collected at stratum corneum and becomes a second drug reservoir, this movement carries on and the drug moves further into the skin. Finally it gets absorbed into the systemic circulation. This process results in a delay from the time of application to the desired minimum effective concentration (MEC). This delay varies between drugs. The time to reach steady-state plasma concentrations varies and may require a few patches before the steady state is reached.

Transport of drug across the skin

- Diffusion through stratum corneum:
  - Major route via lipid-rich, intercellular pathway.
  - Minor transport via hair follicles and sweat ducts.
- Physicochemical characteristics of drug required for passive transdermal diffusion:
  - Low molecular weight.
  - High lipophilicity.
  - Low melting point.

Common drugs used are

- Opioid for analgesia:
  - Fentanyl
  - Buprenorphine
- Hormone replacement therapy:
  - Oestradiol and progesterone, ethinyloestradiol, norelgestromin for contraception
  - Testosterone for hypogonadism
- Cardiovascular system:
  - Clonidine for hypertension
  - Glyceryl trinitrate for angina
- Others:
  - Lidocaine and dexamethasone
  - Hyoscine for motion sickness
  - Nicotine for smoking cessation

Transdermal delivery systems

- The reservoir or membrane-controlled system: there is a reservoir which holds the drug in a gel or solution. This is then delivered through a fixed rate-controlling membrane between the drug reservoir and the skin.
- The matrix system: this holds the drug in an adhesive polymer matrix, from which the drug is continuously released into the skin. The dose of drug delivered depends on the amount of drug held in the matrix and the area of the patch applied to the skin.

Advantages

- Compared to the enteral routes:
  - First-pass metabolism is avoided and
  - Can be used when the enteral route is not available.
- Compared to the IV routes—convenient and simple:
  - No need for IV access.
  - Patients are mobile.
  - Avoids needle-related injury to patient and staff.

Advantages of iontophoresis over conventional skin patches

- Iontophoresis uses a small electric current to transport ionized drug molecules actively across the skin and then into the systemic circulation.
- Iontophoresis (electric current) also increases though reversibly, the permeability of skin to the drug—electro-osmosis.
- Other features: drug diffusion happens only when current is flowing and a fixed dose of drug is delivered per activation.

Factors influencing drug delivery by iontophoretic transdermal system (ITS)

- Surface area of skin in contact with electrode compartment.
- Duration of electric current.
- Intensity of electric current.
- Chemical properties of drug.
- Drug formulation.

Further reading

Grond, S., Hall, J., Spacek, A., et al. Iontophoretic transdermal system using fentanyl compared with patient-controlled intravenous analgesia using morphine for postoperative pain management. *British Journal of Anaesthesia* 2007; **98**:806–15.

Margetts, L. and Sawyer, R. Transdermal drug delivery: principles and opioid therapy. *Continuing Education in Anaesthesia, Critical Care & Pain* 2007; **7**:171–17.

Power, I. Fentanyl HCl iontophoretic transdermal system (ITS): clinical application of iontophoretic technology in the management of acute postoperative pain. *British Journal of Anaesthesia* 2007; **98**:4–11.

Role of cell salvage in anaesthesia

Cell salvage is a process in which patients' own (lost) blood is collected, processed, and transfused back (autologous blood transfusion) into the patient with important reductions in costs and complications. Allogenic blood transfusion has been associated with increased risk of tumour recurrence, postoperative infection, acute lung injury, perioperative myocardial infarction, postoperative low cardiac output failure, and increased mortality.

Principles

Three phases of collection, washing, and re-infusion:
- **Collection**: blood from the operative field is collected by a dedicated suction device for which a predetermined amount of heparinized saline is added and filtered during the process of collection. This blood is centrifuged to separate the RBCs which are then washed.
- **Washing** of RBCs (across a semipermeable membrane) is to filter out free Hb, plasma, white cells, platelets, and heparin.
- **Re-transfusion**: washed RBCs are then suspended in saline (to achieve a haematocrit of 60–70%) and then transfused back to the patient (within 6 hours).

Complications

- Non-immune haemolysis.
- Air embolism.
- Febrile non-haemolytic transfusion reaction.
- Coagulopathy.
- Contamination with drugs, cleansing solutions, and infectious agents, and incomplete washing leading to contamination with activated leucocytes, cytokines, and other microaggregates.
- These risks can be reduced with education, training, technical advances, and increasing experience.
- With large volume blood transfusion there is a risk of coagulopathy and hence such patients should be monitored with dynamic coagulation testing like thromboelastography or coagulation tests like prothrombin time, fibrinogen, levels and platelets.

Benefits

- Aim is to reduce or ultimately eliminate the need for allogenic transfusions and the associated infectious and non-infectious risks associated with it.
- It has been shown to be beneficial in many studies—improved post-oesophagectomy survival, very successful in major joint replacements in orthopaedics.
- The AAGBI suggested the use of intraoperative cell salvage when the anticipated blood loss is expected to >1000 ml or >20% of the estimated blood volume, patients with low Hb, multiple antibodies, or rare blood types, and, of course, patients who refuse allogenic blood transfusions.

Uses

- **Obstetrics**: cell salvage has been controversial due to the potential risk of amniotic fluid embolism (AFE).
    - Two recent systematic review suggests use of cell salvage is safe in the obstetric setting.
    - NICE guidelines (2005) concluded that cell salvage with leukocyte-depletion filters (LDF) is safe.

- **Orthopaedics**: the evidence suggests use in revision arthroplasty reduces the requirement of allogenic transfusions and some evidence of reduction in postoperative infections as well.
- **Cardiac surgery**: use of blood with LDF has been shown to reduce the microemboli and lipid load of cell salvaged blood and shown an improvement in lung function but has not had any effect on length of stay or mortality.
- **Malignancy**: has been previously contraindicated due to the risk of tumour dissemination. No randomized control trials available but some prospective studies are available.
- **Infection/sepsis**: contraindicated due to faecal contamination in spite of using high-volume saline washes and LDF.
- Special situations:
  - Jehovah's Witness: very important if there is refusal of blood transfusion. It is vital to discuss and take specific Jehovah's Witness consent preoperatively.
  - Radical prostatectomy.
  - Living donor liver transplants.
  - Renal cell carcinoma and gynae-oncological procedures.
- In conclusion, use of cell salvage has been shown to be effective in reduction of allogenic transfusions and reduction of costs in cardiac and orthopaedic surgical settings.

Further reading

Ashworth, A. and Klein, A.A. Cell salvage as part of a blood conservation strategy in anaesthesia. *British Journal of Anaesthesia* 2010; **105**:401–16.

Sedation in children and young people: current recommendations

Sedation is being increasingly used in the paediatric population and to reflect the changing trend, NICE has prepared a guideline for the healthcare professionals who are involved with the care of children and young people who need sedation for diagnostic or therapeutic procedures—*Sedation in children and young people* (Clinical Guideline 112) published in December 2010.

When should sedation be used?

Sedation should be considered in the following situations: painful procedures, frightening situations, children with behavioural problems, or in children and young people who are ill. NICE also suggests that sedation, in comparison to anaesthesia, may be a better use of NHS resources.

Levels of sedation (based on American Society of Anesthesiologists (ASA) definitions):

- **Minimal sedation**: a drug-induced state where patients are awake but calm and respond normally to verbal commands. The cognitive function and coordination may be impaired but ventilatory and cardiovascular functions are unaffected.
- **Moderate sedation**: drug-induced depression of consciousness during which patients are sleepy but respond purposefully to verbal commands (known as conscious sedation in dentistry, see below) or light tactile stimulation (reflex withdrawal from a painful stimulus is not a purposeful response). No interventions are required to maintain a patent airway. Spontaneous ventilation is adequate. Cardiovascular function is usually maintained.
- **Conscious sedation**: drug-induced depression of consciousness, similar to moderate sedation, except that verbal contact is always maintained with the patient. The term is commonly used in dentistry.
- **Deep sedation**: drug-induced depression of consciousness during which patients are asleep and cannot easily be roused but do respond purposefully to repeated or painful stimulation. The ability to maintain ventilatory function independently may be impaired. Patients may require assistance to maintain a patent airway. Spontaneous ventilation may be inadequate. Cardiovascular function is usually maintained.

Key priorities for implementation (as recommended by NICE)

- Trained healthcare professionals should carry out pre-sedation assessments and document these in the healthcare record.
- Two trained healthcare professionals should be available during the procedure.
- Immediate access to monitoring and resuscitation equipment should be available.
- Suitability for sedation should be assessed with psychological and developmental status in mind.
- Seek specialist advice if the child is a neonate, ASA ≥3 or there is any concern about potential airway or breathing problem.

Preparation for sedation

- Confirm and document the fasting status of the child.
- Fasting is not necessary for minimal or moderate sedation where the child or young person in verbal contact.

- The 2–4–6 rule for any sedation in which verbal contact is lost is used: 2 hours for clear fluids, 4 hours for breastfeed, and 6 hours for solids.
- Psychological preparation: give age-appropriate information to children and their parents/carers about the procedure, sedation, environment, and how to cope with the procedure.

Choosing sedation technique

Painless imaging
- For children and young people who are unable to tolerate a painless procedure consider either chloral hydrate or midazolam which have a high margin of safety.
- If not sufficient, consider propofol or sevoflurane which have a lower margin of safety.
- Do not routinely use ketamine or opioids for these procedures.

Painful procedures
- Consider using a local anaesthetic as well as a sedative.
- For minimal or moderate sedation consider using nitrous oxide (with oxygen) and midazolam (oral or intranasal).
- If the above is unsuitable, consider using ketamine, IV midazolam with/without fentanyl.
- If the above are unsuitable, consider using propofol with/without fentanyl.

Dentistry
- In addition to local anaesthesia, consider nitrous oxide (with oxygen) or midazolam.
- If the above are not suitable or sufficient consider referral to a specialist team for alternatives.

Endoscopy
- Consider using midazolam for upper gastrointestinal endoscopy.
- Consider adding fentanyl (or alternative opioid) to midazolam for lower gastrointestinal endoscopy.

Monitoring during sedation

Continuously monitor, interpret, and respond to changes in all situations following:
- Moderate or deep sedation—depth of sedation, respiration, oxygen saturations, heart rate, pain, coping, and distress.
- For deep sedation additional monitoring such as 3-lead ECG, end-tidal capnometry ($ETCO_2$), and BP (monitor every 5 min).
- Ensure monitored data is documented in the healthcare record contemporaneously.
- After the procedure, continue monitoring until the child or young person has a patent airway, shows protective airway and breathing reflexes, is haemodynamically stable, and is easily roused.

After sedation

Discharge criteria
- Ensure that all of the following are met before discharge: heart rate, respiratory rate, BP, and temperature are all returned to baseline levels.
- The child or young person is awake or returned to baseline level of consciousness and there is no risk of further reduction in level of consciousness.
- Pain, nausea, and vomiting have been adequately managed.
- Consider referring to an anaesthesia specialist if the child is not able to tolerate the procedure under sedation.

Sedation in critical care

More recent studies have shown that lower doses and daily interruption in the delivery of sedation, along with other important shifts in management, result in better patient outcomes and help cut down on time spent on ventilators and on time spent in ICUs.

Further reading

NICE. *Sedation in children and young people* (Clinical Guideline 112). London: NICE, 2010. Available at: http://www.nice.org.uk/CG112

Failed spinal anaesthesia: mechanisms, management, and prevention

Incidence

Reports of failed spinal anaesthesia and published failure rates in large series of spinal anaesthesia range from 0.46–17%. The failure rate of spinal as an incidence of 1% is attainable. In order to maximize the benefit of spinal anaesthesia and minimize the incidence of failure it is important to be aware of the potential pitfalls so that clinical practice can be tailored to their avoidance.

Mechanism

- Failed lumbar puncture:
  - Poor positioning, incorrect insertion.
  - Knowledge of anatomy to visualize your needle—use of ultrasound increasingly popular.
- Solution injection errors—low doses affect duration and quality more than spread.
- Loss of injectate occurs either:
  - When the syringe is not properly fitted to the needle hub.
  - When the tip of the pencil-point needle has hole on the side and is quite long. So the hole can be partly through the duramater and partly still in the epidural space.
- Inadequate spread—inadequate spread may be limited by:
  - Anatomical abnormalities such as pronounced curvature of lumbar spine leading to trapping of the local anaesthetic caudally.
  - May be septae in the intrathecal space which gives a unilateral block.
  - Decreased spread if hyperbaric solutions used.
- Ineffective drug action:
  - Wrong drug.
  - Denatured local anaesthetic or additives have changed the pH of solution.
  - Very rarely abnormalities in the sodium channels make people resistant.

Management of failed spinal
- Anxiolysis:
  - Anxious patients are more likely to react to sensation.
  - Sedation or light general anaesthesia is required.
- Checking the block:
  - Check motor block then cold/pin prick:
    - Difficult to assess the quality as opposed to level of block—pinch or toothed forceps, without asking patient
  - Slow onset block less likely to be effective especially if >15 min:
    - No block.
    - Inadequate spread.
    - Unilateral block.
    - Patchy block.

No block:
- Repeat the spinal block cautiously:
  - A second dose may be too small and again inadequately low sensory level of anaesthesia, or
  - Too large leading to an inappropriately high block level, or
  - The risk of neurotoxic effects of local anaesthetic.
  - And with a partial block will not feel any direct nerve damage by needle.

- Combine spinal technique: Using CSE is preferable to repeat spinal as CSE will be safer as cautious low dose spinal could be extended using the epidural catheter.
  - Repeat the spinal block cautiously:
    - A second dose may be too small and again inadequately low sensory level of anaesthesia, or
    - Too large leading to an inappropriately high block level, or
    - The risk of neurotoxic effects of local anaesthetic.
    - And with a partial block will not feel any direct nerve damage by needle.
- Inadequate block
  - Head-down tilt.
  - Flex hips and knees.
- Patchy block likely misplaced injection or inadequate dose—offer general anaesthesia or conversion to general anaesthesia
  - Caution for second dose:
    - A second injection of local anaesthetic after failed spinal should be performed when:
      - Complete failure or
      - Patient with incomplete failure
  - Repeat injection is performed the total amount of local anaesthetic should not exceed a dose the reasonable dose for a single injection.

Further reading

Fettes, P.D.W., Jansson, J.R., and Wildsmith, J.A. Failed spinal anaesthesia: mechanisms, management, and prevention. *British Journal of Anaesthesia* 2009; **102**:739–48.

Loo, C.C. and Irestedt, L. Cauda equina syndrome after spinal anaesthesia with hyperbaric 5% lignocaine: a review of six cases of cauda equina syndrome reported to the Swedish Pharmaceutical Insurance 1993–1997. *Acta Anaesthesiology Scandinavia* 1999; **43**:371–9.

Steiner, L.A., Hauenstein, L., Ruppen, W., et al. Bupivacaine concentrations in lumbar cerebrospinal fluid in patients with failed spinal anaesthesia. *British Journal of Anaesthesia* 2009; **102**:839–44.

Ultrasound-guided or peripheral nerve stimulation for peripheral nerve blocks

Despite the growing interest in the use of ultrasound (US) imaging to guide performance of regional anaesthetic procedures such as peripheral nerve blocks, controversy still exists as to whether US is superior to previously developed nerve localization techniques such as the use of a peripheral nerve stimulator (PNS).

Modern clinical ultrasound equipment typically operates in the 2.5–20 MHz frequency range.

- The higher the frequency the better the spatial resolution, but at the expense of reduced depth penetration.
- Lower frequencies provide better depth penetration but at lower spatial resolution. Additional features, such as pulsed wave and colour Doppler imaging, allow the identification of vessels and the blood velocities in those vessels.
- Modern US equipment is cheaper and more portable and produces better quality imaging than that used in previous studies. State-of-the-art diagnostic US equipment has multiple probes and software packages, and costs from £100,000 to £150,000.
- But a modern portable US machine, which might be used for regional anaesthesia and peripheral arterial and central venous cannulation, would have a single variable frequency linear array transducer (5–10 MHz).

Ultrasound-guided or peripheral nerve stimulation for peripheral nerve blocks?

- Previous comparative studies have been small.
- Meta-analysis of 13 RCTs (946 patients):
    - Outcomes.
    - Block failure rate.
    - Procedure time.
    - Onset time.
    - Block duration.
    - Complications.
- Block failure: significantly lower with US (relative risk (RR) 0.41). Block failure defined as needing supplemental analgesia rescue block or general anaesthesia, significantly lower risk in US group.
- Procedures carried out quicker although not by a clinically significant amount—mean 1 min quicker with US.
- Onset faster (nearly a third faster) with US; with longer duration, US also reduced a risk of vascular puncture—mean 29% faster with US.
- Block duration: 25% increased duration with US.
- Complications:
    - No major complications with either.
    - No difference in nerve damage.
    - Less vascular puncture with US (RR 1.6).

Who should use the ultrasound technique for nerve block?

The study concluded that US is definitely better for beginners, inexperienced performers, and supervising trainees. An experienced anaesthetist may produce quicker onset, longer lasting blocks; more studies are needed for:
- Those experienced in use of the machine and probe.
- Those on a regional anaesthesia course performed under supervision.
- Trainee learning as part of competency based training programme.

Use of ultrasound in anaesthesia

- Vascular access
- Peripheral nerve blocks
- Epidural space depth
- Perioperative cardiac US (echo)
- FAST scanning in trauma
- Pneumothorax

Further reading

Abrahams, M.S., Aziz, M.F., Fu, R.F., et al. Ultrasound guidance compared with electrical neurostimulation for peripheral nerve block: a systematic review and meta-analysis of randomized controlled trials. *British Journal of Anaesthesia* 2009; **102**:408–17.

Marhofer, P. and Harrop-Griffiths, W. Nerve location in regional anaesthesia: finding what lies beneath the skin; *British Journal of Anaesthesia* 2011; **106**(1):3–5.

NICE. *Ultrasound-guided regional nerve block*. London: NICE, 2009. Available at: http:// http://www.nice.org.uk/IPG285

Rapid sequence induction and intubation: current controversy

Rapid sequence induction and intubation (RSI) is a procedure used to secure an airway which is at a high risk of aspiration. The concept has evolved with the introduction of suxamethonium (1951), the description of cricoid pressure (1961), to the first description of RSII with all the components in 1970.

Classically RSII has been described as pre-oxygenation, rapid injection of a predetermined dose of thiopentone sodium, immediately followed by suxamethonium and tracheal intubation with cuffed ETT without any intermittent positive pressure ventilation (IPPV). We will review this to highlight the controversy and changing opinion about certain essential components of RSII.

Induction drug: which drug?

The ideal drug should achieve fast and reliable onset of primary end-point loss of consciousness (LOC) which should result in avoiding awareness. It should cause least haemodynamic instability and improve intubating conditions. Thiopentone has been the traditional drug of choice but thiopentone can cause haemodynamic instability in high doses especially in trauma patients. It is also used in obstetric patients in whom any hypotension can cause adverse effects on the fetus. In both these patients we have traditionally advocated and used RSII.

Other induction agents like:
- Etomidate: good haemodynamic stability profile but adrenocortical suppression even with single dose.
- Midazolam: good haemodynamic stability but slow onset and prolonged effect.
- Ketamine good haemodynamic stability, delayed onset, and undesirable side effects.
- Propofol causes haemodynamic instability as much as thiopentone but has much better intubating conditions.

What dose?

Traditionally all the drugs are given with a pre-calculated dose followed rapidly by the neuromuscular relaxant but many clinicians with experience titrate the dose of the induction agent to the primary end-point which is LOC. Titration also helps to prevents overdosing and haemodynamic instability without compromising on the primary end-point LOC. Advocates of the traditional method argue that titration increases the duration of the induction period and hence the risk period but the group who titrate the induction agent argue that though it increases the induction time the at-risk period still remains the same.

Suxamethonium: the optimal dose?

Suxamethonium is an essential part of RSII on the road to a secure airway for a profound and reliable relaxation. In their original study, Stept and Safar used 100 mg/70 kg of suxamethonium 2–3 min after pre-treatment with curare for RSII. Most studies have considered the optimal dose to be 1 mg/kg if no precurarization is used and 1.5 mg/kg if pre-curarization is used. Pre-curarization (for defasciculation) is not as popular in the UK as much as in North America. Defasciculation has been used in elective situations but in emergency situations it may delay RSII due to the calculations required. The dose of rocuronium for defasciculation is 0.03 mg/kg (2 mg/70 kg) and it should be given 3 min before suxamethonium. Defasciculation may cause pharyngeal muscle weakness, loss of oesophageal sphincter tone, and may cause pulmonary aspiration. Defasciculation has been recommended in patients with penetrating eye injuries and patients with increased intracranial pressure.

Opioids

Classically not used as older opioids had slower onset and longer duration. But newer opioids like alfentanil (20–30 mcg/kg) and remifentanil (1 mcg/kg) are quicker onset and quicker offset. The addition of opioids may reduce the dose of induction agents and make the entire process haemodynamically stable. The disadvantage on the other hand is in the possibility of respiratory depression in a difficult intubation situation and that opioids can cause chest wall rigidity and vocal cord closure.

Non-depolarizing relaxants

When suxamethonium is contraindicated, non-depolarizing relaxants are used. The primary disadvantage of this situation is the much slower onset time and the resulting risk for aspiration. On the other hand, with the use of rocuronium (0.6–1.5 mg/kg) it has become much faster onset with intubating conditions similar to that of suxamethonium. Further, with availability of sugammadex it is now possible to use in patients with a difficult airway.

Manual ventilation

Classically IPPV is not performed with RSII for fear of gastric insufflation, regurgitation, and aspiration. The view has been that people with normal airways who are pre-oxygenated adequately do not need PPV due to the short duration of apnoea. But many clinicians do use IPPV with RSII. If the peak airway pressures are kept <20 cm (with cricoid pressure 40 N) then gastric insufflation is rarely seen with IPPV. IPPV may, in fact, be beneficial in patients who are obese, pregnant, children, and critically ill who can become hypoxemic during the process.

Cricoid pressure

This was described originally by Sellick in 1961. Application of cricoid pressure is one of the most important parts of RSII. The limitation of the manoeuvre has been its timing and force of application. It is recommended to apply pressure of 10 N in awake patients and then increased to 30 N on loss of consciousness. When less force is used there is risk of regurgitation but use of high force can distort the view at laryngoscopy. If the cricoid pressure is applied, premature application can lead to retching and vomiting, and may also limit the efficiency of mask ventilation when needed.

The difficulty in establishing a standard rapid sequence induction protocol has been due to the changing opinion regarding the traditional components of the technique.

Hence, the controversy for RSII concerns:
- The choice of induction drug, the dose, and the method of administration. Some experts prefer the traditional rapid injection of a predetermined dose while others use the titration to LOC technique.
- The timing of neuromuscular blocking drug (NMBD) administration is different in both techniques. Whereas the NMBD should immediately follow the induction drug in the traditional technique, it is only given after establishing LOC in the titration technique.
- There is controversy regarding the dose of succinylcholine, traditionally 1–2 mg/kg but for some the current recommendation is a 1.0–1.5 mg/kg dose.
- Prevention of fasciculation before succinylcholine was traditionally recommended but due to risk of complication is avoided.
- The jury is out regarding the use of rocuronium as a rapid sequence drug with the availability of sugammadex.
- Traditionally manual ventilation before tracheal intubation was not recommended due to gastric insufflation, but for some experts its use is currently acceptable and even recommended by some to avoid hypoxemia and to 'test' the ability to mask ventilate.

- As there is no scientific evidence of benefit and risk of possible complications, cricoid pressure remains controversial.
- There is still controversy regarding the best position and whether the head-up, head-down, or supine position is the safest during induction of anaesthesia in full-stomach patients.

Further reading

El-Orbany, M. and Connolly, L.A. Rapid sequence induction and intubation; current controversy. *Anesthesia & Analgesia* 2010; **110**:1318–25.

The current findings of The Centre for Maternal and Child Enquiries (CMACE)

CMACE is an independent charity dedicated to improving the health of mothers, babies, and children.

What is CMACE?

CMACE replaces the Confidential Enquiry into Maternal and Child Health (CEMACH) which identifies deaths of women in the UK during pregnancy and within 42 days of giving birth that are directly or indirectly related to the pregnancy. The circumstances surrounding these deaths are then examined and guidance provided to help improve the care of women presenting with similar conditions in the future. The report considers deaths over a 3-year period and the most recent report to CEMACH, the 'Confidential Enquiry into Maternal Deaths' (CEMD) reported triennially on deaths in pregnancy or following delivery in England and Wales and provided 54 years of valuable continuous data in this area.

Definitions

Maternal death: deaths of women while pregnant or within 42 days of delivery, from any cause related to or aggravated by the pregnancy or its management, but not from accidental or incidental causes.

Direct maternal death: death resulting from obstetric complications of the pregnant state (pregnancy, labour and puerperium), from interventions, omissions, incorrect treatment, or from a chain of events resulting from any of the above.

Indirect maternal death: death resulting from previous existing disease or disease that developed during pregnancy and which was not due to direct obstetric causes, but which was aggravated by the physiological effects of pregnancy.

Late maternal death: death occurring between 42 days and 1 year after termination of pregnancy, miscarriage, or delivery that is due to direct or indirect maternal causes.

Mortality rates

In the triennium 2006–2008, 261 women in the UK died directly or indirectly related to pregnancy. The current report identifies 261 deaths, with 107 directly and 154 indirectly related to pregnancy. The overall maternal mortality rate was 11.39 per 100,000 maternities. Direct deaths decreased from 6.24 per 100,000 maternities in 2003–2005 to 4.67 per 100,000 maternities in 2006–2008 ($p = 0.02$) which is a statistically significant decline in the overall UK maternal mortality rate. This decline is predominantly due to the reduction in deaths from thromboembolism and, to a lesser extent, haemorrhage.

The mortality rate related to sepsis increased from 0.85 deaths per 100,000 maternities in 2003–2005 to 1.13 deaths in 2006–2008, and sepsis is now the most common cause of direct maternal death. Cardiac disease is the most common cause of indirect death; the indirect maternal mortality rate has not changed significantly since 2003–2005. This Confidential Enquiry identified substandard care in 70% of direct deaths and 55% of indirect deaths.

Numbers of maternal deaths reported to the Enquiry by cause

Cause of direct deaths	2000–02	2003–05	2006–08
Sepsis	13	18	26
Pre-eclampsia and eclampsia	14	18	19
Thrombosis, thromboembolism	30	41	18
Amniotic fluid embolism	5	17	13
Early pregnancy	15	14	11
Haemorrhage	17	14	09
Anaesthesia	6	6	7
Indirect causes: cardiac	44	48	53
Other indirect causes	50	50	49
Indirect causes: neurological	40	37	36

Seven women died as a direct result of anaesthesia and poor perioperative anaesthetic management in 2006–2008. In addition to these there are a further 18 deaths where anaesthesia was considered to have contributed to the fatal outcome. Further, there are 12 women with severe pregnancy-induced hypertension or sepsis for which appropriate referral was not considered.

Why do mothers die?

Most deaths worldwide occur due to haemorrhage, obstructed labour, infection, eclampsia, and complications of abortion. In the UK, these problems combined accounted for only 14% of deaths.

Why is the mortality not decreasing?

There are number of risk factors which influence this:

- There is increasing maternal age.
- Increasing migrant population with cultural and language difference.
- Morbid obesity.
- Cardiovascular disease and corrected heart surgeries.
- Smoking.
- Poor overall health.

Death related to anaesthesia and contributed due to poor anaesthetic management

In this triennium, two women died from failure to ventilate the lungs, four from postoperative complications, and one from leucoencephalitis. Two of the seven women were obese.

Difficult airway: failure to ventilate the lungs

At induction of general anaesthesia:

- Patient for urgent care was for Category 2 Caesarean section with working epidural. Subsequently there was a sustained fetal bradycardia, which escalated the urgency of Caesarean section to Category 1. The epidural had not been topped up to provide surgical anaesthesia for Caesarean section because the anaesthetist planned to top the epidural up in theatre.
- This lead to Caesarean section under general anaesthesia. Following which there was failed intubation and the failed intubation guideline was not used.
- If the epidural had been topped up when it was decided she was to have a Caesarean section, general anaesthesia may not have been required.

In intensive care:
- Tracheostomy tube came out in a critical care ward and she had a known airway problem and known difficulty with her tracheostomy.
- A clear strategy of management for this scenario was required in advance, including the use of small tracheal tubes and quick referral for senior help out of hours.

Postoperative complications
Four women died after complications in the postoperative period:
- One death occurred due to opiate overdose in a woman receiving PCA.
- A second death from acute circulatory failure due to blood incompatibility after a blood transfusion.
- There was another woman who died from cardiac arrest while recovering from general anaesthesia following surgical abortion. She was given syntometrine intravenously, which may have caused the cardiac arrest in a woman with cardiac irritability secondary to substance abuse.

Anaesthesia: specific recommendations

- The failed tracheal intubation is a core skill which should be rehearsed and practised regularly.
- The recognition and management of severe, acute illness in a pregnant woman requires multidisciplinary teamwork.
- An anaesthetist and critical care specialist should be involved early.
- Obstetric and gynaecology services, particularly those without an on-site critical care unit, must have a defined local guideline to obtain rapid access to, and help from, critical care specialists.

Lessons for the anaesthetist

Service provision
- All women including those in early pregnancy require the same high standard of anaesthetic care (including recovery period).
- Trainee anaesthetists must be able to obtain prompt advice and help from a designated consultant at all times.
- Morbidly obese women should not be anaesthetized by trainees without direct supervision.
- Trainees across all specialities may not have the experience or skill to recognize a seriously ill woman. If in doubt, refer to senior colleagues.

General measures
- Local guidelines are a useful way of improving the care of women with high-risk pregnancies and the effective management of obstetric emergencies.
- Appropriate prevention of thromboembolic disease.
- Multidisciplinary approach to high-risk patients. Morbidly obese women should also be reviewed by an anaesthetist during pregnancy so that potential problems can be identified and appropriate management plans made and discussed.
- Recognition of the implications of substance misuse. Smoking and ischaemic heart/respiratory disease; alcohol and liver disease; IV drug use and difficult venous access; risk of endocarditis; and challenging postoperative analgesia.

Recognition and management of the sick mother
- It is essential to recognize important clinical signs, including maternal tachycardia to aid early recognition of serious illness. The normal physiological changes of pregnancy may be misinterpreted when managing sick pregnant women. During late pregnancy and labour, cardiac

output is increased and a woman may be seriously ill before she becomes hypotensive. At this point she will have little physiological reserve and may deteriorate rapidly if action is not taken.
- All healthcare professionals who care for pregnant and recently delivered women should be well aware of the infection control policy, and the signs and symptoms of sepsis in view to urgently assess and treat.
- The sick mother should be referred early for anaesthetic or intensivist consultations, especially in conditions where presentation may be atypical but rapidly progressive, as noted by the Emergent Theme Briefing on sepsis. Early detection of severe illness is challenging. This requires need to improve education and training.
- Modified early warning scoring systems for all acute obstetric admissions including early pregnancy.
- Reduced exposure of junior medical staff to illness. Introduction of simulator-based training may be appropriate.
- Maternity teams should demonstrate competence in scenario-based training.
- Protocols for management on major obstetric emergencies should be subject to regular review.
- All staff (including temporary) involved in care of seriously sick women should have competency-based training recorded.

What is the modified early obstetric warning scoring system (MEOWS)?

MEOWS is a method to graphically record observations of various measurements to identify abnormal scores that will determine a change in outcome. The observations include:

- Neurological state: mental response
- Pulse rate
- Systolic BP
- Respiratory rate
- Temperature
- Urine output

Further reading

Centre for Maternal and Child Enquiries (CMACE). Saving Mothers' Lives: reviewing maternal deaths to make motherhood safer: 2006–08. The Eighth Report on Confidential Enquiries into Maternal Deaths in the United Kingdom. *BJOG: An International Journal of Obstetrics & Gynaecology* 2011; **118**(Suppl. 1):1–203.

Kinsella, S.M. Anaesthetic deaths in the CMACE (Centre for Maternal and Child Enquiries) Saving Mothers' Lives report 2006–08. *Anaesthesia* **66**:243–46.

Index

abdominal aortic aneurysm (AAA)
    repair 187–91
    ECG abnormality 73, 76
abdominal wall anatomy 270
Accident and Emergency 213–18
acute renal failure, rhabdomyolysis 216–17
adrenal cortex, aldosterone 154–5
adrenalectomy, phaeochromocytoma 248, 297
adrenaline 248–9
    infusion 16
airway, spinal stenosis 117
airway management, thyroidectomy 33
airway obstruction, immediate postoperative period 34
albumin, low 139, 273
alcoholism 5
    and anaesthesia 335
    multiple medical issues 234–8
    perioperative management 238
aldosterone, functions 154–5
aldosterone antagonists 155
alkaline phosphatase 6
allodynia 147
anaemia
    investigations 51, 115
    renal failure 44
anaesthesia circuits 45
antepartum haemorrhage (APH) 100–1
anticoagulants 230–1, 315
antidepressants, neuropathic pain 148
antiepileptics, neuropathic pain 148
antithrombin 299
antithyroid drugs 83
aortic cross-clamping 191
aortic stenosis 290
Apfel score, PONV 241
apnoea
    child 75
    suxamethonium apnoea 78
apnoea test 81
aqueous humour. IOP 179–80
arteriovenous oxygen content difference 16
aseptic meningitis 166
aspiration
    chest X-ray 146
    pathophysiology 146
aspiration pneumonia 145
atracurium, renal failure 44
atrial fibrillation, ECG abnormality 139
atrioventricular conduction block (AVB) 76
atrioventricular node 42

atropine
    dose 198
    oculocardiac reflex 58
autoimmune connective tissue disease 283
autonomic neuropathy 168, 173–5
    renal failure 44
autonomic NS 173–4
AV block, 3rd-degree AV block 77
awareness under anaesthesia 36–9
    high risk groups 38
    implicit and explicit awareness 38
    incidence 38
    suxamethonium apnoea 78

Bazette's formula, QT interval 42
Beer—Lambert law 84
beta-2-agonists 132
beta-blockers 189
Bier's block 97–8
bilirubin metabolism 63
    hepatorenal syndrome 63
    jaundice 64, 314
    liver failure 63–4
bleeding, post-tonsillectomy bleeding 219–20
blood clotting 229–30
blood pressure
    damping 302
    invasive pressure monitoring 301
    measurement 277
Bohr effects, double 322
bone, intraosseous (IO) needle insertion 61
bone anatomy 61
botulism 165
brachial plexus block 97
brain, blood supply 201
brainstem death 81
breathing circuits 45
    fresh gas flow (FGF) requirements 46
    Mapleson circuits 45
    Mapleson E (Ayres T-piece) 45
        Jackson—Rees modification 45–6
bronchial carcinoma, chest X-ray 95, 97
bronchoconstriction 131
bronchodilators
    administration 52
    classification 132
    measuring PFTs 71
bronchomotor tone 131
bronchospasm 132
bundle branches 42
bupivacaine toxicity 182

Index

burns
    emergencies 193
    TBSA 193

C-reactive protein (CRP) 6, 139
Caesarean section
    apnoeic child 75
    general anaesthesia 78, 101
    pre-eclampsia 171
calcitonin 129
calcitriol 129
calcium homeostasis 129
cancer pain 147
cancer surgery 281
can't intubate-can't ventilate 198
capacitance 26, 231
capnography 85
carbamazepine, dose 149
carbon dioxide
    measurement 84–5
    no end-tidal 196
carcinoid syndrome 157
cardiac arrest, local anaesthesia 153
cardiac circulation 226
cardiac conduction 42
    atrioventricular node 42
    bundle branches 42
    cardiodefibrillator, insertion 42
    long QT syndrome 42
    nodes 42
    QT interval, Bazette's formula 42
    sinoatrial node 42
    ventricular depolarization 42
cardiac tamponade 315–16
cardiodefibrillator, insertion 42
carotid arteries 201
carotid endarterectomy 193–6
    hypertension 195
cauda equina syndrome 237
cautery, safety mechanisms 27
cell salvage 342
central neuraxial block 315–16
central venous oxygen saturation 16
Centre for Maternal and Child Enquiries (CMACE) 354
cerebral arteries 201
cerebral blood flow 203
cerebral oximetry, near infrared spectrometry (NIRS) 195
cerebral perfusion pressure 195, 203
    hyperperfusion 196
cervical plexus block 195
cervical spine (C-spine), clearing 37, 267
chest tube insertion/removal, pneumothorax 121–2
child
    apnoea 75

    sedation 344
    upper respiratory tract infection 329–30
chronic obstructive pulmonary disease (COPD) 189–90
    cause 52
    chest X-ray 71
chronic pain see neuropathic pain
Circle of Willis anatomy 201
clinical trials 83–4
clopidogrel 91
    coronary stent 91, 92
    discontinuing 93
Clostridium tetani 263
clotting 229–30, 298
coagulation cascade 297
coeliac plexus procedure 98–9
    complications 100
colectomy 49–52
    bronchodilators 52
    ECG assessment 52
    epidural analgesia 53
    obstructive lung disease 52
    pulmonary function tests 49, 52
    respiratory disease 51
    right ventricular hypertrophy (RVH) 52
    spirometry 51
Colles' fracture 97
complete heart block (CHB) 76
complex regional pain syndrome (CRPS) 148
connective tissue disease 283
context-sensitive half-life 107
coronary arteries, anatomy 226
coronary perfusion 227
coronary stent
    clopidogrel 91, 92
    risk of thrombosis 92
cranial nerves, Guillain—Barre syndrome 56
craniotomy 3–7
    chest X-ray 6
    ECG 6
    flow-volume loop 6
creatine levels, and glomerular filtration rate (GFR) 71
creatinine levels 214–17
cricothyroidotomy 198
critical illness
    nutrition 247
    nutritional supplements 248
critical illness neuropathy 123

dabigatran 338
damping 302
dead space, measurement 23
deep vein thrombosis (DVP) 229
    prophylaxis 315
defibrillators 231
    ICDs 232
    monophasic vs biphasic 232

360

Index

dental clearance, day-care 255–60
diabetes insipidus 257
diabetes mellitus, autonomic neuropathy 168, 1735
diaphragm, rupture 321
diaphragm anatomy 319–21
diathermy
   bipolar diathermy 27
   cautery, safety mechanisms 27
   and pacemaker 92–3
   principle 26
   unipolar diathermy 27
digoxin, and hypomagnesaemia 139
dobutamine, infusion 16
dopamine, infusion 16
Doppler echocardiography 291
Doppler effect 133
Doppler principle 133
double Bohr effect 322
double lumen tubes (DLTs) 43, 284
Douleur neuropathique 99
drug, half-life, context-sensitive 107
drug overdose 214–18
drug trials 83–4

Eaton—Lambert myasthenic syndrome 107, 144
ECG abnormality 54–5
   absent P waves 139
   atrial fibrillation 139
   following AAA repair 73, 76
   Guillain—Barré syndrome 164
   hyperkalaemia 214–16
   permanent pacing 77, 91
   sinus rhythm with LBBB 309
   supraventricular tachycardia (SVT) 59
   Wolff—Parkinson—White syndrome (WPW) 58–9
echocardiography 283
   assessment of ventricular function 52
   Doppler 291
   types 134
eclampsia 157, 169–70
ECMO 18
elective or emergency case 5
electricity 26–7
   diathermy principle 26
   effects on body 26
   microshock 26
electroconvulsive therapy (ECT) 292–4
emergency surgery, epilepsy 307–12
epidural analgesia 53
   MASTER trial 72
epidural block, post-dural puncture headache 265
epilepsy
   emergency surgery 307–12
   status epilepticus 311–12
evidence-based medicine (EBM) 275
eye anatomy 104

eye blocks 105
eye injury 223–4, 310–12

failed intubation, obstetric anaesthesia 75–6
fascia iliaca compartment block 178
fast tracking in anaesthesia 336
femoral nerve block 178
femoral triangle 177
fentanyl, renal failure 44
fetal distress 75
fetal haemoglobin 322
Fick principle 16
fire injuries 8–14
   burns 12–14
   carbon monoxide poisoning 12–13
   disorientation 12
   Henry's law 13
   inhalational injury 11–12
   oxygen saturation 12
   oxygen therapy, hyperbaric 13
flow
   laminar and turbulent flow 158, 249
   and pressure 158
flow loops, lung volumes 23–4
fluids, septic shock 16
flupenthixol 257
fondaparinox 315
forced expiration measurements 23
   FEV_1/FVC ratio 23
fractures, mandible, ORIF 35
fuel cells 65
functional residual capacity (FRC) 22

G proteins 131
gabapentin 299–300
   dose 149
gamma—aminobutyric acid (GABA) 25
   effects of thiopentone 25
gas flow 159
gastric emptying, delayed, renal failure 44
gastric tonometry 17
'Gillick' competence 167
glomerular filtration rate (GFR) 283
   and creatine levels 71
goitre 31, 33
Guillain—Barré syndrome 54–5, 163–8
   chest x-ray 164
   differential diagnosis 56
   ECG 164
   ICU 166

haemoglobin, fetal 322
haemostasis 297
Hagen—Poiseuille equation 158–9, 249
head injury 267
   and autoregulation 204

Index

headache, post-dural puncture 265
heart, circulation 226
heart block
 classification 76
 complete 76
 new-onset 3rd-degree AV block 77
heat moisture exchange (HME) filters 325
Heliox 250
heparin, aortic cross-clamping 191
hepatorenal syndrome 63
hiatus hernia 137–41
high frequency oscillatory
 ventilation (HFOV) 18
hip replacement 89–94
HIV patient 288–90
homonymous hemianopia 7
5-HT receptors 156
humidity, absolute/relative 324
hydrocortisone, perioperative cover 72
hygrometers 34
hyperaldosteronism 155
hyperalgesia 147
hyperbaric oxygen 64–5
 applications 64
 fuel cells 65
 oxygen content of gases 65
hypercalcaemia 130
hyperkalaemia 214–18
hyperparathyroidism, renal failure 44
hyperpathia 148
hyperperfusion syndrome 196
hyperphosphataemia, renal failure 44
hypertension
 AAA repair 190
 carotid endarterectomy 195
 postoperative 285
 in pregnancy 169
 renal failure 44
 thyroidectomy 33
hyperthyroidism 82, 83
hypnotics 107
hypoalbuminaemia 139, 273
 sigmoid colon carcinoma 71
hypocalcaemia 34, 130
 thyroidectomy 34
hypokalaemia 238
hypomagnesaemia, and digoxin 139
hypotension, post carotid
 endarterectomy 196
hypothalamus, and pituitary gland 296
hypothermia 39, 109
 CV effects 39
 definitions 39
 perioperative 109–10
hypovolaemia, and thiopentone 25
hypoxia, laryngospasm, day-care 198

immunoglobulins, vs plasmapheresis 167
immunosuppression, and prolonged
 bleeding time, renal failure 44
implantable cardiodefibrillators (ICDs) 42, 232
inductance 26, 231
induction, rapid sequence induction and
 intubation 351
induction agents 351
infrared spectrometry 84
inotropes, septic shock 16
intercostal nerve block 151–3
intercostal nerves, anatomy 151
intracranial pressure
 monitoring 267
 and volume 205
intracranial tumour 5
intracranial vascular aneurysm 202
intraocular pressure 179
intraoperative SVT 34
intraosseous (IO) needle insertion
 complications 61
 contraindications 61
 correct placement 61
 resuscitation 61
intrapleural block 124–5
intrauterine growth restriction (IUGR) 170
intravenous RA, Bier's block 97–8
invasive pressure monitoring 301
iontophoretic transdermal system (ITS), drug
 delivery 341
IPPV, and RSII 352
ischaemic heart disease 140
 renal failure 44
ITU management 57

jaundice 313–14
 bilirubin metabolism 64, 314
 causes 64
Jehovah's witness 167, 343
jet ventilation 22

laminar and turbulent flow 158, 249
LANSS, neuropathic pain 98–9
laparoscopy procedure 140
laryngeal anatomy 127–8
laryngoscopy 221
 priorities 75
laryngospasm, day-care 196
laser measurements 208
levobupivacaine, coeliac plexus
 procedure 98–9
lithium 257–8
liver failure, pharacological effect 63–4
local anaesthesia 181
 cardiac arrest 153
 classification 181

Index

and pH 181–2
toxicity 153–4, 179
long QT syndrome
  cause 42
  treatment 42
lung specimens 243
lung volumes 22–7
  closing capacity 23
  dead space measurement 23
  FEV_1/FVC ratio 23
  flow loops 23–4
  forced expiration measurements 23
  functional residual capacity (FRC) 22
  respiratory function tests 22
lungs, function 131–3

magnesium 206
  normal levels 207
  toxicity 207
mandible fracture, ORIF 35
Mapleson circuits 45
  Jackson—Rees modification 45–6
Mapleson E (Ayres T-piece) circuit 45
MASTER trial, epidural analgesia 72
maternal deaths, Centre for Maternal and Child Enquiries (CMACE) 354–7
mean corpuscular volume (MCV) 5
meta-analysis 276
metabolic alkalosis 189
mexiletine, dose 149
microlaryngeal tube 221
microvascular decompression (MVD) 21
mixed venous oxygen saturation 16
Mobitz type 1 and 2 block 76
modified early obstetric warning scoring system (MEOWS) 357
Monro—Kellie doctrine 205
morphine, renal failure 44
multiple medical issues 234–8
muscle relaxants, renal failure 44
myasthenia 106
myasthenia gravis 144
myasthenic syndromes 107
myocardial blood supply 226–7
myopathy 165
  in ICU 123

near infrared spectrometry (NIRS) 195
neuralgia, post-herpetic 62
neuraxial block, central 315–16
neuromuscular junction 106, 165
neuropathic pain 98–9, 143, 147
  treatment 148
neuropathy
  acute polyneuropathy 56

critical illness 123–4
peripheral 123
nitric oxide, inhaled 18
noradrenaline, infusion 16
null hypothesis 84
nutrition, enteral vs parenteral 248
nutritional status, critical illness 247
nutritional supplements, critical illness 248

obesity
  morbid 20
  pathophysiology 9–10
  thyroidectomy 33
obstetric anaesthesia
  failed intubation 75–6
  MEOWS 357
obstetric haemorrhage 100
obstructive lung disease 52, 71
obstructive sleep apnoea 242
octreotide 157
oculocardiac reflex (OCR) 58
one lung ventilation
  de-saturation 43
  indications 43
  physiological changes 43
one-lung anaesthesia 43
  double lumen tubes 43
  physiological changes 43
open reduction and internal fixation (ORIF) 35, 261, 268
ophthalmic nerves, anatomy 104
opiates
  fentanyl 44
  morphine 44
  remifentanil 44
opioids, and RSI 352
orbit, anatomy 104
organ dysfunction, criteria 17
ORIF, mandible fracture 35
oxygen
  100% 65
  hyperbaric oxygen 64–5
oxygen content of gases, determining 65

pacemaker 91–2
  chest X-ray 90
  and diathermy 92–3
  indications 92
pacing
  permanent 77, 91
  temporary 77
parathyroid glands 129
parathyroid hormone 129
parenteral nutrition 248
Patil's test 37
peribulbar eye blocks 105

Index

peripheral nerve blocks, ultrasound-guided 349
peripheral nerve stimulation, peripheral nerve blocks 349
peripheral neuropathy 123, 165
phaeochromocytoma 248, 297
pharmacology of renal failure 44
phenytoin, dose 149
piezoelectric effect 133
pituitary anatomy 296
placenta physiology 321
placental abruption 75
plasma proteins 273
plasmapheresis, vs immunoglobulins 167
plasmin 299
pleural effusion 237
pneumonia, ventilator-associated pneumonia 242
pneumotachograph 159–60
pneumothorax 119, 121–2
  chest tube insertion/removal 121–2, 237–8
  hydropneumothorax 237
poliomyelitis 166
polyneuropathy, acute 56
post-dural puncture headache 265
post-herpetic neuralgia 62
post-tonsillectomy bleeding 219–20
postoperative bleeding, renal failure 44
postoperative nausea and vomiting (PONV) 157, 241
  Apfel score 241
power calculation 84
pre-eclampsia 157, 168–70
prednisolone, side-effects 116
pregabalin, dose 149
prone position
  physiology 228
  surgery 238
  ventilation 17
prostacyclin 299
  inhaled 18
proteins, plasma proteins 273
pulmonary embolism 230
pulmonary fibrosis 116
pulmonary function tests 49, 52, 69, 283
  administration of bronchodilators 71

QT interval, Bazette's formula 42

rapid sequence induction and intubation 351–3
recurrent laryngeal nerve 128
  and vagus nerve 245–6
red cell flow velocity (RCFV) 195
remifentanil, renal failure 44
renal failure 44
  anaemia 44
  autonomic neuropathy 44
  delayed gastric emptying 44
  drugs

  accumulation 44
  clearance 44
  Hoffman degradation 44
  loading dose effects 44
  volume of distribution effects 44
  hyperparathyroidism 44
  hyperphosphataemia 44
  hypertension 44
  ischaemic heart disease 44
  opiates 44
  postoperative bleeding 44
  rhabdomyolysis 216–17
  uraemia (immunosuppression and prolonged bleeding time) 44
renal replacement therapy 218
resistance 26, 231
respiration maintenance, fresh gas flow (FGF) requirements 46
respiratory function tests 22
respiratory tract
  neurotransmitters 131
  receptors 131
resuscitation, antepartum haemorrhage (APH) 101
Reynolds number 159, 249
rhabdomyolysis 216–17
rheumatoid arthritis, spinal stenosis 115
right ventricular hypertrophy (RVH) 52, 71
rivaroxaban 315
rocuronium
  dose 310, 352
  renal failure 44
  and sugammadex 339, 352
rotameter 159

sclerodema 283
sedation 107
  on ICU 108
sedation, children and young people 344–6
  levels 344
seizures, differential diagnosis 7
sepsis, anaesthetic management 331–3
sepsis six 14
septic shock 14–18
  ArdsNet group recommendations 17
  gastric tonometry 17
  lactic acidosis 17
  management 14–15
  oxygen extraction ratio (OER) 16
  ventilation 17–18
serotonin 155–6
sickle cell trait 33
  HbS level 33
  implications 33
sigmoid colectomy 49–53
  abdominal surgery 51
  blood investigations 51

Index

anaemia 51
ECG 52
respiratory status 51
sigmoid colon carcinoma 69–72
   chest X-ray 71
   ECG findings 71
   hypoalbuminaemia 71
   RVH 71
sildenafil 383
sinoatrial node, position 42
skin, transdermal drug delivery 340–1
sleep apnoea, obstructive vs central 242
smoking 256, 334
   abstinence, before surgery 335
   and alcoholism 334
sodium valproate, dose 149
spinal anaesthesia, failed, mechanisms, management and prevention 347–8
spinal cord lesions 165
spinal stenosis, elective decompression 113–18
   airway 117
   extubation 118
spirometry 51
spontaneous breathing trial (SBT) 18
squint correction 54, 57
   bradycardia 58
   oculocardiac reflex 58
steroids 284
   perioperative cover 72
strabismus, correction 54, 57
stridor, causes 246–7
stroke, carotid endarterectomy 193–4
sub-Tenon's eye blocks 105
subarachnoid haemorrhage (SAH) 202
sugammadex 339, 352
sulphasalazine, side-effects 116
supraventricular tachycardia (SVT)
   causes 59
   intraoperative 34
suxamethonium
   alternative 310
   dose 197, 351
   and IOP 310
   RSI 350
suxamethonium apnoea 78
systemic inflammatory response syndrome (SIRS) 331–3

temperature, and humidity 324
temperature measurement 108
   core 40, 109
temporary pacing 77
TENS 62–3
tension pneumothorax 121
tetanus 263
thermistors 108
thermocouples 108
thiopentone 24–5
   advantages in eye injury 310
   effects on cerebral blood flow 25
   effects on respiratory system 25
   gamma—aminobutyric acid (GABA) 25
   hypovolaemia 25
   and porphyria 25
   structure 24
thyroid goitre 34
thyroid hormones, synthesis, transport, control 82–3
thyroidectomy 31–4
   airway management 33
   blood results 33
   cardiovascular instability 33
   chest X-ray abnormalities 34
   deviated trachea 33
   ECG 34
   hypertension 33
   hypocalcaemia 34
   intraoperative SVT management 34
   investigations 82
   sickle cell trait, positive 33
   supraventricular tachycardia (SVT) 34
   thyroid status 33
   WPW syndrome 33
tibia
   intraosseous (IO) needle insertion 61
   ORIF 268
tissue hypoperfusion, organ dysfunction 17
tonsillectomy, postoperative bleeding 219–20
tourniquets 183
tranexamic acid 323
transcranial Doppler 195
transcutaneous nerve stimulation (TENS) 62–3
transdermal drug delivery 340–1
transducer 302
transfusion, trigger 191
transient ischaemic attacks (TIAs) 193–4
transurethral resection of prostate (TURP) 168, 172
transverse abdominis plane (TAP) block 271–3
trigeminal ganglion, anatomy 20
trigeminal nerve 20–1
   eye nerve supply 104
trigeminal neuralgia 20
   alcohol injection 21
   gamma-knife treatment 21
   glycerol injection 21
   International Headache Society 20
   macrovascular decompression (MVD) 21
   microvascular decompression (MVD) 21
   pathophysiology 20–1
   treatment options 21
turbulent flow 158
TURP syndrome 172

Index

ultrasound 133–4
  NICE guidelines 134
  transverse abdominis plane (TAP) block 271–3
ultrasound-guided peripheral nerve blocks 349–50
unipolar diathermy 27
upper respiratory tract infection, child 329–30
uraemia, immunosuppression and prolonged bleeding time 44
uterine blood flow 322

vagus nerve, and recurrent laryngeal nerve 245–6
vecuronium, renal failure 44
venlaxafine 257
ventilation, dry gases 324
ventilator-associated pneumonia 242
ventricular depolarization 42
Virchow's triad 229

WBC count 115
Wolff—Parkinson—White syndrome (WPW) 34
  ECG abnormality 58–9
  pathophysiology 34
  supraventricular tachycardia (SVT) 33, 34

ziconotide 337